CURRENT CONCEPTS IN GENERAL THORACIC SURGERY

Edited by **Lucio Cagini**

Current Concepts in General Thoracic Surgery
http://dx.doi.org/10.5772/3070
Edited by Lucio Cagini

Contributors

Michele Scialpi, Teresa Pusiol, Irene Piscioli, Alberto Rebonato, Lucio Cagini, Lucio Bellantonio, Marina Mustica, Francesco Puma, Luca Brunese and Antonio Rotondo, Noritoshi Nishiyama, Jacopo Vannucci, Cristian Rapicetta, Massimiliano Paci, Tommaso Ricchetti, Sara Tenconi, Salvatore De Franco and Giorgio Sgarbi, Constance K. Haan, Naohiro Kajiwara, Masatoshi Kakihana, Jitsuo Usuda, Tatsuo Ohira, Norihiko Kawate and Norihiko Ikeda, Antonio F. Corno, B. Goslin and R. Hooker, José Francisco Valderrama Marcos, María Teresa González López and Julio Gutiérrez de Loma, Christodoulos Kaoutzanis, Tiffany N.S. Ballard and Paul S. Cederna, Slobodan Milisavljević, Marko Spasić and Miloš Arsenijević, Nicolas J. Mouawad, Ajay Gupta, Hiroshi Makino, Hiroshi Yoshida and Eiji Uchida, Christopher Rolfes, Stephen Howard, Ryan Goff and Paul A. Iaizzo

Published by InTech
Janeza Trdine 9, 51000 Rijeka, Croatia

Publishing Process Manager Oliver Kurelic
Technical Editor InTech Prepress, Novi Sad
Cover InTech Design team

Additional hard copies can be obtained from orders@intechopen.com

Current Concepts in General Thoracic Surgery, Edited by Lucio Cagini
p. cm.
ISBN 978-953-51-0870-2

For EU product safety concerns:
IN TECH d.o.o., Prolaz Marije Krucifikse Kozulić 3, 51000 Rijeka, Croatia,
info@intechopen.com or visit our website at intechopen.com.

Meet the editor

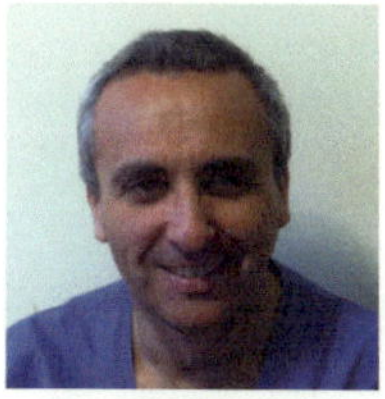

Lucio Cagini M.D. graduated with a medical degree in 1986 at the University of Perugia and subsequently majored in General Surgery and General Thoracic Surgery. His professional growth has been characterized by frequent and prolonged periods of work and study abroad and in Italy, in centres such as the Royal Brompton Hospital in London and the Istituto Europeo di Oncologia in Milan. He has acted as first surgeon for hundreds of surgical procedures in general and in thoracic surgery. He is author of many scientific papers regarding his fields of research; pulmonary metastases, tumour growths factors, the body reaction to surgical stress, thoracic trauma and surgical techniques. At present he is Assistant Professor of Thoracic Surgery at the University of Perugia.

Contents

Preface

The Aim of "Current Concepts of General Thoracic Surgery" is to provide a brief overview of several topics in this field. It includes a collection of contributions from many outstanding Authors who provide their knowledge and experience from many countries around the world. We apologize for the chapters reviewed that have were not chosen for publication in this book; however, according to the single centres experience, the final result offers thorough and precious information on the several topics evaluated by the Authors. The wide range of subjects discussed goes from CT assessment of solitary pulmonary and metastatic nodules to prospective studies of drug delivery in thoracic surgery including surgical risk prediction, stress reaction, robotic pulmonary and cardiac procedures, vascular and thoracic reconstruction techniques, thoracic trauma and mediastinal fistula. I believe that this book represents an enhancement in the knowledge and in the involvement of individuals dedicated to these areas of study. It is my duty and pleasure to thank colleagues who helped me in the interesting and stimulating review process; Dr. Stefano Pasquino for cardiac surgery and Professor Francesco Puma for his many worthwhile suggestions.

Lucio Cagini
Thoracic Surgery Unit, Department of Surgical, Radiologic, and Odontostomatologic Sciences, University of Perugia, S. Maria della Misericordia Hospital, Perugia, Italy

Chapter 1

Malignant Pulmonary Solitary Nodules: High Resolution Computed Tomography Morphologic and Ancillary Features in the Differentiation of Histotypes

Michele Scialpi, Teresa Pusiol, Irene Piscioli, Alberto Rebonato, Lucio Cagini, Lucio Bellantonio, Marina Mustica, Francesco Puma, Luca Brunese and Antonio Rotondo

Additional information is available at the end of the chapter

http://dx.doi.org/10.5772/54671

1. Introduction

Solitary pulmonary nodule (SPN) or "coin lesion" is a rounded lesion that does not exceed 3 cm in diameter, completely surrounded by normal lung parenchyma without other concomitant anomalies (not associated with atelectasis or adenopathy), and often asymptomatic. Lesions bigger than 3 cm are more properly called masses and are often malignant [1,2].

SPNs can be found randomly in the course of imaging exams conducted at the level of the neck, upper limbs, chest, abdomen, and are described in approximately 0.9-2% of all chest X-rays [3].

Since the early 80's the advent of computed tomography (CT) has resulted in a large increase in the frequency of detection of SPN. In the clinical practice it is important to determine the radiological and pathological features of benign and malignant tumors for an accurate management [4-13].

According to the literature the overall prevalence of SPNs ranged between 8% and 51% [14,15]. The American College of Chest Physicians (ACCP) does not recommend the implementation of screening for lung cancer in the general population because the implementation of these tests is not so far proved able to achieve a reduction of mortality rates [16].

Because the diagnosis and treatment of early stage lung cancer allows more favourable results, a close monitoring for identified lesions is recommended [17].

A SPN can be attributed to various causes. The first step in the clinical evaluation of these lesions is to define the benignity or malignancy. The most common benign etiologies include infectious granulomas and hamartomas, while the most frequent malignant etiologies include primary lung cancer and lung metastases [2].

The clinical relevance of accurately subtyping lung cancers was initially challenged by the advent of novel therapeutic options (targeted therapies, such as erlotinib/gefitinib and bevacizumab, or third-generation chemotherapeutic agents, such as pemetrexed), which are effective in specific lung cancer subtypes, and needed for a more detailed histological definition of non-small-cell lung cancer (NSCLC), separating at least squamous-cell carcinoma (SQC) from non-SQC. This event led pathologists to concentrate their efforts on the accurate diagnosis of small cell lung carcinoma (SCLC), because further subtyping of NSCLC was an optional and clinically unimportant diagnostic exercise. The generic diagnosis of NSCLC gained popularity originally for cytological samples and later for small biopsies. Currently, on cytological or small biopsy samples, most pathologists are able to correctly distinguish SCLC from NSCLC, and within the NSCLC group to identify well-differentiated or moderately differentiated SQC or adenocarcinoma (ADC). [18,19]

However, a high percentage of cases continues to be simply diagnosed as NSCLC, especially when lacking clear-cut morphologic signs of differentiation. From a practical standpoint, the call back to histological categorization of NSCLC raises several types of questions. Although NSCLC subtyping may be relatively easy and feasible on surgical specimens, there are objective difficulties in examining small biopsies and cytology samples. These techniques often are the only ones for the final diagnosis of lung cancer, as most patients are not candidates for radical surgery. When dealing with these small samples, pathologists may be faced with a higher degree of uncertainty because of the frequent lung tumor heterogeneity and the higher prevalence of poorly differentiated NSCLC among clinically advanced and unresectable cases[18,19]. A useful tool to identify squamous or glandular differentiation and to characterize poorly differentiated NSCLC may be to incorporate ancillary techniques, such as immunohistochemistry. This approach seems the most promising one, although the accuracy, sensitivity, and specificity of the diverse immunohistochemical markers remain to be further defined. Thyroid transcription factor (TTF-1) and/or cytocheratin 7 (CK7) for ADC and p63 and high-molecular weight cytokeratins (HMWCKs) for SQC are the most specific and currently validated immunohistochemical markers that may be suitable for refining most diagnoses even when dealing with quantitatively limited material, such as cytological samples or small-sized biopsies [20,21]. When the pathologist is not able to perform a precise histotype diagnosis, the high-resolution computed tomography (HRCT) may be proposed as further diagnostic approach for determining the lung histotype maligancies with single polmonary nodule presentation [21].

The aim of our study is to assess whether morphological characteristics of a SPN and ancillary signs allow to differentiate between the following lung malignancies: bronchioloalveolar carcinoma (BAC) classified in according to the new criteria, variants of ADC and SCLC.

2. Materials and methods

2.1. Patients

From January 2007 to June 2011 we retrospectively reviewed the HRCT examinations of 33 patients (14 females and 19 males) with SPN presentation and histologic diagnosis of SCLC (n = 5), invasive lepidic ADCs (formerly diagnosed nommucinous BAC with > 5 mm invasion) (n=7), invasive mucinous ADCs (formerly diagnosed mucinous BAC)(n=2) and other variants invasive ADCs (acinar, papillary, solid predominant with mucin production, colloid and enteric variants) (n= 19). SQC, large cell carcinoma, adenosquamous carcinoma and sarcomatoid carcinoma cases were excluded.

The mean age in the three type of SPNs (SCLC, BACs and ADCs) were: 60 years ± 6 (SCLC), 67,2 years ±8,2 (BACs) and 71, 3 years ± 8,5 (ADCs) respectively.

2.2. Histological analysis

The histological diagnosis was performed in accordance with the examination of lobectomy in all cases of ADCs and transbronchial biopsy in 5 SCLC. The classification of ADCs tumors was performed in accordance with the criteria of International Association for the Study of Lung Cancer/American Thoracic Society/European Respiratory Society International Mutlidisciplinary Classification of Lung Adenocarcinoma [22]. The following immunostaining analysis were performed in all cases of ADCs: TTF1, CK7, P63 and HMWCKs. The immunostaining of synaptophysin and CD56 was performed in all cases of SCLC.

2.3. HRCT technique

The examinations were performed with three different CT scanners: 16-slices CT (Light Speed Pro 16, GE, Milwaukee, USA), 16-slices CT (Toshiba Aquilion, Japan) and 64-slices CT (Philips *Medical Systems, Best, the* Netherlands) by direct volumetric acquisition with high spatial resolution CT (HRCT) in a single inspiratory breath with the patient in a supine position. The technical parameters expected to acquire volumetric reconstruction, are the following: collimation: 1.0-1.25mm, kV: 135, mA: 300, scan time: 0.7 sec / rotation, table speed of 17.85 mm / sec. High-*spatial*-frequency *(*bone*)* reconstruction algorithm was used. Using the axial images the multiplanar reconstructions (MPRs) with high diagnostic quality were obtained.

2.4. Image analysis

All HRCT images of each SNP were read in consensus by two experienced radiologists (M.S., A.R.) in chest CT with respect to morphology and ancillary signs. Size , margins/countours, calcifications, central necrosis or cavitation and air bronchogram were evaluated for the morphologic assessment [23]. Furthermore, in association with the morphological study the following ancillary signs were assessed: pleural connecting striae and ground glass opacity (GGO).

The percentage of ancillary signs and the morphologic appearance were evaluated for the differential diagnosis.

3. Results

Lesion size ranging from 8 mm to 25 mm (mean 20 mm ±10,4 SD) for SCLC, 15 mm to 30 mm (mean 22,5 ± 5,7 SD) for BACs , 10 mm to 29mm (mean 21,2 ± 5,9 SD) for ADCs.

In the table are reported the data related to the morphologic features and to the ancillary signs with relatives percentages of the three histotype malignant nodules.

Morfologic features: calcifications within the SPN were absent in all case of SCLC and BACs and found in 1/19 (5,2%) cases of ADCs variants; cavitation was observed in 1/5 (20%) cases of SCLC; margins/countours (irregular or spiculated, multilobulated, frayed) were revealed in SCLC, BACs and variants of ADC in 4/5 (80%) 9/9 (100%) 15/19 (79%) and air bronchogram was revealed in SCLC, BACs and variants of ADC in 2/5 (40%) 5/9 (60%) 8/19 (42%) respectively.

Ancillary signs: air bronchogram and pleural connecting striae were found in SCLC, BACs and variants of ADC in 2/5 (40%), 5/9 (60%), 8/19 (42%) and 3/5 (80%), 9/9 (100%) 17/19 (89%) respectively.

The representative HRTC features for the three type of SPNs for SCLC, BACs and variants of ADC are reported in figures 1,2, figures 3-5 and figures 6-9 respectively.

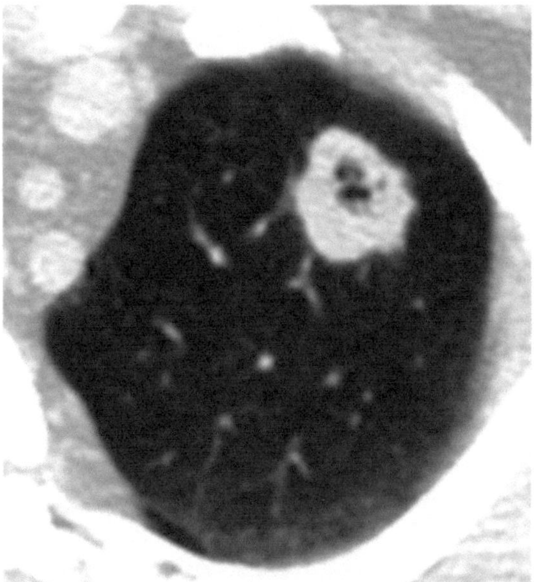

Figure 1. Small cell lung carcinoma in a 59 year-old man. HRCT shows spiculated and lobulated nodule with cavitations in the upper left lobe.

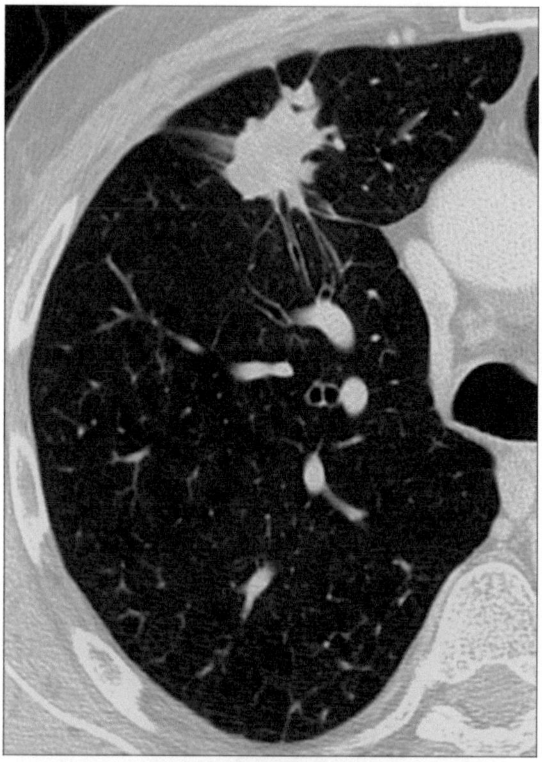

Figure 2. Small cell lung carcinoma in a 69 year-old man.
HRCT shows spiculated nodule with pleural connecting striae in the ventral segment of the upper right lobe.

HRCT features	SCLC (size ranging from 8 mm to 25 mm (mean 20 mm ±10,4 SD) (n=5)	BAC (size ranging , 15 mm to 30 mm (mean 22,5 ± 5,7 SD) (n=9)	ADCs size ranging 10 mm to 29mm (mean 21,2 ± 5,9 SD) (n=19)
Calcifications	**0/5 (0%)**	**0/9 (0%)**	**1/19 (5,2%)**
Cavitations	**1/5 (20%)**	**0/9 (0%)**	**0/19 (0%)**
Margins (irregular or spiculated, multilobulated)	**4/5 (80%)**	**9/9 (100%)**	**15/19 (79%)**
Air bronchogram	**2/5 (40%)**	**5/9 (60%)**	**8/19 (42%)**
Pleural connecting striae	**3/5 (80%)**	**9/9 (100%)**	**17/19 (89%)**
Ground-glass opacity	**1/5 (20%)**	**9/10 (90%)***	**5/19 (26,3%)**

*In 1 case of invasive mucinous adenocarcinoma (formerly diagnosed mucinous bronchiolo-alveolar carcinomas) the GGO appearance was not revealed.

Table 1. HRCT morphologic and ancillary of 5 small cell lung carcinomas (SLCL), 7 invasive lepidic adenocarcinomas (formely diagnosed bronchiolo-alveolar carcinomas pattern, with > 5 mm invasion), 2 invasive mucinous adenocarcinomas (formerly diagnosed mucinous bronchiolo-alveolar carcinomas) and 19 other variants invasive ADCs (acinar, papillary, solid predominant with mucin production, colloid and enteric variants).

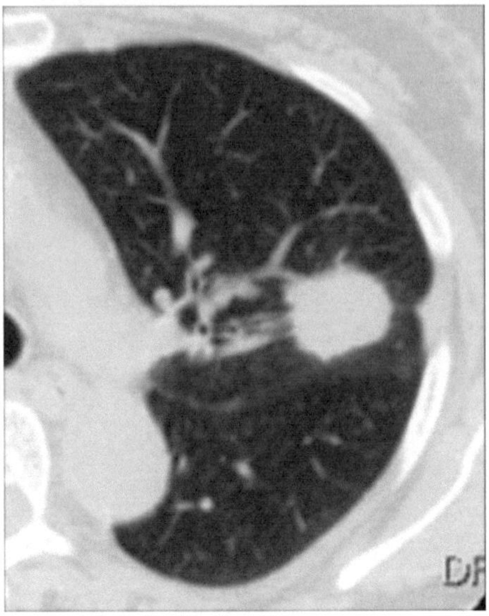

Figure 3. Invasive mucinous adenocarcinoma (formerly diagnosed mucinous bronchiolo-alveolar carcinoma) in a 74 year-old female.
HRCT shows spiculated nodule with pleural connecting striae in the dorsal segment of the left upper lobe.

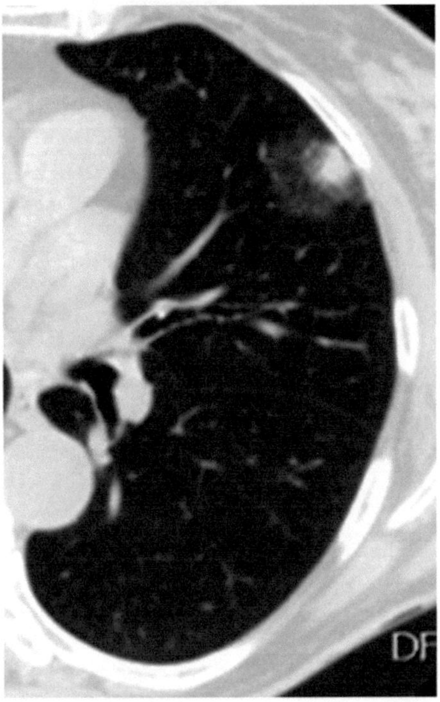

Figure 4. Invasive lepidic adenocarcinoma (formely diagnosed bronchiolo-alveolar carcinoma pattern, with > 5 mm invasion) in a 75 year-old female. HRCT shows nodule with irregular contours and GGO in the ventral segment of the left upper lobe .

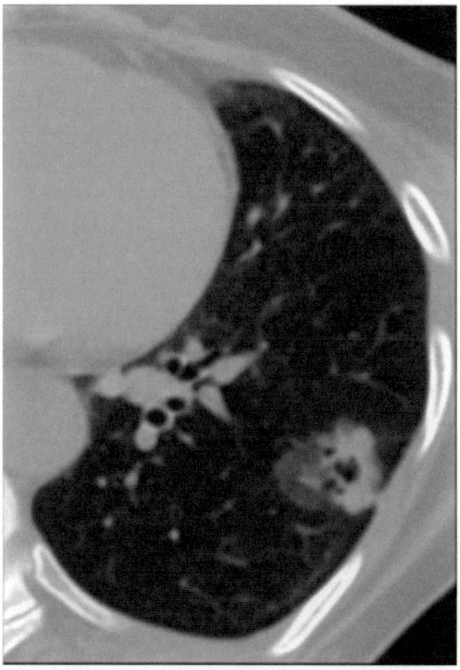

Figure 5. Invasive lepidic adenocarcinoma (formely diagnosed bronchiolo-alveolar carcinoma pattern, with > 5 mm invasion) in a 75 year-old female. HRCT shows lobulated nodule with air bronchogram and GGO in the left lower lobe.

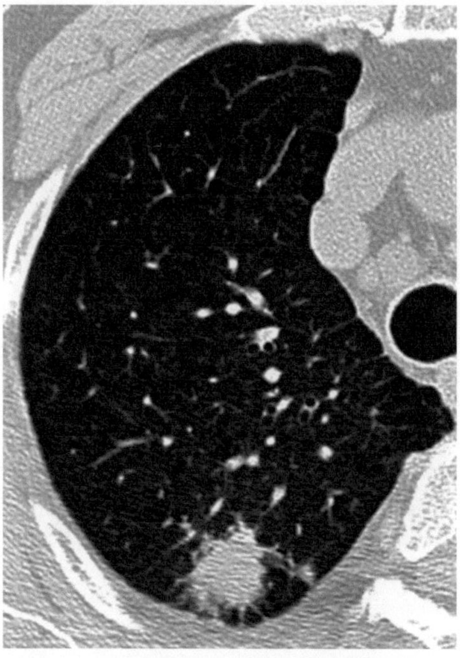

Figure 6. Invasive variant enteric adenocarcinoma in a 76 year-old man. HRCT shows spiculated nodule with pleural connecting irregular striae in the dorsal upper right lobe.

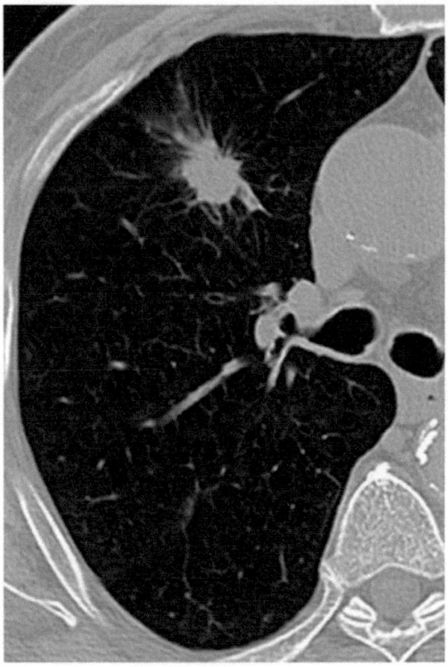

Figure 7. Invasive variant enteric adenocarcinoma in a 79 year-old man.
HRCT shows spiculated nodule with pleural connecting striae and GGO in the ventral upper righ lobe.

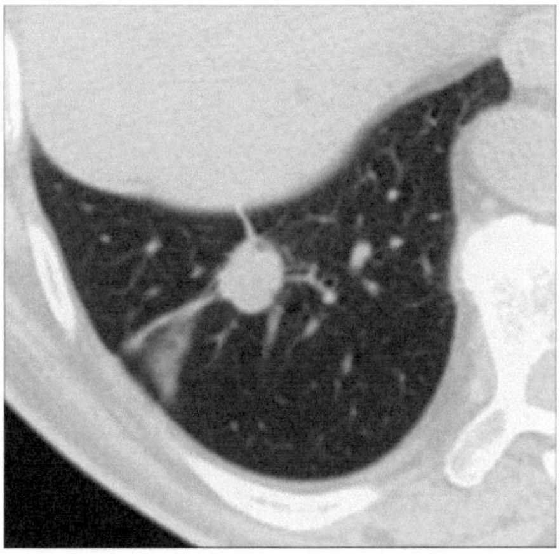

Figure 8. Invasive variant colloid adenocarcinoma in a 64 year-old man.
HRCT shows lobulated spiculated nodule with pleural connecting striae and GGO in the left lower lobe.

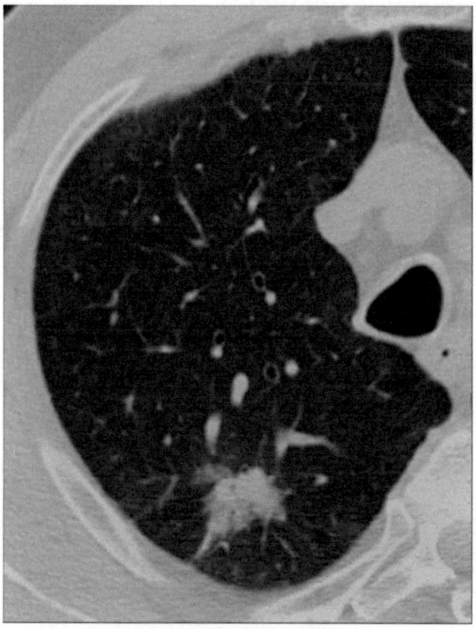

Figure 9. Invasive variant enteric high grade-fetal adenocarcinoma in a 64 year-old man.
HRCT shows spiculated nodule with pleural connecting striae and GGO in the dorsal upper right lobe.

4. Discussion

Adenocarcinoma is the most common histologic subtype of lung cancer in most countries, accounting for almost half of all lung cancers [24]. A widely divergent clinical, radiologic, molecular, and pathologic spectrum exists within lung adenocarcinoma. As a result, confusion exists, and studies are difficult to compare. Despite remarkable advances in understanding of this tumor in the past decade, remains a need for universally accepted criteria for adenocarcinoma subtypes, in particular tumors formerly classified as BAC [18,19].

As the SPN may be the expression of multiple pathologic entities, the incidental finding of SPN by CT raises the issue of differential diagnosis between benign and malignant nodules. Moreover the importance of differential diagnosis between malignant histotypes can affect the prognosis and management of these patients.

A number of terms have been used to describe lung ADC by CT imaging. In particular, for tumors that present as small nodules, the terms used have reflected the various ground glass (nonsolid), solid, or part-solid appearances that can occur. Largely based on the Fleischner Society glossary of terms [21] and the recently suggested guidelines by Godoy and Naidich [25] for subsolid nodules, we propose the following definitions: (1) a pure ground-glass nodule (GGN) (synonym: nonsolid nodule) as a focal area of increased lung attenuation within which the margins of any normal structures, e.g., vessels, remain outlined, (2) a solid nodule as a focal area of increased attenuation of such density that any normal structures, e.g., vessels, are completely obscured, and (3) part solid nodule (synonym: semisolid nodule) as a focal nodular opacity containing both solid and ground-glass components [21,25]. The Fleischner Society glossary of terms for thoracic imaging defines a nodule on a CT scan as "a rounded or irregular opacity, well or poorly defined, measuring up to 3 cm in greatest diameter" in any plane [21]. If the opacity is greater than 3 cm, it is referred to as a mass [21]. The 3 cm cut-off is in keeping with our concept of the maximum accepted size for the pathologic diagnosis of AIS and MIA. The term subsolid nodule has also entered common radiologic usage, referring to both part-solid nodules and a pure GGN [25]. Optimal evaluation of subsolid nodules requires thin-section CT scans (<3 mm thickness) to assess the solid versus ground-glass components [20,21].

The aim of our study is to assess the morphologic and ancillary HRCT features of the histotypes of malignant SPNs considering that often histological and/or cytological material may be unsatisfactory and immunoistochemical techniques may be not performed.

In our study the calcifications within the SPN were absent in all cases of SCLC and BACs and found in one case of ADCs.

The margins were irregular or spiculated, multilobulated in 4/5 (80%) of SCLC, in 9/9 (100%) of cases previously diagnosed as BACs, and in 15/19 (79%) of other variants of ADCs.

The opacity-like bullous, a sign of the presence of air bronchogram, does not help us in making any differential diagnosis, being present in 40% (2/5) of SCLC in 42% (8/19) of variants of ADCs and in 60% (5/9) of formerly diagnosed BACs. The occurrence of cavitations, expression of the speed of growth of the tumor cell and indicative of the presence of necrosis [26,27], was detected only in one aggressive forms of SCLC (20%). In all cases of all variants of ADCs and in cases previously diagnosed as BACs the cavitations were absent.

The SPN may be connected to the pleura by striae or streaks defined as linear density that extends to the pleura and were the result of a fibrosis in the pulmonary peripheral lung. The striae connecting pleura or pleural effusion tags are found with high frequency in the three tumor subtypes, ranking as a sign that directs us to a differential diagnosis of malignancy without giving specific indications about the histotype tumor (80% SCLC, 89% variants of ADCs, 100% formerly diagnosed BACs).

The ground glass perinodular opacity were areas of increased attenuation of hazy lung with preservation of bronchial and vascular margins [29] and intranodular air bronchogram were the result of asymptomatic growth with the larger bronchi free of malignancies. The ground glass opacity (GGO) instead is significantly more present in the lesions slower growing and less invasive locoregional (26,3 % variants of ADCs and 90% formerly diagnosed BACs) than lesions infiltrative rapidly (only 20% of SCLC).

In conclusion, ancillary signs (pleural striae and GGO) in association with air bronchogram are suggestive of diagnosis of the invasive lepidic ADCs (formerly diagnosed nommucinous BAC with > 5 mm invasion) and can be considered in the differential diagnosis of malignat SNPs histotypes (SCLC and ADCs)

Author details

Michele Scialpi, Alberto Rebonato, Lucio Bellantonio and Marina Mustica
Department of Surgical, Radiologic, and Odontostomatologic Sciences, Complex Structure of Radiology 2, University of Perugia, S. Maria della Misericordia Hospital, S. Andrea delle Fratte, Perugia, Italy

Teresa Pusiol
Institute of Anatomic Pathology, S. Maria del Carmine Hospital, Rovereto (Trento), Italy

Irene Piscioli
Institute of Radiology, Budrio Hospital, Bologna, Italy

Lucio Cagini and Francesco Puma
Department of Surgical, Radiologic, and Odontostomatologic Sciences, Thoracic Surgery Unit, University of Perugia, S. Maria della Misericordia Hospital, S. Andrea delle Fratte, Perugia, Italy

Luca Brunese
Department of Health Science, University of Molise, Campobasso, Italy

Antonio Rotondo
Department of Clinical and Experimental Medicine and Surgery "F. Magrassi," University of Naples, Naples, Italy

5. References

[1] Tuddenham Wj: Glossary of terms for thoracic radiology: recommendations of Nomenclature Committee of Fleischner Society - *AJR* 1984; 143(3):509-517.

[2] Ross H. Albert, John J. Russell: La valutazione di un nodulo solitario del polmone - *Minuti* Sett. 2010 Anno XXXIV - n.8.

[3] Holin S.N., Dwork R.E., Glaser S., et al.: Solitary pulmonary nodules found in a community-wide chest roentgenographic survey - *Am Tuberc Pulm Dis.* 1959; 79:427-439.

[4] Bartolotta TV, Midiri M, Scialpi M, Sciarrino E, Galia M, Lagalla R. Focal nodular hyperplasia in normal and fatty liver: a qualitative and quantitative evaluation with contrast-enhanced ultrasound. Eur Radiol. 2004 Apr;14(4):583-91.

[5] Scialpi M, Pierotti L, Piscioli I, Brunese L, Rotondo A, Yoon SH, Lee JM. Detection of small (<=20 mm) pancreatic adenocarcinoma: histologic grading and CT enhancement features. *Radiology.* 2012;262(3):1044.

[6] Brancato B, Crocetti E, Bianchi S, Catarzi S, Risso GG, Bulgaresi P, Piscioli F, Scialpi M, Ciatto S, Houssami N. Accuracy of needle biopsy of breast lesions visible on ultrasound: audit of fine needle versus core needle biopsy in 3233 consecutive samplings with ascertained outcomes. *Breast.* 2012;21(4):449-54.

[7] Tranfaglia C, Cardinali L, Gattucci M, Scialpi M, Ferolla P, Sinzinger H, Palumbo B (111)in-pentetreotide spet/ct in carcinoid tumours: is the role of hybrid systems advantageous in abdominal or thoracic lesions? *Hell J Nucl Med.* 2011;14(3):274-7.

[8] Pusiol T, Zorzi MG, Morichetti D, Piscioli I, Scialpi M. Uselessness of radiological differentiation of oncocytoma and renal cell carcinoma in management of small renal masses. *World J Urol.* 2011 May 21.

[9] Brancato B, Scialpi M, Pusiol T, Zorzi MG, Morichetti D, Piscioli F. Needle core biopsy should replace fine needle aspiration cytology in ultrasound-guided sampling of breast lesions. *Pathologica.* 2011;103(2):52.

[10] Pusiol T, Zorzi MG, Morichetti D, Piscioli I, Scialpi M. Uselessness of percutaneous core needle renal biopsy in the management of small renal masses. *Urol Int.* 2011;87(1):125-6.

[11] Pusiol T, Zorzi MG, Morichetti D, Piscioli I, Scialpi M. Uselessness of percutaneous core needle renal biopsy in the management of small renal masses. *Urol Int.* 2011;87(1):125-6.

[12] Pusiol T, Zorzi MG, Morichetti G, Piscioli I, Scialpi M. Synchronous nonfunctional duodenal carcinoid and high risk gastrointestinal stromal tumour (GIST) of the stomach. Eur Rev Med *Pharmacol Sci.* 2011;15(5):583-5.

[13] Pusiol T, Franceschetti I, Scialpi M, Piscioli I, Sassi C, Parolari AM. Incidental Necrotizing Paratubal Granuloma Associated with Multiple Neoplasms. *J. Gynecol Surg.* 2011, 27(1): 29-32.

[14] Gohagan J., Marcus P., Fagerstrom R., et al.: Baseline findings of a randomized feasibility trial of lung cancer screening with spiral CT scan vs chest radiograph: the Lung Screening Study of National Cancer Institute - *Chest.* 2004;126(1):114-121.

[15] Swensen S.J., Jett J.R., Hartman T.E., Midthun DE, Sloan JA, Sykes AM, Aughenbaugh GL, Clemens MA: Lung cancer screening with CT: Mayo Clinic experience - *Radiology.* 2003; 226(3):756-761.

[16] Bach P.B., Silvestri G.A., Hanger M, Jett JR., for the American College of Chest Physicians: Screening for lung cancer: ACCP evidence-based clinical practice guidelines - 2nd ed. *Chest* 2007; 132(3 suppl):69S-77S.

[17] Steele J.D.: The solitary pulmonary nodule. Report of a cooperative study of resected asymptomatic solitary pulmonary nodules in male - *J Thorac Cardiovasc Surg.* 1963;46:21-39.

[18] World Health Organisation Classification of Tumours, Pathology & Genetics, Tumours of the Lung, Pleura, Thymus and Heart. Edited by Travis WD, Brambilla E, Muller-Hermelink HK, Harris CC. Lyon, France: IARC Press, 2004.

[19] Travis WD, Colby TV, Corrin B, et al. Histological Typing of Lung and Pleural Tumors. Berlin: Springer, 1999.

[20] Lee HY, Goo JM, Lee HJ, et al. Usefulness of concurrent reading using thin-section and thick-section CT images in subcentimetre solitary pulmonary nodules. *Clin Radiol* 2009;64:127–132.

[21] Hansell DM, Bankier AA, MacMahon H, et al. Fleischner Society: glossary of terms for thoracic imaging. *Radiology* 2008;246:697–722.

[22] Travis WD, Brambilla E, Noguchi M, Nicholson AG, Geisinger KR, Yatabe Y, Beer DG, Powell CA, Riely GJ, Van Schil PE, Garg K, Austin JH, Asamura H, Rusch VW, Hirsch FR, Scagliotti G, Mitsudomi T, Huber RM, Ishikawa Y, Jett J, Sanchez-Cespedes M, Sculier JP, Takahashi T, Tsuboi M, Vansteenkiste J, Wistuba I, Yang PC, Aberle D, Brambilla C, Flieder D, Franklin W, Gazdar A, Gould M, Hasleton P, Henderson D, Johnson B, Johnson D, Kerr K, Kuriyama K, Lee JS, Miller VA, Petersen I, Roggli V, Rosell R, Saijo N, Thunnissen E, Tsao M, Yankelewitz D. International Association for the Study of Lung Cancer/American Thoracic Society/European Respiratory Society International Multidisciplinary Classification of Lung Adenocarcinoma. *J Thorac Oncol.* 2011;6(2):244-85.

[23] Travis WD, Linnoila RI, Tsokos MG, Hitchcock CL, Cutler GB Jr, Nieman L, Chrousos G, Pass H, Doppman J, Neuroendocrine tumors of the lung with proposed criteria for large-cell neuroendocrine carcinoma. An ultrastructural, immunohistochemical, and flow cytometric study of 35 cases. *Am J Surg Pathol.* 1991;15(6):529-53.

[24] Curado MP, Edwards B, Shin HR, et al. Cancer Incidence in Five Continents, Vol. IX. Lyon: IARC Scientific Publications, 2007.

[25] Godoy MC, Naidich DP. Subsolid pulmonary nodules and the spectrum of peripheral adenocarcinomas of the lung: recommended interim guidelines for assessment and management. *Radiology* 2009;253:606– 622.

[26] Pentheroudakis G, Kostadima L, Fountzilas G, Kalogera-Fountzila A, Klouvas G, Kalofonos C, Pavlidis N. Cavitating squamous cell lung carcinoma-distinct entity or not? Analysis of radiologic, histologic, and clinical features. *Lung Cancer* 2004;45:349–355.

[27] Onn A, Choe DH, Herbst RS, Correa AM, Munden RF, Truong MT, Vaporciyan AA, Isobe T, Gilcrease MZ, Marom EM. Tumor cavitation in stage I non-small cell lung cancer: epidermal growth factor receptor expression and prediction of poor outcome. *Radiology* 2005;237:342–347.

[28] Travis WD, Garg K, Franklin WA, Wistuba II, et al. Evolving concepts in the pathology and computed tomography imaging of the lung adenocarcinoma and bronchioloalveolar carcinoma. *J Clin Oncol* 2005; 23: 3279-87.

Chapter 2

Primary Lung Cancer Coexisting with Lung Metastases from Various Malignancies

Noritoshi Nishiyama

Additional information is available at the end of the chapter

http://dx.doi.org/10.5772/46066

1. Introduction

Various tumors metastasize to the lung, and they are often detected as multiple nodules. Advances in computed tomography (CT) have made it possible to detect small tumors. Even for multiple pulmonary nodules with previous malignancy, surgical removal is often required when the primary sites are well controlled and no other sites are involved. However, preoperative differential diagnosis of coexisting primary lung cancer is usually difficult for such small nodules [1].

Here, three cases of lung metastases that coexisted with primary lung cancer, confirmed by postoperative histological examination, are presented. In addition, a case with a proven lung cancer that coexisted with small nodules in the ipsilateral lung, one of which was pathologically diagnosed as a metastasis from rectal cancer, is presented. Further, the importance of active tissue diagnosis including surgery is discussed.

2. A: Lung metastases from various malignancies coexisting with primary lung cancer

2.1. Case 1

A 53-year old woman was diagnosed by needle biopsy as having a myxoid liposarcoma in the right thigh. A chest CT scan revealed small bilateral pulmonary nodules, which were diagnosed as pulmonary metastases; and the patient underwent two courses of preoperative chemotherapy with ifosfamide and adriamycin. There was a partial response to the chemotherapy for both the primary tumor and pulmonary metastases. Surgical resection of the primary tumor in the right thigh and bilateral pulmonary metastasectomy via sequential small axillary thoracotomies under video assistance (one in the right lower lobe and one in the left upper lobe measuring 3 and 5 mm, respectively, and two in the left lower lobe measuring 5 and 8 mm) (Figure 1) was simultaneously performed in January 2008.

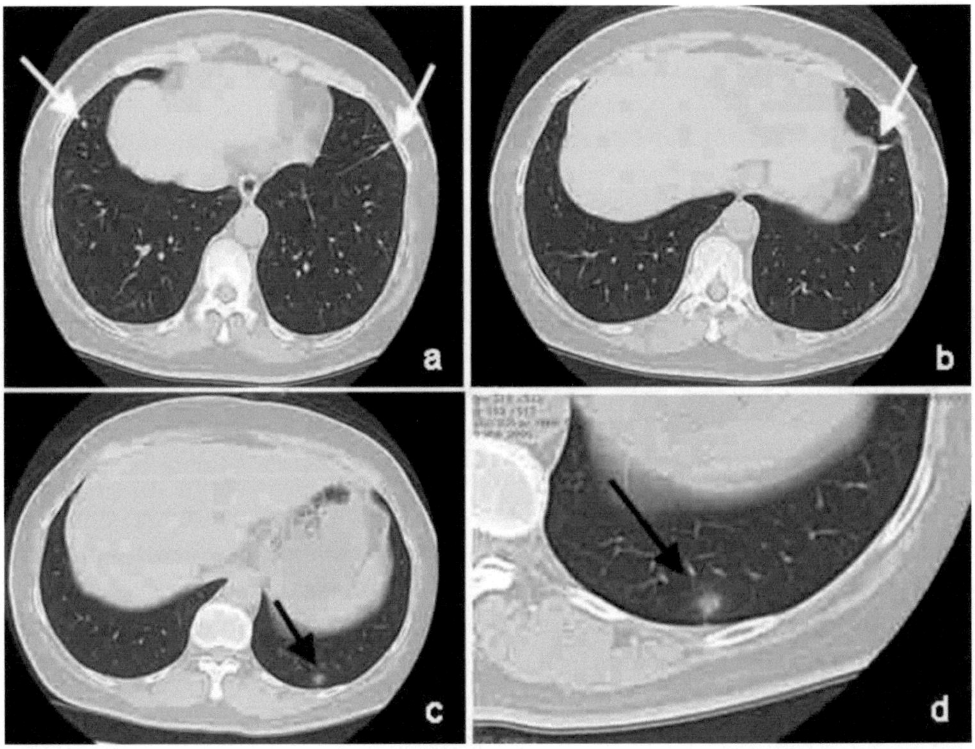

Figure 1. Preoperative chest computed tomography (CT) images showing tumors (arrows): one in the right lower lobe and one in the left upper lobe measuring 3 and 5 mm, respectively (**a**, white arrows), and two in the left lower lobe measuring 5 and 8 mm (**b**, white arrow; **c**, black arrow). (**d**) Magnified image of (**c**). Postoperative pathological examination revealed that the tumor shown in panels (**c**) and (**d**) was a well differentiated adenocarcinoma. (From Nishiyama, Iwata, Nagano et al. Lung metastases from various malignances combined with primary lung cancer. Gen Thorac Cardiovasc Surg 2010; 58: 539. With permission)

A postoperative pathological examination revealed that one of the resected pulmonary tumors in the left lower lobe, measuring 8 mm in diameter, was a well differentiated adenocarcinoma (Noguchi type F) [2], and there were no viable tumor cells in the remaining three nodules; the resected tumor in the right thigh was finally diagnosed as a myxoid liposarcoma. Carcinoembryonic antigen (CEA), squamous cell carcinoma-related antigen (SCC), cytokeratin 19 fragment (CYFRA), and Sialyl Lewis^x (SLX) were within normal ranges. No distant metastasis was found, and the patient was diagnosed with clinical stage IA primary lung cancer [3].

The risks and benefits for lobectomy and observation were explained to the patient. After informed consent was obtained, a left lower lobectomy via a left axillary thoracotomy was performed 17 days after the initial surgery. The patient recovered uneventfully, and a postoperative pathological examination revealed no lymph node metastasis. She was discharged with a treatment plan involving postoperative adjuvant chemotherapy for the liposarcoma.

2.2. Case 2

A 70-year old woman was referred to our hospital in June 2008 for further treatment of pulmonary metastases due to colon cancer. A chest CT scan revealed bilateral small pulmonary nodules: three in the right upper lobe and two in the left upper lobe (Figure 2). The patient underwent right hemicolectomy for stage IIIB transverse colon cancer in October 2005, followed by adjuvant chemotherapy with oral tegafur and leucovorin for 18 months postoperatively. Bilateral pulmonary metastases appeared in June 2007, but were markedly diminished in January 2008 when chemotherapy with 17 courses of 5-fluorouracil (5-FU), leucovorin and oxaliplatin was completed. However, the tumors re-grew and were diagnosed in May 2008. Serum CEA and CA 19-9 were within normal ranges. Bilateral pulmonary metastasectomy via sequential small axillary thoracotomies under video assistance (three in the right upper lobe measuring 12, 12 and 20 mm, and two in the left upper lobe measuring 5 and 12 mm) was carried out in June 2008.

A postoperative pathological examination revealed that one of the resected pulmonary tumors in the left upper lobe, measuring 5 mm in diameter, was Noguchi type B bronchioloalveolar carcinoma [2]. The remaining four tumors were diagnosed as metastatic tubular adenocarcinoma from colon cancer. No distant metastasis was found, and the patient was diagnosed with clinical stage IA primary lung cancer [3]. She recovered uneventfully and was discharged with a plan of postoperative adjuvant chemotherapy for the colon cancer.

2.3. Case 3

A 69-year old man was referred to our hospital in October 2011 for further treatment of pulmonary metastases due to renal cell carcinoma. He underwent left nephrectomy for a left renal cell carcinoma (T1a, G1, INFα) in June 2007. A chest CT scan revealed two small pulmonary nodules in segments S8 and S9 of the right lower lobe that appeared in

November 2010 and increased in size in September 2011 (Figure 3). Serum CEA, CYFRA and SLX were within normal ranges, but SCC was slightly elevated to 2.1 ng/ml (normal range < 1.5 ng/ml). Although lung metastases were suspected, tissue diagnosis through bronchoscopy was unsuccessful and pulmonary metastasectomy via a small axillary thoracotomy was conducted under video assistance in October 2011.

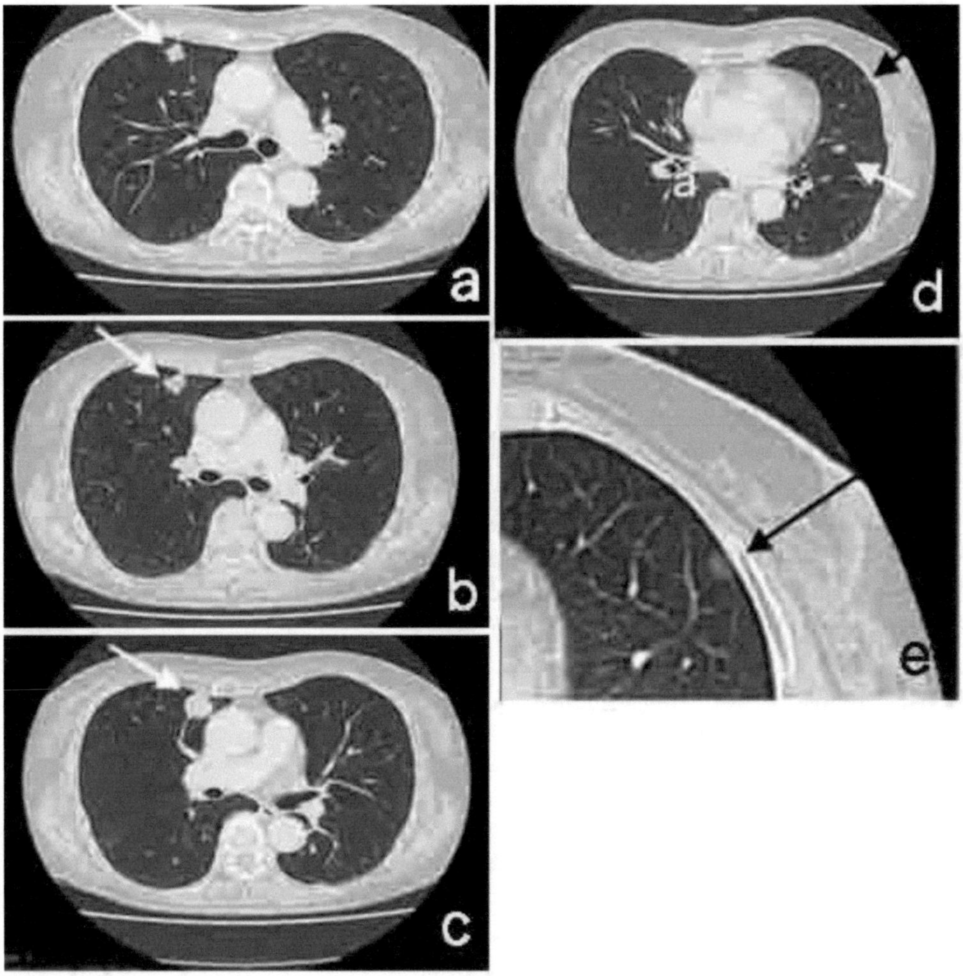

Figure 2. Preoperative chest CT images showing tumors (arrows): three in the right upper lobe measuring 12, 12 and 20 mm (**a**, **b**, **c**, white arrows), and two in the left upper lobe measuring 5 mm (black arrow) and 12 mm (white arrow) (**d**). **(e)** Magnified image of panel (**d**) (black arrow). Postoperative pathological examination revealed that the tumor shown in panel (**e**) was a Noguchi type B bronchioloalveolar carcinoma. The remaining four tumors were diagnosed as metastatic tubular adenocarcinoma from colon cancer. (From Nishiyama, Nagano, Izumi et al. Lung metastases from various malignances combined with primary lung cancer. Gen Thorac Cardiovasc Surg 2010; 58: 540. With permission)

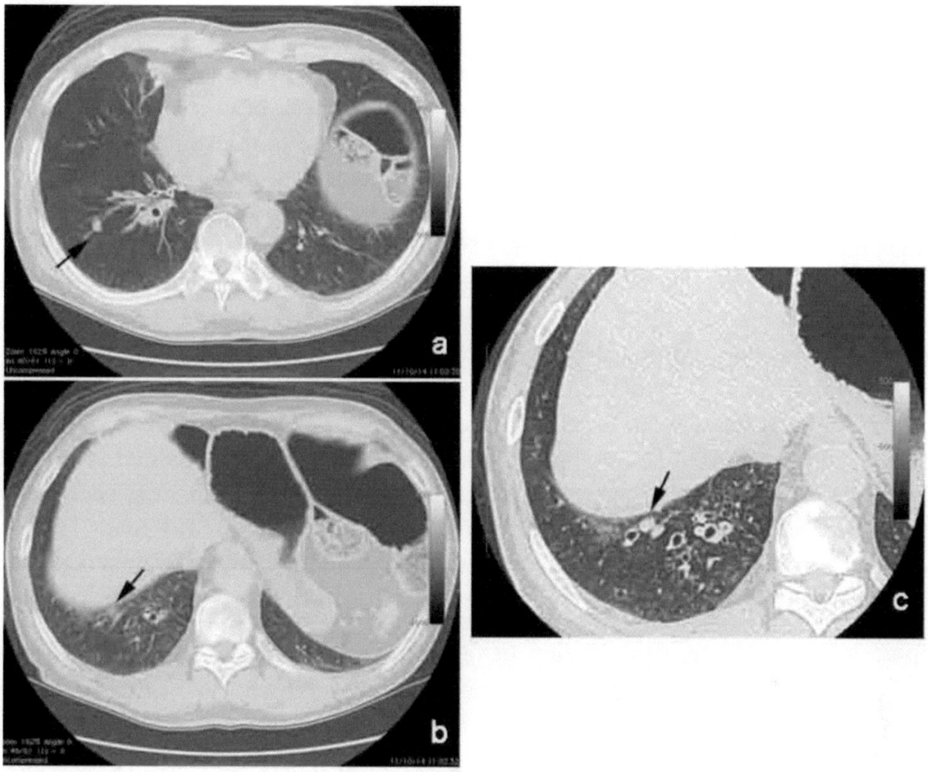

Figure 3. Preoperative chest CT images showing tumors in the right lower lobe (black arrows): one in the S8 segment measuring 8 mm (**a**), and the other in the S9 segment measuring 7 mm (**b**). (**c**) Thin slice image of (**b**). An intra-operative pathological examination revealed that the tumor in the S9 segment was adenocarcinoma and postoperative pathological examination revealed that the tumor shown in panel (**a**) in the S8 segment was a metastatic clear cell carcinoma from renal cell carcinoma.

An intra-operative pathological examination revealed that one of the pulmonary tumors in segment S9 measuring 7 mm in diameter was adenocarcinoma and a right lower lobectomy was performed. A postoperative pathological examination revealed that the tumor in segment S9 was Noguchi type A bronchioloalveolar carcinoma [2], and the other tumor measuring 8 mm in segment S8 of the resected lobe was metastatic clear cell carcinoma from renal cell carcinoma. No lymph node metastasis or distant metastasis was found, and the patient was diagnosed with clinical stage IA primary lung cancer [3]. He recovered uneventfully and was discharged with a plan of postoperative adjuvant chemotherapy for the renal cell carcinoma.

3. B: Primary lung cancer coexisting with lung metastases from other malignancies

3.1. Case 4

A 62-year old man was referred to our hospital for further examination of a suspicious primary lung cancer in the left upper lobe, measuring 23 mm in diameter on a chest CT. In addition, the chest CT scan revealed other two nodules, one beside the tumor in the left upper lobe measuring 5 mm and the other in the left lower lobe measuring 10 mm (Figure 4). The patient had undergone surgery for stage IIIA rectal cancer followed by postoperative adjuvant chemotherapy 6 years ago, and stage IA gastric cancer 3 years ago. Trans-bronchial curettage cytology of the larger tumor in the left upper lobe revealed adenocarcinoma. CEA 13.2 ng/ml, SCC 2.0 ng/ml and SLX 47 U/ml (normal range <5.0 ng/ml, 1.5 ng/ml and 38 U/ml, respectively) serum tumor markers were elevated. Clinical diagnosis of primary lung cancer was established by cytology and chest CT, leaving a differential diagnosis of pulmonary metastasis from rectal cancer or gastric cancer. Preoperative tissue diagnosis of the other two nodules was unobtainable because of small lesions. The patient was advised on the risks and benefits of surgery for disease with metastases from lung cancer, rectal cancer or gastric cancer. After obtaining informed consent the patient underwent left upper lobectomy with mediastinal lymph node dissection, combined with partial resection of the left lower lobe in April 2008.

A postoperative pathological examination using immunohistological staining revealed the tumor and the nodule in the left lower lobe as being poorly differentiated adenocarcinoma, which was cytokeratin (CK) 7 positive and CK 20 negative, CEA positive, surfactant apoprotein negative and thyroid transcription factor-1 (TTF-1) positive. Metastasis in the resected hilar lymph node was also diagnosed. Definitive pathological diagnosis of primary lung cancer with pulmonary metastasis in the ipsilateral lung and hilar lymph node metastasis (pT4N1M0, stage IIIA) [3] was established. The remaining nodule besides the tumor in the left upper lobe was diagnosed as metastasis from rectal cancer, and was CK 7 negative and CK 20 positive, CEA positive, surfactant apoprotein negative and TTF-1 negative. The patient recovered uneventfully and was discharged with a treatment plan involving postoperative chemotherapy for lung cancer.

4. Discussion

Recent advances in CT have obviously contributed to the diagnosis of small pulmonary nodules and ground-glass opacity components which indicate possible primary lung cancer [4]. The preoperative differential diagnosis of either metastatic or primary lung cancer is usually difficult, because with the exception of surgery, it is not possible to obtain sufficient tissue from these small neoplasms. A retrospective assessment of case 1 suggested that a careful review of the CT scans could lead to a diagnosis of possible primary lung cancer because they demonstrated an unclear-bordered nodule with pleural indentation. In addition, the nodule, which was different from the others, did not reduce in size after chemotherapy. A retrospective assessment of the tumor in case 2, which was diagnosed as bronchioloalveolar carcinoma, revealed unclear-bordered ground-glass opacity (GGO) indicating possible primary lung cancer. A retrospective assessment of the tumor in case 3, which was diagnosed as adenocarcinoma, indicated a relatively clear-bordered nodule underlining the difficulty of distinguishing primary lung cancer and lung metastasis from other malignancies in the preoperative differential diagnosis of this small nodule.

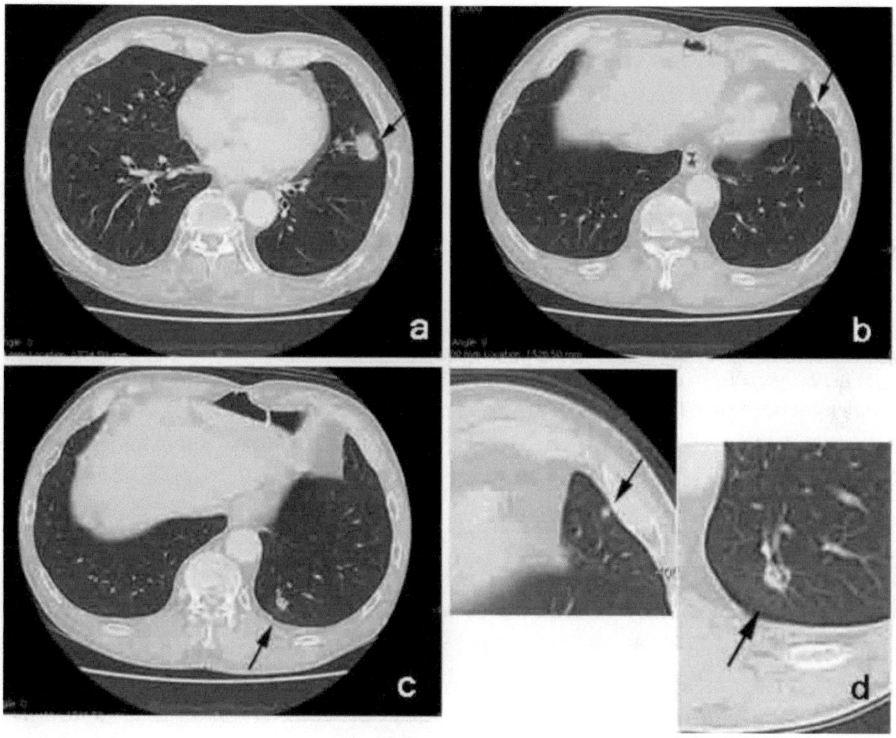

Figure 4. Preoperative chest CT images showing tumors (black arrows): a primary lung cancer in the left upper lobe measuring 23 mm in diameter (**a**) and two nodules, one beside the tumor in the left upper lobe measuring 5 mm (**b**) and the other in the left lower lobe measuring 10 mm (**c**). (**d**) magnified image of (**b**) (the left side) and (**c**) (the right side). Postoperative immunohistological examination revealed the tumor shown in panel (**b**) was a lung metastasis from rectal cancer, and the tumor shown in panel (**c**) was metastasis from lung cancer.

Noguchi et al. [2] reported on the pathological features of small adenocarcinomas of the lung in 1995, in which Noguchi type A and B tumors had a 100% postoperative 5-year survival rate. Advances in CT imaging since the early 1990s have led to considerably more accurate diagnoses of GGO lesions, corresponding to such early-stage lung cancer [5]. Recently, a new classification of lung adenocarcinoma has been proposed that takes into consideration their clinical outcomes, and Noguchi type A and B tumors correspond to adenocarcinoma in situ [6,7].

When nodules are removed and diagnosed as primary lung cancer coexisting with lung metastasis from other malignancies, additional treatment should be considered according to the prognosis of each disease (i.e., primary lung cancer and primary tumor metastasized to the lung). In case 1, although the general prognosis of a myxoid liposarcoma with multiple lung metastases is still unclear [8], excellent effects of preoperative chemotherapy (demonstrated pathologically as no remaining viable tumors in the lungs) prompted us to recommend completion lobectomy with the intent of a precise diagnosis including lymph node dissection. In case 2, the primary lung cancer was preinvasive [2,6] and required no further resection. In case 3, lobectomy was performed with an intra-operative diagnosis of adenocarcinoma, and was sufficient treatment for the remaining single metastasis from the renal cell carcinoma in the same lobe.

Recently, the appropriateness of sublobar resection has been investigated for such small lung cancers, because they are likely to have no lymph node metastases [9-11]. Following a careful reassessment of preoperative CT images including the presence of GGO and the size and pathological features of the tumor, the necessity of additional pulmonary resection with lymph node dissection should be considered.

In contrast, proven primary lung cancer sometimes appears with small nodules in the same lobe or other lobes. As shown in case 4, the stage of the lung cancer depends on the definitive tissue diagnosis of the small nodules. In addition, we experienced a case of a primary adenocarcinoma in the right upper lobe, with a small nodule in the left lower lobe that was diagnosed as cryptococcosis. Therefore, importance of active tissue diagnosis including surgery should be emphasized, especially in patients with previous malignancies. On the other hand, for indeterminate lung tumors with a strong suspicion of lung cancer, lobectomy followed by thorough pathological examination is required in some conditions, because of difficulties in pre- or intra-operative tissue diagnosis when the lesion is deeply located near the major pulmonary vessels [12]. Even such tumors could present with other pulmonary nodules.

In all situations, once definitive diagnosis has been established, additional treatment including additional surgery or chemotherapy should be considered depending on the prognosis of each disease (i.e., primary tumor metastasized to the lung and primary lung cancer).

5. Conclusion

In surgery for pulmonary tumors, possible coexistence of lung metastasis from various malignancies and primary lung cancer should be considered. When resected tumor is diagnosed as primary lung cancer coexisting with lung metastasis from other malignancies, the necessity for additional treatment should be considered, depending on the prognosis of each disease (i.e., primary lung cancer and primary tumor metastasized to the lung).

Author details

Noritoshi Nishiyama
Department Thoracic Surgery, Osaka City University Graduate School of Medicine, Osaka, Japan

6. References

[1] Nishiyama N, Iwata T, Nagano K, Izumi N, Tsukioka T, Tei K, et al (2010) Lung metastases from various malignancies combined with primary lung cancer. Gen Thorac Cardiovasc Surg. 58: 538-541.

[2] Noguchi M, Morikawa A, Kawasaki M, Matsuno Y, Yamada T, Hirohashi S, et al (1995) Small adenocarcinoma of the lung: histologic characteristics and prognosis. Cancer. 75: 2844-2852.

[3] Sobin LH, Gospodarowicz MK, Wittekind CH, eds (2009) UICC (International Union Against Cancer) TNM classification of malignant tumors. 7th ed. New York: Wiley-Blackwell.

[4] Yankelevitz D, Henschke CI (2004) State-of-the-art screening for lung cancer. Part 2. CT screening. Thorac Surg Clin. 14: 53-59.

[5] Yoshida J (2007) Management of the peripheral small ground-glass opacities. Thorac Surg Clin. 17:191-201.

[6] Travis WD, Brambilla E, Noguchi M, Nicholson AG, Geisinger KR, Yatabe Y et al (2011) International association for the study of lung cancer / American thoracic society / European respiratory society International multidisciplinary lung adenocarcinoma classification. J Thorac Oncol. 6: 244-285.

[7] Russell PA, Wainer Z, Wright GM, Daniels M, Conron M, Williams RA (2011) Does lung adenocarcinoma subtype predict patient survival?: a clinicopathologic study based on the new international association for the study of lung cancer / American thoracic society / European respiratory society International multidisciplinary lung adenocarcinoma classification. J Thorac Oncol. 6: 1496-1504.

[8] Nicolas M, Moran CA, Suster S (2005) Pulmonary metastasis from liposarcoma: a clinicopathologic and immunohistochemical study of 24 cases. Am J Clin Pathol. 123: 262-275.

[9] Asamura H, Nakayama H, Kondo H, Tsuchiya R, Shimosato Y, Naruke T (1996) Lymph node involvement, recurrence, and prognosis in resected small, peripheral, non-small

cell lung carcinomas: are these carcinomas candidates for video-assisted lobectomy? J Thorac Cardiovasc Surg. 111: 1125-1134.

[10] Takizawa T, Terashima M, Koike T, Akamatsu H, Kurita Y, Yokoyama A (1997) Mediastinal lymph node metastasis in patients with clinical stage I peripheral non-small cell lung cancer. J Thorac Cardiovasc Surg. 113: 248-252.

[11] Okada M, Nishio W, Sakamoto T, Uchino K, Yuki T, Nakagawa A, et al (2005) Effect of tumor size on prognosis in patients with non-small cell lung cancer: the role of segmentectomy as a type of lesser resection. J Thorac Cardiovasc Surg. 129: 87-93.

[12] Nishiyama N, Nagano K, Izumi N, Tei K MD, Hanada S, Komatsu H, et al (2011) Lobectomy for indeterminate lung tumors with a strong suspicion of lung cancer. Ann Thorac Cardiovasc Surg Nov 30. [Epub ahead of print]

Chapter 3

The Acute Stress Reaction to Major Thoracic Surgery

Lucio Cagini, Jacopo Vannucci, Michele Scialpi and Francesco Puma

Additional information is available at the end of the chapter

http://dx.doi.org/10.5772/54667

1. Introduction

The aim of this revue is to examine the current literature on the physio-pathological mechanism liable for the inflammatory reaction after major surgical injury and the nature and development of the related morbidity. We describe the endocrine and metabolic changes that occur as consequences of major thoracic surgery and the clinical implications of these reactions. The understanding of the stress response mechanism and the early detection of it's clinical manifestations will aid in recognizing and probably help in correcting deviations from the norm.

Major surgical procedures represent an important insult for the homeostasis and determine a systemic inflammatory response syndrome, evolved to ensure survival, characterized by changes in haemodynamic, endocrine and immune functions directed towards preservation of the blood supply to essential organs. [1]

The first description of the clinical manifestations of such responses was presented in 1942 by Cuthbertson [2] who described a biphasic immune, inflammatory and metabolic response to injury. However during the last 20 years, as knowledge has continuously accumulated, it has become clear that the physiologic response to injury is not as simple as initially described and represents a rather complex physiological phenomenon, yet even today it is not completely understood.

The data we recently published confirmed the generalized tendency to accumulate large volumes of fluids in the postoperative days after pulmonary lobectomy. Fluid retention with weight gain was evident despite a negative intra-operative fluid balance, peri-operative strict fluid restriction, early mobilization and an encouraged intake of oral fluids as part of a normal diet. [3]

As reported by several authors following lung resection, multiple factors such as thoracotomy, rapid fluid infusion, and manipulation of the lung result in an increase of the extravascular lung water. Fluids from the interstitial space transudate into the alveolar space severely impairing gas diffusion and facilitating the occurrence of pulmonary edema.

2. Overview

Generally speaking the term ''inflammatory reaction'' refers to events which occur in tissues in response to a pathogenic stimulus. It consists of a series of specific immunological reactions that are protective, aimed at promoting survival. In the case of specific pathogenesis (bacteria, viruses), the inflammatory response is tightly linked to immune-mediated reactions and specifically cellular activation (lymphocytes, antibodies, macrophages, mast cells). Whereas if the stimulus is non-specific (neoplastic disease, surgical stress), the systemic inflammatory response relies on the innate defence mechanisms.

Post injury stress or inflammatory response, is the name given to the hormonal and metabolic changes which follow an anesthetized (e.g. surgery) or unanesthetized (e.g. trauma) injury [4]. It includes an adaptive set of events, a predictable well orchestrated reaction, that has evolved to maximize an organism's healing potential and it is not unique to humans but is found in all vertebrate animals [1].

In evolutionary term it seems likely that the stress response developed as a survival mechanism to allow injured animals to sustain themselves until their injures were healed, by catabolising their own stored body fuels and retaining salt and water. However it has been argued that such response is unnecessary in current surgical and anaesthetic practice [4].

During the last century, scientific efforts to clarify aspects of non-cellular inflammatory responses have revealed some special molecules that play an important role in local and systemic alterations in the affected individual: histamine, prostanoids leukotrienes, platelet activating factor, bradykinin, nitric oxide, neuropeptides and cytokines.

The cytochines are a group of low molecular-weight proteins released in inflammatory and immune reactions which include interleukins, interferons, tumor necrosis factor, growth factors and chemokines. They are produced by activated leucocytes, fibroblasts and endothelia cells as an early response to tissue injury and have a major role in mediating immunity and inflammation. [5] They have local effects of mediating and maintaining the inflammatory response to tissue injury and after major surgery the main cytochines released are interleukin-1 (IL-1], tumor necrosis factor-alfa (TNF alfa) and IL-6 [4, 5].

The activation of the cytokine cascade is accompanied by the release of soluble cytokine receptors with significant growth factor functions, and by the activation of the massive neuro-endocrine-hormonal flux involving the production and secretion of catecholamines, antidiuretic hormone, cortisol, insulin, glucagon and growth hormone. The natural final goal is the retention of water and sodium; if the body is going to conserve water and sodium as a response to the surgical trauma, that would imply that smaller quantities of these elements should suffice to maintain homeostasis [6].

Localized inflammation is a physiological protective response which is generally tightly controlled by the body at the site of injury. Loss of this local control or an overly activated response results in an exaggerated systemic response which is clinically identified as systemic inflammatory response syndrome (SIRS). Compensatory mechanisms are initiated in concert with SIRS and outcome (resolution, multiple organ dysfunction syndrome or death) depends on the balance of SIRS and such compensatory mechanisms. No direct therapies have been successful to date in influencing outcome [7].

The outcome of the inflammatory response may be altered in several conditions; in particular following major thoracic surgery preexisting diseases (such as chronic obstructive pulmonary disease, renal failure, coronary artery disease, diabetes, hypertension), type and quantity of fluid infused, lung manipulation, anesthetic agents and single lung ventilation may interact with the inflammatory response and affect the ability of an individual to mount an appropriate stress response. Some patients develop an exaggerated response that results in what is commonly referred to as systemic inflammatory response syndrome (SIRS), on the contrary after an illness that depletes the organism, outcome may result in generally compromised organ function that is known most commonly by the multiple-organ dysfunction syndrome (MODS) or, more generically, chronic critical illness.

3. The biphasic reaction

This reaction characterized by a biphasic immune, inflammatory and metabolic response was described for the first time in 1942 by Cuthbertson [2] and some decades later some detail was added by Moore [8].

In the first phase the major points are the attempt to limit the blood loss by the activation of the responses that must ensure survival following injury; i.e. peripheral vasoconstriction, the derived hypothermia, the translocation of blood and substrate from the peripheral to vital organs (heart and central nervous system) circulation, retention of salt and water and decreases of energy expenditure. The length of this phase of the response that in Cuthbertson's description lasted 24 hours, can be restricted by appropriate treatment of the trigger. The activation of these conservative mechanisms occur in anesthetized or unanesthetized injury. In the former (elective major surgery) the beginning may be represented by the dilatation of the venous capacitance system produced by the commonly used anesthetic induction agents which decreases the blood return to the heart diminishing the cardiac output [1] or by the cytochines produced by activated leucocytes, fibroblasts and endothelia cells at the site of the surgical insult. [5]

In case of unanesthetized injury the neuro-endocrine-hormonal response is activated by afferent neuronal impulses from the site of injury that travel along sensory nerve roots through the dorsal root of the spinal cord to the medulla to activate the hypothalamus [4]. In this early stage of shock, adequate fluid therapy comprise of goal-directed filling [9] to prevent evolution to multiple organ dysfunction syndrome (MODS).

The second phase of the response is termed the hypermetabolic phase and is driven and is proportional to the degree of initial injury [1]. It is characterized by the peak, on the second postoperative day, of all the mediators of inflammation, and by the activity of the reparative cells, in particular white blood cells (WBCs). The energy needs come from catabolism of both skeletal and visceral muscle with release into the circulation of protein and amino acids resulting in loss of body cell mass that primarily reflects a decrease in skeletal muscle mass. The cardiovascular system plays a critical role in this phase; the vasculature dilates to improve flow and substrate delivery. Vascular leak allows fluid and substrate to flow towards the avascular area of injury and to remove waste products. [1]

The resultant tachycardia and elevated cardiac output boosts myocardial oxygen consumption, and increase in resting energy expenditure and in total body oxygen consumption and $CO2$ production.

The net effect is an increased catabolism with increased substrate availability for energy production, and sodium and water retention to maintain fluid volume and haemodynamic stability [4, 10]. Sodium and water are retained avidly in the first few days, and convalescence and recovery are heralded by a return of the capacity to excrete any salt and water overload acquired during the earlier phase [11].

Following major surgery the well known clinical manifestations of this hypermetabolic phase include tachycardia, hyperthermia (representing hypermetabolism), hyperglycemia, leukocytosis, micro-albuminuria and edema (from capillary leak). This phase continues for several days and ceases with the transition from catabolism to anabolism, resolution of vasodilatation, and edema. At this point fluids are reabsorbed and eliminated with diuresis. All these facts support the concept that parts of intra-operatively administered fluids are redistributed into the interstitial and intracellular spaces, which undergo reabsorption in the postoperative period [12].

4. The endothelial surface layer and the pathogenesis of extra vascular water

The current basic research has brought fascinating insights to the function of the endothelial vascular barrier and, in particular, to the functional changes that lead to vascular leakage.

The etiopathogenesis of extravascular water is explained very clearly by S.R. Walsh et al in an interesting manuscript "Perioperative fluid restriction reduces complications after major gastrointestinal surgery" [6]. They reported that the body's fluid and electrolyte balance is maintained within a tightly defined range and this is achieved mainly by the kidney, under the influence of antidiuretic hormone and the renin--angiotensin—aldosterone axis, which influence sodium and water excretion and retention as necessary to maintain the volume and osmolality of the extracellular fluid. The mechanism involves a daily obligatory sodium loss of about 100 mmol and a daily maintenance sodium requirements of about 1.0--1.2 mmol/kg. Daily water requirements are between 25 and 35 mL/kg. The surgical trauma causes an intense distortion of the normal physiology. Preoperative fasting, intraoperative bleeding, and insensible losses combine to produce extracellular volume depletion. Leukocyte activation increases capillary wall permeability, allowing seepage of proteins, water, and electrolytes out of capillaries into tissues, further depleting the intravascular space. The increase in capillary permeability is sufficient to allow the passage of large albumin molecules into the interstitium at a faster rate than the lymphatic system can drain it. The resulting accumulation of albumin increases the oncotic pressure of the interstitium, serving to draw further water and sodium from the intravascular space. [6]

A new insight in the mechanism liable for the fluid's transendothelial permeability came from the comprehension of the endothelial surface layer (ESL) and the role of endothelial glycocalyx as reported by Strunden [13]. Every healthy vascular endothelium is coated by transmembrane syndecans and membrane-bound glypicans containing heparan sulphate and chondroitin sulfate side chains, which together constitute the endothelial glycocalyx [14,15]. Bound plasma proteins, solubilized glycosaminoglycans, and hyaluronan are loading the glycocalyx to the endothelial surface layer (ESL), which is subject of a periodic constitution and degradation. Under physiologic conditions, the ESL has a thickness of approximately 1 µm and binds approximately 800 ml of blood plasma, so plasma volume can be divided into a circulating and non circulating part [15,16]. Accordingly, the glycocalyx seems to act as a molecular filter, retaining proteins and increasing the oncotic pressure within the endothelial surface layer.

A number of studies identified various agents and pathologic states impairing the glycocalyx scaffolding and ESL thickness.

In a genuine pig heart model, Chappell et al. demonstrated a 30-fold increased shedding of heparan sulphate after postischemic reperfusion [17]. These data were approved by a clinical investigation, which showed increased plasma levels of syndecan-1 and heparan sulphate in patients with global or regional ischemia who underwent major vascular surgery [18].

Beside ischemia/reperfusion-injury, several circulating mediators are known to initiate glycocalyx degradation. Tumor necrosis factor-(a), cytokines proteases, and heparanase from activated mast cells are well-described actors in systemic inflammatory response syndrome leading to reduction of the ESL thickness, which triggers increased leucocyte adhesion and transendothelial permeability [17,19, 20].

Interestingly, hypervolemia represents one of the several factors able to cause glycocalyx impairment mediated by liberation of atrial natriuretic peptide as shown by Bruegger D in the recent manuscript "Atrial natriuretic peptide induces shedding of endothelial glycocalyx in coronary vascular bed of guinea pig hearts" [21].

Therefore hypervolemia resulting from inadequately high fluid administration therefore may cause iatrogenic glycocalyx damage [13].

As shown in basic research, the dramatic consequence of a rudimentary glycocalyx, which loses much of its ability to act as a second barrier, is strongly increased transendothelial permeability and following formation of interstitial edema [17,21]. The relevance of these experimental data were impressively underlined by Nelson et al., who found increased plasma levels of glycosaminoglycans and syndecan-1 in septic patients, whereas median glycosaminoglycan levels were higher in patients who did not survive [13, 22].

5. The pathogenesis of extra vascular lung water (EVLW) and pulmonary edema

The lungs provide valuable insight into dynamic microcirculatory changes during systemic inflammation because they are maximally exposed to the proinflammatory cascade, receiving the entire cardiac output [23]. The pulmonary artery follows the course of bronchial anatomy and carries blood to the alveoli where the gas exchange will occur. The blood pressures in the areas of the small circle are lower than in the large circle. The reason lies in the low impedance and resistance of the pulmonary vessels. In addition, the blood flowing in the pulmonary arterial bed is different in composition than the systemic blood. The laws that balance the content of lung capillaries and the surrounding environment are, however, the same underlying vascular physiology in other districts. These are defined in part by the Starling forces and by variations in capillary permeability. The alveolar ventilation and perfusion are therefore the two transport systems of the gas until the alveolus. The way in which an efficient gas exchange is produced, is subtended by the ratio ventilation / perfusion which brings together (in the ideal condition, therefore purely theoretical) the amount of blood and the volume of air which carry oxygen and carbon dioxide in different moments of shipping.

In this context, all cellular functions, the systemic endocrine regulation, intercellular communication, extracellular matrix features, the neurophysiological control systems and many other functions and properties find space.

The respiratory dynamics are achieved through countless joints, but the basic steps are 6. 1) gas exchange between alveoli and external environment, 2) gas exchange between alveoli and blood, 3) transport of gas from the lungs to the tissues, and viceversa, through blood, 4) gas exchange between blood and interstitium, 5) gas exchange between the cell and interstitium, 6] mitochondrial metabolism [24].

The respiratory unit consists of a respiratory bronchiole, the alveolar ducts and the alveoli. The walls of the alveoli are thin and placed in communication with each other through a network of interconnected capillaries [25]. The thickness of the alveolar walls is accompanied by an equally thickness of the lamina of blood flowing through them. Thanks to this contact, alveolar and blood gases can determine the respiratory exchange. The respiratory membrane therefore represents the interface between the environment and the organism but not only, it is also the site of oxygen flow and discharge of carbon dioxide. The efficiency of the respiratory membrane provides the metabolic capacity and thus cellular function is directly responsible for the availability of the organism to accomplish any aerobic metabolism.

The respiratory membrane is composed of several layers that described, from the inside of the alveolus, are: 1) liquid surfactant, 2) alveolar epithelium, 3) basement membrane, 4) the interstitial space, 5) the capillary basement membrane, 6) epithelium of the capillary. Each of these areas of the respiratory membrane is subjected to different stimulations that vary, depending on the conditions, the efficiency and the speed of the exchanges.

For the air–blood barrier, a minimum volume of interstitial water assures the maximum surface/ thickness ratio to optimise gas diffusion. In the lung the endothelium of the capillary wall is tightly glued to the epithelial wall. Most of the diffusion occurs in the so called ''thin'' portion that accounts for almost 50% of the barrier surface and whose thinness is as low as 0.2–0.3 mm. The thinness of the air–blood barrier reflects a functionally ''dry'' condition. In addition, for the extravascular space of the lung one can speak of a ''minimum'' volume of water. In fact, when fluid fluxes increase due to alteration in fluid dynamics, this results in an impairment of diffusion [26].

The Pathophysiology of fluid and the dynamics of extravascular lung water in the Interstitium After Lung Thoracic Surgery, has been clearly elucidated in a series of manuscripts by Miserocchi and collaborators that we here cite.

The lung's air-blood barrier is 0.2-0.3 microns thin with a "minimum" volume of water reflecting a functionally "dry" condition that ensures a high efficiency of the gas diffusion [27]. Furthermore similarly to the pleural fluid, also lung interstitial fluid is kept at a subatmospheric pressure (also ~ -10 cmH2O) due to the powerful draining action of lymphatics in face of a very low microvascular permeability [26].

Two important molecules, belonging to the proteoglycans (PGs) family, whose role appears crucial to control the extravascular water volume, as they act as highly hydroplhilic link proteins are Perlecan, an heparansulphate PG (MW 0.1-0.5 MDa) placed in the basement membrane that controls the porosity to water and solutes. Versican (MW 0.5 MDa), a large PG bound to hyaluronan (a random coiled molecule), provides rigidity to the tissue by establishing multiple non-covalent links with other molecules of the matrix and with cells [28, 29].

Miserocchi reported that the volume of the extravascular water is strictly controlled so that the lung appears quite resistant to the development of edema. In fact, at least three mechanisms cooperate to allow only minimal variations in extravascular water volume relative to the steady state condition [26].

First, the glycosaminoglycan chains of PGs can bind excess water to form gel-like structures; this results in an increase in the steric hindrance of proteoglycans and corresponding decrease in the porosity of the basement membrane and thus also in microvascular permeability.

Second, the assembly of large matrix PGs within the extracellular matrix provides low tissue compliance and this represents an important "tissue safety factor" against the development of edema. In fact, a minor increase in extravascular water in response to increased microvascular filtration, causes a marked increase in interstitial pressure (e.g., from ~ -10 to ~ 5 cmH2O) [26] that buffers further filtration.

Third, arteriolar vasoconstriction represents an important reflex to avoid or actually decrease capillary pressure when filtration is increased due to an increase in microvascular permeability [31,32]

Fragmentation/degradation of PGs of the basement membrane cause an increase in microvascular permeability of the paracellular pathway as pore size can reach 50-100 nm allowing easy leakage of albumin. Finding of red blood cells in the alveolar fluid reflects major lesions of the air blood barrier. Fragmentation of matrix PGs removes the "tissue safety factor" by causing an increase in interstitial compliance. The loss of integrity of PGs reflects the sustained increase in parenchymal stresses, the weakening of the non-covalent bonds due to increased water binding, and the activation of tissue metalloproteases (32 Miserocchi et al, 2001a). The hypothesis that the activation of tissue metalloproteases leads to the loss of integrity of PGs faces to new therapeutic approachs by drugs able to control this family of proteinases [33,34,35].

The development of severe pulmomary edema is known as a tumultuous event taking place in minutes. Experimental models in animals have allowed us to attribute the sudden increase in extravascular lung water [32] to the loss of integrity of the proteoglycan components of the macromolecular structure of the lung interstitial space.

One shall consider interstitial edema as a sharp edge between tissue repair and severe disease: in fact, the transition from interstitial to severe lung edema occurs through an "accelerated" phase when the loss of integrity of the interstitial matrix proceeds beyond a critical threshold. Interestingly, the same pathophysiological mechanism can be extended to all forms of lung edema, the only difference being the time sequence of fragmentation of the families of PGs. The initial degradation process involves the large matrix PGs in cardiogenic edema, while in the lesional edema model, the initial process involves PGs of the basement membrane. In the hypoxia lung edema model, both PGs families are involved [32]. A further peculiar feature of lung edema is that it develops in a patchy way, thus revealing regional differences in the efficiency of control of extravascular water volume. These differences have been recently documented in a hypoxic edema model [30] and the hypothesis was put forward that alterations in the geometry of the microvascular-alveolar design might favor an imbalance in interstitial fluid dynamics.

6. Clinical considerations

Post operative or post traumatic fluid retention represents a frequent clinical result of the reaction to surgical stress or injury and frequently is underestimated. In clinical practice this condition is not always emphasized and assessed. Because it may show several clinical manifestations, it is not always clinically evident and may be asymptomatic. The incidence of postoperative edema is common, affecting up to 40% of patients [36], and a similar incidence is reported in patients managed in the intensive care unit after surgery [37].

Indeed edema is a frequent manifestation of fluid retention and it is not easily recognized because fluids collect in a dependent position. Furthermore, often, fluid retention, i.e. edema formation and weight gain, even if reported, are not overall considered a marker of impending complications. Even in our previous manuscripts the we did not reported any information on the presence of post operative fluids retention [38,39,40]

This condition has been thoroughly investigated only in the last two decades. Fluids i.e. water and sodium retention have several clinically important consequences. The increase of water in the interstitial space leads to tissue edema, affecting several organ systems. In the gut wall it impairs motility, prolonging gastric emptying times and predisposing the patients to postoperative ileus [41]. Peripheral edema may impair mobility, the hydrostatic pressure exerted on tissue microvasculature harm tissue perfusion and oxygenation slowing down wound healing and predisposing to wound infection, dehiscence, or anastomotic breakdown [42].

However this condition is associated with a worse prognosis. After major abdominal surgery a weight gain of 3-6 kg is typical and associated with increased morbidity including prolonged ileus, sepsis and delayed recovery time [41,42,43]. Lowell et al. showed a weight gain of more than 10% in >40% of patients admitted to the intensive care unit after major surgery and this increase of body weight, representing interstitial edema, correlated strongly with mortality [37].

After thoracic surgery and particularly after major pulmonary resections, besides the activation of the stress response to the surgical injury [4] several factors may induce pooling of water in the lung interstitium. It may be explained by the volume and the type of fluids administered during the surgical procedure, hypoxia, blood loss, the anaesthesia effects [44], one-lung ventilation [45] and lung manipulation. In this setting the incidence of post-pneumonectomy pulmonary edema may be as high as 12—15% [45]; and this condition may be very dangerous because the increase of extra-vascular lung water can severely impair gas exchange and oxygenation.

Indeed a cornerstone to prevent and treat the reaction to stress of patients in the operating room and in the immediate postoperative period is appropriate types of fluid and volume therapy. In this setting, in clinical practice sometimes an exact determination of fluid balance may be cumbersome and independent risk factors for an increased need for peri-operative fluid replacement are advanced age, diabetes mellitus, chronic obstructive pulmonary disease, and chronic renal failure, so minimizing interstitial fluid accumulation in these patients is particularly important.

The British Consensus Guidelines on Intravenous Fluid Therapy for Adult Surgical Patients' [46] reported that the most reliable method to estimate fluid balance in surgical patients is considered daily weighing, with fluid replacement being based on clinical observation of fluid loss. But daily fluid balance may be inaccurate due to "perspiratio insensibilis", poor quantitation of oral fluid intake and/or urine collections [3].

Fluid loss from insensible perspiration also is often overestimated in many patients, although loss of only 1 ml/kg per hour occurs even when the abdominal cave is opened [47]. Daily weighing may be cumbersome in clinical practice, not so accurate as expected or even unfeasible in the early PODs due to the presence of chest drains and difficulties in maintaining an upright position. Furthermore this measure do not include a determination of the capillary permeability and postoperative fluid retention is reported despite fluid-restriction regime. Undoubtedly, there are other factors, not sufficiently investigated, that could cause this event [3].

Urine production and insensible perspiration are physiologically replaced by free water absorbed from the gastrointestinal system and primarily affect the extravascular space, if they are not pathologically increased. Because the physiologic replacement is limited in fasted patients, it has to be compensated artificially by infusing crystalloids. During surgery, trauma or septic shock additional fluid loss (blood loss, vascular leakage) affects mainly the intravascular compartment [48]. Consequently, the first type of fluid loss is attenuated by slow redistribution between intracellular, interstitial, and intravascular space and causes dehydration, whereas the second type of loss leads to acute hypovolemia. [21]

Preoperative hypovolemia after an overnight fasting period, as reported [49,50], cannot be explained by the considerations above and does not occur regularly in all patients [51]. Fluid reloading is unjustified, at least in cardiovascular healthy patients before low-invasive surgery [51]. Mediated by increased liberation of atrial natriuretic peptide, undifferentiated fluid loading can cause glycocalyx degradation, increase vascular permeability, promote tissue edema formation and therefore may constitute a starting point of the vicious circle of vascular leakage and organ failure [52].

Several facts support the concept that parts of intra-operatively administered fluids are redistributed into the interstitial and intracellular spaces, and undergo reabsorption in the postoperative period [12]. As shown by blood volume measurements, major surgery causes a deficit of 3-6 liters in the perioperative fluid balance. The peak even persists up to 72 hours after trauma or surgery. The common explanation for this phenomenon is a fluid shift into the so-called third space [53,54].

Physiologic fluid shifting from the vessel toward the interstitial space across an intact vascular barrier contains only small amounts of proteins. It does not cause interstitial edema as long as it can be quantitatively managed by the lymphatic system [13]

The transpulmonary thermodilution is an invasive method that allows the estimation of of extravascular lung water (EVLWI) and the extent of capillary leak and fluid overload [55,56]; this technique requires a central venous catheter and a thermistor-tipped arterial thermodilution catheter (Pulsiocath 5F) inserted into the femoral artery and attached to a PiCCOplus® system (Pulsion Medical Systems, Munich, Germany). Therefore this procedure is not feasible in all the surgical and intensive care units.

In clinical practice quantitative and non-invasive methods to estimate fluid retention could be very useful to monitor patients susceptible of fluid compartmentalisation after major surgery and early detection may reduce the risks associated with this condition.

In our experience we investigated, following pulmonary lobectomy, fluid retention by the methods commonly utilized to evaluate body fluids. We found a significant postoperative weight gain, the mean increase in body weight was 2.7 kg ([1.9– 3.4]; $p < 0.001$] on postoperative day 2.

Fluid balance was calculated from the day of operation up to the discharge. Bioimpedance analysis(BIA)-derived parameters resistance(R) and reactance(Xc) is a reproducible, non-invasive method, used in various clinical settings to estimate total body water (TBW). It s based on the different conductive and resistive properties when a small electric current is applied to tissues in vivo [57]. Natriuretic peptides, B-type (BNP), are vasoactive hormones involved in the regulation of blood pressure and volume homeostasis. Alterations in the natriuretic peptide system have been described in several conditions associated with abnormal regulation of body fluids and blood pressure control [58].

In our experience, the three methods used to assess fluid gain consistently showed a significant fluid retention over the course of the study. BIA is a bed side tool allowing non-invasive, early, informative and convenient assessment of fluid retention independent of intake. The time course of BIA in our study is consistent with the results reported by Itobi et al. following major abdominal surgery [36]. Besides, as reported by the Danish Study Group on Peri-operative Fluid Therapy [43], BIA is a more sensitive indicator of fluid overload than body weight and clinical examination. In our patients, preoperative BNP was within the normal range, whereas, in the postoperative observation, plasma BNP rapidly increased and remained above the normal range for the whole study period as reported by several Authors. Nojiri et al. [22]

7. Conclusion

Fluids compartmentalization in mammalians and its dynamics is an evolving topic for several reasons. All subjects in biology, medical sciences and clinical practise finally come to interface H_2O balance. The basic research recently moved important steps but this trend has not been followed by applicative research yet. Such discrepancy shows the need of investigation on novel techniques to translate into the clinical practice the ever greater knowledge on body fluids. The possible application and measurement of extravascular water in different systems and organs will possibly open scientific and clinical opportunities. Some devices are already available but some less invasive, reproducible and specific instruments have to be developed. Furthermore, among all the molecules that can bring information on homeostasis, no specific one is so far recognized and further investigations are thus required.

Author details

Lucio Cagini, Jacopo Vannucci and Francesco Puma
Thoracic Surgery Unit, Department of Surgical, Radiologic, and Odontostomatologic Sciences
University of Perugia, S. Maria della Misericordia Hospital, Perugia, Italy

Michele Scialpi
Section of Diagnostic and Interventional Radiology, Department of Surgical, Radiologic, and Odontostomatologic Sciences University of Perugia, S. Maria della Misericordia Hospital, Perugia, Italy

8. References

[1] Kohl BA, Deutschman CS. The inflammatory response to surgery and trauma. Curr Opin Crit Care. 2006 Aug;12(4):325-32.

[2] Cuthbertson DP: Post-shock metabolic response. Lancet 1942, , i: 433-447.

[3] Cagini L, Capozzi R, Tassi V, Savignani C, Quintaliani G, Reboldi G, Puma F: Fluid and electrolyte balance after major thoracic surgery by bioimpedance and endocrine evaluation. European Journal of Cardio-thoracic Surgery 40 (2011) e71—e76.

[4] Holte K, Sharrock NE, Kehlet H. Pathophysiology and clinical implications of perioperative fluid excess. Br J Anaesth 2002;89:622—32.

[5] P, Hall GM. Cytokines in anaesthesia. Br J Anaesth. 1997 Feb;78(2):201-19.

[6] Walsh SR, Tang TY, Farooq N, Coveney EC, Gaunt ME: Perioperative fluid restriction reduces complications after major gastrointestinal surgery. Surgery. 2008 Apr; 143(4):466-8.

[7] M. G. Davies, P.-0. Hagen. Systemic inflammatory response syndrome. British Journal of Sugery 1997,84, 920-935.

[8] Moore FD, Olsen KH, McMurrey JD. The body cell mass and its supporting environment. Philadelphia: WB Saunders; 1978.

[9] Rivers E, Nguyen B, Havstad S, Ressler J, Muzzin A, Knoblich B, Peterson E, Tomlanovich M: Early goal-directed therapy in the treatment of severe sepsis and septic shock. The New England journal of medicine 2001, 345(19):1368-1377.

[10] Desborough JP. The stress response to trauma and surgery. Br J Anaesth 2000;85:109—17.

[11] Lobo DN, Macafee DA, Allison SP. How perioperative fluid balance influences postoperative outcomes. Best Pract Res Clin Anaesthesiol 2006;20:439—55.

[12] Rosenthal MH. Intraoperative fluid management-what and how much? Chest 1999;115(5 suppl.):106S—12S.

[13] Strunden MS, Heckel K, Goetz AE, Reuter DA. Perioperative fluid and volume management: physiological basis, tools and strategies. Ann Intensive Care. 2011 Mar 21;1(1):2.

[14] Pries AR, Kuebler WM: Normal endothelium. Handb Exp Pharmacol 2006, 1:1-40.

[15] Pries AR, Secomb TW, Gaehtgens P: The endothelial surface layer. Pfluger Arch 2002, 440:653-66.

[16] Rehm M, Haller M, Orth V, Kreimeier U, Jacob M, Dressel H, Mayer S, Brechtelsbauer H, Finsterer U: Changes in blood volume and hematocrit during acute preoperative

volume loading with 5% albumin or 6% hetastarch solutions in patients before radical Hysterectomy. Anesthesiology 2001, 95:849-56.
[17] Chappell D, Jacob M, Hofmann-Kiefer K, Bruegger D, Rehm M, Conzen P, Welsch U, Becker BF: Hydrocortisone preserves the vascular barrier by protecting the endothelial glycocalyx. Anesthesiology 2007, 107:776-84.
[18] Rehm M, Bruegger D, Christ F, Conzen P, Thiel M, Jacob M, Chappell D, Stoeckelhuber M, Welsch U, Reichart B, Peter K, Becker BF: Shedding of the endothelial glycocalyx in patients undergoing major vascular surgery with global and regional ischemia. Circulation 2007, 116:1896-906.
[19] Chappell D, Westphal M, Jacob M: The impact of the glycocalyx on microcirculatory oxygen distribution in critical illness. Curr Opin Anaesthesiol 2009, 22:155-62.
[20] Bernfield M, Gotte M, Park PW, Reizes O, Fitzgerald ML, Lincecum J, Zako M: Functions of cell surface heparan sulfate proteoglycans. Annu Rev Biochem 1999, 68:729-77.
[21] Bruegger D, Jacob M, Rehm M, Loetsch M, Welsch U, Conzen P, Becker BF: Atrial natriuretic peptide induces shedding of endothelial glycocalyx in coronary vascular bed of guinea pig hearts. Am J Physiol Heart Circ Physiol 2005, 289:H1993-9.
[22] Nelson A, Berkestedt I, Schmidtchen A, Ljunggren L, Bodelsson M: Increased levels of glycosaminoglycans during septic shock: relation to mortality and the antibacterial actions of plasma. Shock 2008, 30:623-7.
[23] Schrier RW, Wang W: Acute renal failure and sepsis. The New England journal of medicine 2004, 351(2):159-169.
[24] Guyton AC, Hall JE. Medical Physiology. Edises ed 2002, 442.
[25] Nagaishi C. Functional anatomy and histology of the lung. Baltimore: University Park Press; 1972.
[26] Miserocchi, G. (2009). Mechanisms controlling the volume of pleural liquid and extravascular lung water. Eur Respir Rev, Vol. 18, pp. 244–52.
[27] Conforti, E., Fenoglio, C., Bernocchi, G., Bruschi, O. & Miserocchi, G. (2002). Morphofunctional analysis of lung tissue in mild interstitial edema. Am J Physiol (Lung Cell Mol Physiol), Vol. 282, pp. L766-L774.
[28] Roberts, C.R., Wight, T.N. & Hascall, V.C. (1997). Proteoglycans. In: The LUNG scientific foundations., Crystal, R.G. West, J.B., Weibel, E.R. & Barnes, P.J. pp. 757-767, Lippincott-Raven Pub, New York.
[29] Miserocchi G, Beretta E. (2012) Pathophysiology of Extravascular Water in the Pleural Cavity and in the Lung Interstitium After Lung Thoracic Surgery. Topics in Thoracic Surgery, Prof. Paulo Cardoso (Ed.), ISBN: 978-953-51-0010-2, InTech.
[30] Rivolta, I., Lucchini, V., Rocchetti, M., Kolar, F., Palazzo, F., Zaza, A. & Miserocchi, G. (2011). Interstitial pressure and lung oedema in chronic hypoxia. *Eur Respir J*, Vol. 37, pp. 943–949.
[31] Negrini, D. (1995). Pulmonary microvascular pressure profile during development of hydrostatic edema. *Microcirculation*, Vol. 2, pp. 173-180.

[32] Miserocchi G, Negrini D, Passi A, et al. Development of lung edema: interstitial fluid dynamics and molecular structure. News. Physiol Sci 2001; 16: 66–71.

[33] Balducci C, Lilli C, Stabellini G, Marinucci L, Giustozzi G, A Becchetti A, Cagini L, Locci P. Human desmoid fibroblasts: matrix metalloproteinases, their inhibitors and modulation by Toremifene BMC Cancer. 2005; 5: 22.

[34] Lilli C, Marinucci L, Bellocchio S, Ribatti D, Balducci C, Baroni T, Cagini L, Giustozzi G, Locci P. Effects of transforming growth factor-beta1 and tumour necrosis factor-alpha on cultured fibroblasts from skin fibroma as modulated by toremifene. Int J Cancer. 2002 Apr 20;98(6):824-32.

[35] Locci P, Bellocchio S, Lilli C, Marinucci L, Cagini L, Baroni T, Giustozzi G, Balducci C, Becchetti E. Synthesis and secretion of transforming growth factor-beta1 by human desmoid fibroblast cell line and its modulation by toremifene. J Interferon Cytokine Res. 2001 Nov;21(11):961-70.

[36] Itobi E, Stroud M, Elia M. Impact of oedema on recovery after major abdominal surgery and potential value of multifrequency bioimpedance measurements. Br J Surg 2006;93:354—61.

[37] Lowell JA, Schifferdecker C, Driscoll DF, Benotti PN, Bistrian BR. Postoperative fluid overload: not a benign problem. Crit Care Med 1990;18:728—33.

[38] Puma F, Capozzi R, Daddi N, Ragusa M, Cagini L, Quintili A, Vannucci J. Experience with the autologous pulmonary vein for pulmonary arterioplasty. Eur J Cardiothorac Surg. 2011 Sep;40(3):e107-11. Epub 2011 Jun 15.

[39] Cagini L, Vannucci J, Scialpi M, Puma F. Diagnosis and Endovascular Treatment of an Internal Mammary Artery Injury. J Emerg Med. 2012 May 10.

[40] Ragusa M, Vannucci J, Cagini L, Daddi N, Pecoriello R, Puma F. Left main bronchus resection and reconstruction. A single institution experience. J Cardiothorac Surg. 2012 Apr 10;7:29.

[41] Lobo DN, Bostock KA, Neal KR, Perkins AC, Rowlands BJ, Allison SP. Effect of salt and water balance on recovery of gastrointestinal function after elective colonic resection: a randomised controlled trial. Lancet 2002;359:1812—8.

[42] Brandstrup B. Fluid therapy for the surgical patient. Best Pract Res Clin Anaesthesiol 2006;20:265—83.

[43] Brandstrup B, Tønnesen H, Beier-Holgersen R, Hjortsø E, Ørding H, Lindorff- Larsen K, RasmussenMS, LanngC,Wallin L, Iversen LH,GramkowCS,Okholm M, Blemmer T, Svendsen PE, Rottensten HH, Thage B, Riis J, Jeppesen IS, Teilum D, Christensen AM, Graungaard B, Pott F, Danish Study Group on Perioperative Fluid Therapy. Effect of intravenous fluid restriction on post- operative complications: comparison of two perioperative fluid regimens: a randomized assessor-blinded multicenter trial. Ann Surg 2003;238:641—8.

[44] Slinger P. Post-pneumonectomy pulmonary edema: is anaesthesia to blame? Curr Opin Anaesthesiol 1999;12:49—54.

[45] Jordan S, Mitchell JA, Quinlan GJ, Goldstraw P, Evans TW. The pathogen- esis of lung injury following pulmonary resection. Eur Respir J 2000;15:790—9.

[46] Powell-Tuck J, Gosling P, Lobo DN, Allison SP, Carlson GL, Gore M, Lewington AJ, Pearse RM, Mythen MG. British Consensus Guidelines on Intravenous Fluid Therapy for Adult Surgical Patients (GIFTASUP). Lon- don: NHS National Library of Health. http://www.ics.ac.uk/downloads/ 2008112340_GIFTASUP%20FINAL_31-10-08.pdf.

[47] Lamke LO, Nilsson GE, Reithner HL: Water loss by evaporation from the abdominal cavity during surgery. Acta Chir Scand 1977, 413:279-84.

[48] Chappell D, Jacob M, Hofmann-Kiefer K, Conzen P, Rehm M: A Rational approach to perioperative fluid management. Anesthesiology 2008, 109:723-40.

[49] Larsen R: Anästhesie. München: Urban & Fischer Elsevier GmbH; 2008.

[50] Rossaint R, Werner C, Zwißler B: Die Anästhesiologie. Heidelberg: Springer Medizin Verlag; 2008.

[51] Jacob M, Chappell D, Conzen P, Finsterer U, Rehm M: Blood volume is normal after preoperative overnight fasting. Acta Anaesthesiol Scand 2008, 52:522-9.

[52] Kamp-Jensen M, Olesen KL, Bach V, Schütten HJ, Engquist A: Changes in serum electrolyte and atrial natriuretic peptide concentrations, acid-base and haemodynamic status after rapid infusion of isotonic saline and Ringer lactate solution in healthy volunteers. Br J Anaest 1990, 64:606-10.

[53] Rehm M, Orth V, Kreimeier U, Thiel M, Mayer S, Brechtelsbauer H, Finsterer U: Changes in blood volume during acute normovolemic hemodilution with 5% albumin or 6% hydroxyethylstarch and intraoperative retransfusion. Anaesthesist 2001, 50:569-79.

[54] Rehm M, Orth V, Kreimeier U, Thiel M, Haller M, Brechtelsbauer H, Finsterer U: Changes in intravascular volume during acute normovolemic hemodilution and intraoperative retransfusion in patients with radical hysterectomy. Anesthesiology 2000, 92:657-64.

[55] Sakka SG, Ruhl CC, Pfeiffer UJ, Beale R, McLuckie A, Reinhart K, Meier- Hellmann A: Assessment of cardiac preload and extravascular lung water by single transpulmonary thermodilution. Intensive care medicine 2000, 26(2):180-187.

[56] Phillips CR, Chesnutt MS, Smith SM: Extravascular lung water in sepsis associated acute respiratory distress syndrome: indexing with predicted body weight improves correlation with severity of illness and survival. Critical care medicine 2008, 36(1):69-73.

[57] Ackland GL, Singh-Ranger D, Fox S, McClaskey B, Down JF, Farrar D, Sivaloganathan M, Mythen MG. Assessment of preoperative fluid depletion using bioimpedance analysis. Br J Anaesth 2004;92:134—6.

[58] Maisel AS, Krishnaswamy P, Nowak RM, McCord J, Hollander JE, Duc P,Omland T, Storrow AB, Abraham WT,Wu AH, Clopton P, Steg PG,Westheim A, Knudsen CW, Perez A, Kazanegra R, Herrmann HC, McCullough PA, Breathing Not Properly Multinational Study Investigators. Rapid measurement of B-type natriuretic peptide in the emergency diagnosis of heart failure. N Engl J Med 2002;347:161—7.

[59] Nojiri T, Maeda H, Takeuchi Y, Funakoshi Y, Kimura T, Maekura R, Yamamoto K, Okumura M. Predictive value of B-type natriuretic peptide for postoperative atrial fibrillation following pulmonary resection for lung cancer. Eur J Cardiothorac Surg 2010;37:787–91.

Chapter 4

Short and Long Term Results of Major Lung Resections in Very Elderly People

Cristian Rapicetta, Massimiliano Paci, Tommaso Ricchetti,
Sara Tenconi, Salvatore De Franco and Giorgio Sgarbi

Additional information is available at the end of the chapter

http://dx.doi.org/10.5772/50987

1. Introduction

Improvement in health care has lead to increased life expectancy through the chronicization of formerly fatal diseases. On the other hand, increasing duration of exposure to risk factors means that the incidence of lung cancer increases in proportion to age, and is actually the first cause of death for malignancy in the world.

Consequently, a growing number of very elderly people, aged 80 or more, are presenting with a resectable lung tumour. The increased prevalence of cardiovascular and pulmonary comorbidity and consequently poor performance status often make patients unfit to surgery, which remains the treatment of choice for early stages Non-Small Cell Lung Cancer (NSCLC) [1, 2]. Increasing age is often associated with lower likelihood of treatment and more liberal use of radiation therapy than of surgery [3].

1.1. Background

In a recent paper Janssen and Kunst found that in 2050 predicted life expectancy for people reaching 80 years will be 9.16 years for men and 12.65 for women [4], which clearly overcome the prognosis of lung cancer. Therefore, cancer-related mortality will likely have a even more great impact on octogenarians survival.

Although several studies have shown that long term survival after surgery can be achieved in a significant proportion of octogenarians. However the minimal prognosis of untreated or palliated early stage lung cancer (1.5 years) forces to go beyond palliative cares [5].

Recently, even more Authors reported results after surgery in very elderly patients: unfortunately many studies consist of retrospective, non-randomized studies on small number of patients making difficult to define risk factors for complications and mortality.

Considering the improvement in preoperative functional assessment, anaesthetic care, pain relief, postoperative facilities and modern surgical techniques, it is possible that more octogenarians could be successfully operated, but an accurate selection of patients is mandatory to avoid excessively high incidence of complications and mortality. Moreover long term results such as respiratory function and quality of life (QOL) is as well as important in decision making process to schedule or deny surgery: even less data are available in this field, particularly comparing surgery to medical therapies (chemo- and radiotherapy).

Established that surgery is undoubtedly the best therapy for early stage lung cancer to date, especially in terms of local control of disease, this chapter aims to analyse short (complications, mortality) and long-term (respiratory function) of very elderly people. Analysing results in a large cohort of patients and reviewing literature we try to suggest proper selection criteria to surgery in these patients, considering risk/benefit of alternative treatment modalities.

2. Report of a single institution experience

My colleagues and I reported some years ago our results in a large series of octogenarians consecutively operated on between January 1990 through December 2005 [6]. Life expectancy in the province is greater than the national average and octogenarians have always represented a significant percentage of patients with resectable lung cancer.

2.1. Material and methods

The lung cancer database of a single centre (Thoracic Surgery Unit at the University Hospital of Siena) was retrospectively reviewed to identify all patients aged >= 80 years who underwent lung resection for NSCLC with curative intent in the period considered above. We tried to limit the period of study to 1990, mainly because the very few octogenarians treated before 90's and secondly to eliminate bias due to patients selection, clinical staging and functional assessment through decades.

All patients were extensive evaluated throughout medical history, physical examination, routine blood tests, electrocardiogram, echocardiography, blood gas analysis, spirometry and calculation of diffusion capacity of the lung for carbon monoxide (DLCO). Second level tests were performed when indicated: cardio-respiratory test and/or lung perfusion scintigraphy in case of poor pulmonary function at basal spirometry (predicted post-operative FEV1% less than 40%, computed on the basis of pulmonary segments to be removed); cardiac stress tests and eventually coronary angiography were performed in presence of clinical symptoms of angina pectoris, significant ischemic signs at basal electrocardiogram, or segmental cardiac discinesia at basal echocardiography.

Clinical staging was based on chest CT-scan, bronchoscopy, CT-scan of chest, abdomen and brain and bone scintigraphy. Mediastinoscopy was electively performed in case of enlarged mediastinal lymphnodes at CT scan (short axis > 1 cm) with irregular pattern of post-contrast perfusion. PET was not routinely used due to unavailability in the hospital of Siena but was performed in the last seven consecutive patients resulting positive only in the site of primary tumour. Whenever possible, a preoperative diagnosis was done, even by transpleural methods (Fine Needle trans-thoracic Aspiration - FNA).

Indication to surgery was established on the basis of features of disease (determining resectability), and features of the patient (determining operability). Efforts spent to achieve accurate preoperative staging were finalized to select early clinical stages (I-II). Operability of the patients was judged in a multidisciplinary setting including pneumologist and anaesthesiologist. Decision was based on functional status and comorbidities: we did not considered an age-limit as a contraindication per se to surgery. Our surgical policy favoured lobectomies over sublobar resections and whenever possible we tried to avoid pneumonectomy. Sublobar resection was preferred by the attending surgeon in case of poor respiratory function and/or severe cardiovascular comorbidities, and was considered a compromise: anatomical segmentectomies were however preferred to wedge resections and were considered adequate for stage I peripherally located tumours.

None of the patients received neoadjuvant therapy for at least two reasons: first, patients in advanced clinical stages (III or IV) were denied to surgery in favour of low dose chemo or radiation therapy and best supportive care; second, postoperative risk of major lung resection after induction chemotherapy was judged excessively high in such patients

Adjuvant therapy was administered in case of unforeseen lymph nodal disease or residual disease. Radiotherapy was preferred, although 4 patients in very good health conditions could tolerate chemotherapy.

Postoperative complications were classified as minor (non life-threatening) or mayor (potentially life-threatening), according to gravity of the disease and its mortality in literature and in our population.

Data recorded included demographic and clinical features of population (gender, age, smoking history, performance status, preoperative pulmonary function tests, comorbidities, use of induction therapies), as well as perioperative data (type of lung resection, operative mortality - defined as death within 30 days from surgery or during the same hospitalization, complications, length of in-hospital stay, admission to ICU, histology, pathologic stage and the use of adjuvant therapy.

Follow up included total-body CT scan and serum cancer markers every 6 months for first 2 years, then chest CT scan every 12 months until the fifth years. Bronchoscopy and recently, PET-scan were performed only in case of suspected local or distance recurrent disease.

Deaths included all causes but we differentiated only cancer and non-cancer related deaths.

Binary logistic regression analysis was used to discriminate independent risk factors for mayor complications and 30-days mortality after surgical resection. Long term survival curves were computed by the Kaplan-Meier method and compared with Log-rank test. Cox regression analysis was used to determine significance of prognostic factors for long term survival.

2.2. Results

In the period considered, 96 octogenarians affected by NSCLC underwent surgery with curative intent (5.6% of 1711 lung resections performed during the same period).

Over the years an increase of percentage of octogenarians having a pulmonary resection for NSCLC was observed (from 2.7% in 1990 to 14% in 2005): it reflects the considerations expressed above and it is likely that there will be a growing trend of such percentages in next years.

Population was predominantly male (84), with age ranging from 80 to 89 (median, 82 years).

Data of population is shown in Table I: some of the data are worthy of note: almost all patients (90%) had a history of cigarette smoking with 40 median pack-years and almost half of them (48.9%) presented comorbidities, mainly cardiopulmonary. Thirteen patients had a history of coronary artery disease, defined as a history of prior myocardial infarction, prior coronary stenting or by-pass or angina pectoris. Despite this percentages, almost all the octogenarians (94 – 97.9%) were Eastern Cooperative Oncology Group (ECOG) status 0 or 1.

The surgical procedures performed included 59 standard lobectomies, 4 extended lobectomies, (one upper sleeve lobectomy, 3 en block chest wall resections), 13 wedge resections (2 performed by VATS), 9 pneumonectomies, 7 segmentectomies and 4 bilobectomies. Patients with $pO_2<65$ mmHg or a $pCO_2>45$ mmHg and/or MVV or an $FEV_1<$ 50% of predicted were scheduled for sublobar resection.

The histological examination of the resected specimens revealed NSCLC in all patients: one of the aims of preoperative histological biopsy was to exclude histology with proven poor survival (small-cell carcinoma).

Regarding pathologic stage, 61 (63,5%) patients were confirmed to be in stage IA or IB: concordance with clinical staging was not so high but it should be taken into account unavailability of modern diagnostic tools for staging. Adjuvant chemotherapy was administered in 6 patients and radiotherapy in 2 patients due to unforeseen pathological N2 disease or unexpected residual microscopic disease.

One or more complications developed in 42 patients for a total morbidity of 44%. Five patients suffered multiple complications. Mayor complications lead to death 9 of 17 patients (52.9%) resulting in an overall mortality rate of 9.4% (Table 2).

The median postoperative hospitalization was 8 days, not significantly longer than in younger patients (7 days) although 7 patients were discharged after more than 2 weeks. Eighty patients (83%) were discharged home without need of further rehabilitation; only 10 patients (9.6%) were discharged to a convalescent care facility.

It must be underlined that no patient suffered permanent or prolonged disability after lung resection although post-thoracotomy pain syndrome was present in a small percentage after several months (14% after 1 year), causing significant discomfort.

Mean age (years)	81.5 ± 1
Sex (M/F)	84/12
Smokers	86 (90%)
Comorbidities	47 (49%)
> 1 comorbidity	13 (13.5%)
Respiratory parameters	
FEV1 (% of predicted)	75.8% ± 16.2%
CO diffusion (% of predicted)	76.5% ± 20.7%
PaO2 (mm Hg)	75.1 ± 11.4
Pathological stage	
I	61 (63.5%)
II	17 (17.7%)
*III**	17 (17.7%)
IV§	1 (1%)
Surgical procedure	
Lobectomy	68 (70.8%)
Sublobar resection	19 (19.8%)
Pneumonectomy	9 (9.4%)
Extended resection	
Bilobectomy	4 (4.2%)
En-bloc resection with chest wall	3 (3.1%)
Histology	
Adenocarcinoma	42 (43.8%)
Squamous cell carcinoma	48 (50%)
Adenosquamous carcinoma	2 (2.1%)
Large cell carcinoma	4 (4.2%)
Comorbidities	
*Coronary artery disease**	13 (13.5%)
Chronic obstructive pulmonary disease	19 (19.7%)
Vascular disease	13 (13.5%)
Diabetes mellitus	8 (8.3%)
Chronic atrial fibrillation	4 (4.1%)
Heart valve disease	3 (3.1%)
Kidney failure	1 (1%)

FEV_1 = forced expiratory volume in 1 s.

* N2 disease in 12 cases and T3N1 disease in 5 cases

§ contralateral pulmonary metastasis

Table 1. Demographic, clinical, and pathological data of patients

Major complications	N. (%)	30-day mortality (%)
Respiratory failure	3	
ARDS	3	3
Broncho-pleural fistula	2	2
Cardiac failure	2	1
Kidney failure	1	
Pneumonia	1	1
Pulmonary embolism	1	
Stroke	1	1
Pulmonary edema	1	
Hematemesis	1	
IMA	1	1
	17 (17,7)	9 (9)

Table 2. Major complications rate and mortality

Using binary logistic regression analysis, among the pre- and peri-operative covariates analyzed, we found that resection of more than 1 lobe (p=0.008), cardio-respiratory comorbidity (p=0.042), PaO2<75 mmHg (p=0.029) and DLCO<60% (p=0.023) were predictive of major complications with the first risk factor predicting 30-day mortality too (p=0.01). Detailed results are reported in Table 3 and 4.

Covariate	RR	95% CI	*p*
Extended resection*	**10.5**	**1.9–59.7**	**0.008**
Comorbidity	**5**	**1.06–24**	**0.042**
FEV_1 < 60%	0.45	0.08–2.5	0.36
CO diffusion < 60%	**6.24**	**1.28–30.37**	**0.023**
PaO_2 < 75 mm Hg	**5.42**	**1.19–24.65**	**0.029**
Age	0.7	0.46–1.04	0.076
Sex	0.17	0.014–2.21	0.18

*Bilobectomy, pneumonectomy, or en-bloc chest wall resection. CI = confidence interval, FEV_1 = forced expiratory volume in 1 s, RR = relative risk.

Table 3. Predictors of major postoperative complications

Covariate Value	RR	95% CI	*p*
Extended resection	**12.96**	**1.85–90.89**	**0.01**
Comorbidity	6.69	0.69–64.69	0.1
FEV_1 < 60%	1.59	0.2–12.87	0.66
CO diffusion < 60%	3.97	0.52–30.61	0.18
PaO_2 < 75 mm Hg	1.08	0.18–6.36	0.93
Age	0.78	0.47–1.31	0.36
Sex	1.15	0.08–17.36	0.91

Table 4. Predictors of 30-day postoperative mortality

At the mean follow-up of 42 months (range 8 months to 12 years), 46 (47.9%) patients were alive and 50 (52%) had died.

It was surprising that, despite the advanced age, the majority of patients (29/50, 71%) died of cancer, either by local recurrence or distant metastasis.

The 5-year survival rate was significantly different between stage I and stage III (60%vs14%, $p<0.001$) and between stage II and stage III (42%vs14%, $p=0.046$). There was no statistical difference in 5-year survival rate between stage I and stage II ($p=0.39$). The overall 3- and 5-year survival rates were 51% and 34%, respectively, with a median survival of 3.7 years (95% CI, 2.7 to 4.6 years) (Figure 1).

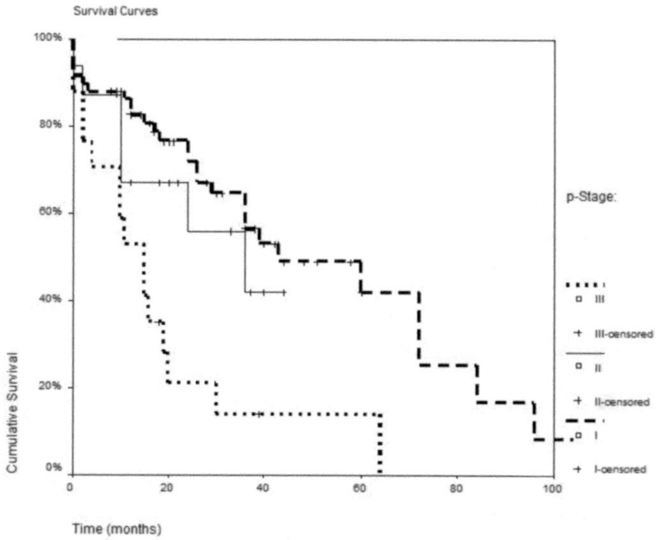

Figure 1. Actuarial survival according to pathological stage.

Using the Cox proportional hazard model of multivariate analysis, only pathological stage of disease resulted as an independent predictor of long term survival ($p=0.003$): stage II or more carries a relative risk of 4.2 to die of disease (Table 5).

Covariate	RR	95% CI	*p*
Pathological stage (II-III Vs I)	**4.2**	**1.74–10.46**	**0.001**
Extended resection	1.2	0.37–3.6	0.81
Comorbidity	16.4	1.1–237.5	0.38
FEV_1	1	0.97–1.03	0.87
DLCO	1	0.98–1.02	0.56
PaO_2	0.95	0.95–1.2	0.295
Age	0.97	0.79–1.2	0.81
Sex	0.61	0.17–2.2	0.44

Table 5. Predictors of long-term survival

2.3. Interpretation of results

Although recent studies have demonstrated acceptable long term survival after lung cancer surgery in octogenarians [7, 8, 9, 10], elderly patients are less likely to have surgical resection [4], because advanced age is an important risk factor for postoperative complications and death, [1, 2]. In fact, despite an improvement in early outcome in the past ten years, the risk of life-threatening complications for octogenarians remains variable: Harvey et al., reported a 1.6% risk in patients 70-79 years old compared to a 17.6% rate in octogenarians [11] and Naunheim et al. [12] reported that even within the octogenarians, increasing age was a negative factor.

The 9.4% operative mortality observed in this series is similar to other reports covering the same time period [13] but was exceedingly higher in patients who required an extended resection (more than one lobe or chest wall and lung en bloc resection), as found also by other Authors. [14, 15].

The mortality rate after pneumonectomy and even after bilobectomy was remarkable: 22% and 25%, respectively: it is well known that operative mortality is substantial in elderly people having extended resection, especially right sided pneumonectomy, with mortality exceeding 20% [1, 16, 17]. Besides, the British Thoracic Society noted that pneumonectomy is associated with a higher mortality risk in the elderly and that age should be a factor in deciding suitability for pneumonectomy.

These results convinced us to consider for surgical operation only octogenarians with lung cancers amenable to be resected by lobectomy. In addition, also pulmonary resections combined with en bloc chest wall removal should be avoided since they carry an increased mortality rate as previously reported by [2, 18]. The mortality rate was instead acceptable after standard lobectomy (8.4%, result in line with those reported in literature) and was null after wedge resection or segmentectomy.

We observed 17 major complications (mainly cardiopulmonary) in 16 patients, and is note worthy that they lead to death in more than half of the cases (9/17, 52.6%).

Cardiac complications developed frequently during the postoperative period. All patients had an echocardiogram but exercise stress testing was only executed in case of symptomatic angina, history of infarction or ECG abnormalities. The efficacy and cost-effectiveness of exercise stress testing or dipyridamole thallium scan as screening tests is controversial, but probably we should use a lower threshold for these second- and third-level investigations in the octogenarians. When they result positive, it is useful to proceed to coronary angiography because patients found to have significant coronary lesions amenable to angioplasty, can be successfully operated on after 2 months (3 cases in our experience). On the other hand, if coronary artery bypass surgery would be required, we prefer to manage the patient nonoperatively with radiotherapy, because we believe that combined heart-lung surgery carries an excessive risk in advanced age people [19].

Long term survival is also of critical importance in this patient population with limited natural life expectancy.

Our overall 5-year survival of 35% is consistent with that reported in similar series over the past decade, with 5-year survival rates ranging from 16% to 55% [7, 8, 9, 10, 20, 21].

As expected pathologic stage was an independent prognostic factor for long-term survival but, differently from previous studies in the octogenarians except for one [14], our survival curves justify surgery also for patients with stage II NSCLC, with 5-year survival rate of 42%. Survival in stage III disease is uniformly very poor in all the series and is significantly lower than in the younger counterparts, probably because a fewer percentage of older patients are able to tolerate extended surgical procedures and complete multimodal treatments. A recent report of Fanucchi and coll. reported a low 5-years survival: Authors correctly recognized that it was due to unexpected high incidence of stage III disease because of inaccurate clinical staging [22].

The QOL and the level of independence after surgery should be a major component in the decision-making process in the elderly.

We did not identify any prolonged disability and the fact that nearly 80% of octogenarians in this cohort were discharged directly to home suggests that most patients were able to resume the preoperative lifestyle.

3. Lung volume reduction era and its importance in lung cancer surgery

In the late 1950s, Brantigan and co-workers were the first to present the modern concept of lung reduction for emphysema, theorizing that by surgically reducing lung volume, part of circumferential pull upon the bronchioles could be restored, diaphragm could be brought higher with more efficient function and size of the thoracic cage could be reduced, allowing for better contraction of the intercostal muscles and ultimately reducing airflow obstruction and relieving dyspnoea [23]. Further results confirmed efficacy of lung volume reduction surgery (LVRS), with outcome improving parallel to refinement of selection criteria, although long-term survival did not seem to be positively affected as symptoms and pulmonary function.

Because lung cancer and emphysema share common risk factors, it is not surprising to find that both conditions are often seen in the same individual as stated in the text. First papers addressing combined adequate cancer resection with volume reduction were published only in 1998 and were based on very small series of patients (5 and 14): all of them did well postoperatively and showed long term benefits in dyspnoea index, FEV1, and 6-minute walk test [24, 25].

In the evaluation of patients candidate for surgery, spirometry is still considered the gold standard: ppoFEV1% is the most powerful predictor of medical postoperative mortality and morbidity as demonstrated by Kearney and coll. [26]. The second-level assessments as inhalation-perfusion lung scintigraphy and cardio-respiratory exercise test may be useful in further evaluation of "critical" patients: however, while they demonstrated valid predictors of postoperative complications, they did not clearly show a higher accuracy than simple ppoFEV1% obtained by calculation of broncho-pulmonary segments removed [27].

McKenna and coll. [28] reported in 1997 that improvement in poFEV1% and dyspnoea score was more evident in patients aged under 70, although the differences were not statistical significant. A growing number of studies in the recent years have reported an improvement of respiratory function after lobectomy in some patients affected by COPD [29], or at least a minimal impairment of respiratory function indicated by better apoFEV% (actual postoperative) than ppoFEV1% (predicted postoperative)[30]. In such cases Authors have hypothesized that lobectomy could have a lung volume reduction surgery (LVRS) effect [31].

This data from literature suggested us that even elderly patients with less severe COPD could get some benefit from resection of emphysematous parenchyma and therefore in the decision making process that lead to schedule an octogenarian to lung surgery, additional considerations should be made in evaluating respiratory function: not only preoperative FEV1% but also ppoFEV1% could be inaccurate in some cases in predicting the real postsurgical pulmonary function loss. Moreover, other studies reported that abnormal pulmonary function (FEV1%<60%) was not associated with mortality [20, 7, 10], with only first study reporting higher incidence of complications.

Curative surgery chance to octogenarians affected by emphysema and lung cancer is therefore to be seriously considered.

4. Long term respiratory function in our series

A previous study conducted Thoracic Surgery Unit at University Hospital of Siena on patients who underwent pneumonectomy demonstrated that a lower preoperative respiratory function was associated to a much lower loss after pneumonectomy [32]: these data, together with some comforting results of bilateral LVRS procedures performed by VATS in the same Institution, stimulated us to analyzed late variation of respiratory parameters in the same cohort of octogenarians presented above. Results were published in 2011 [33].

4.1. Materials and methods

In order to analyze a subgroup as more homogeneous as possible, we considered only patients with COPD (defined by a Tiffenau index < 0.7). Since sublobar resections demonstrated to be well tolerated by elderly patients and resection of more than 1 lobe or combined chest wall resection is not recommended (being associated to major complications and in-hospital mortality) we limited analysis to standard lobectomy. Patients who received adjuvant therapies (anyway a small number) and those who continued smoking were excluded in order to eliminate bias. Spirometry was not routinely repeated at predetermined time and it was decided to consider patients with spirometry executed after 12±3 months from surgery (in absence of local relapsing disease or exacerbation of COPD). Pulmonary Function Test (PFT) were performed after bronchodilator inhalation in order to eliminate the reversible component of airflow impairment Out of the 96 patients 24 fulfilled all inclusion criteria and formed the population of the study.

Obviously removing non-functioning lung tissue does not affect pulmonary reserve, however no patients presented atelectasis or obstructive pneumonia of lobe to be resected.

Predicted Postoperative FEV1% (ppoFEV1%) was computed not simply on the basis of crude amount of segments to be resected: the attenuation value of lung parenchyma (between -600 and -900 Houmsfield Unit) was used to compute the percentage of functioning tissue resected and to correct the predicted-postoperative FEV1, as proposed by WU et al [Wu 1994]. This method had been demonstrated to be a valid substitute of lung perfusion scintigraphy, with a good correlation of values found by the two methods [Yoshimoto 2009]; however in patients with worst respiratory impairment (FEV1<60%) lung perfusion scintigraphy was executed and used to compute ppoFEV1.

Roentgenographic pattern of emphysema (homogeneous Vs upper lobe) was established according to criteria proposed by Goddard and coll. for CT-scan [34]; data were analyzed using unpaired Student t-test for comparison of means of continuous variables between groups, paired t-test was used to assess differences within groups between preoperative and postoperative values.

4.2. Results

Patients were categorized into two groups (Group 1: moderate COPD; Group 2: mild COPD) according to the Global initiative for chronic Obstructive Lung Disease (GOLD) criteria [35]: Group 1 (G1) FEV1% < 80%; Group 2 (G2) FEV1% ≥ 80%). The threshold value coincided with median FEV1% of population, making the two groups equal in terms of number of patients.

There was no difference in gender, age, pathologic stage, comorbidities and histology between the two groups, nor in incidence of major complications (15% Vs 12% - p=0.72) and postoperative ECOG status Considering the whole population (96 patients) which this series of patients came from, overall perioperative and in-hospital death was 6.5% in Group 1 and 11.5% in Group 2 (p=0.35).

Comparing preoperative and postoperative PFT values in both groups, FVC% and RV%, showed significant variations. In G2 a significant loss in DLCO was registered. Interestingly the FEV1% loss was statistically significant only in G2 (88.3 to 73.7, p<0.001): in G1 FEV1% loss was much less remarkable, decreasing from a mean value of 67.8 to 59.1 (p=n.s.).

Variation of FEV1% between the two groups after surgery was -7.9% in Group 1 and -14.9% in Group 2, showing a tendency to significance (p=0.17); also differences in FVC% between the two groups were not remarkable (-13.3% in Group 1 and –6.7% in Group 2 – p=0.33). DLCO% loss was much higher in G2 than in G1 (-22.5 Vs +1.5, p=0.001).

Six patients showed an improvement of actual postoperative FEV1%, ranging from +1.5 to +7.3 compared with the preoperative value. All of these patients had a preoperative FEV1% lower than 60%, a homogeneous or upper lobe pattern emphysema as confirmed by both CT-scan and/or lung perfusion scintigraphy (when available) and had undergone a upper lobectomy. Type of lobectomy had no influence in FEV1% loss in G2 (upper lobectomy: -14.5% - lower lobectomy: -15.6%, p=0.81), as it demonstrated to have in G1 (upper lobectomy: +5.4% - lower lobectomy: -14.5%, p=0.05). (Figure 2).

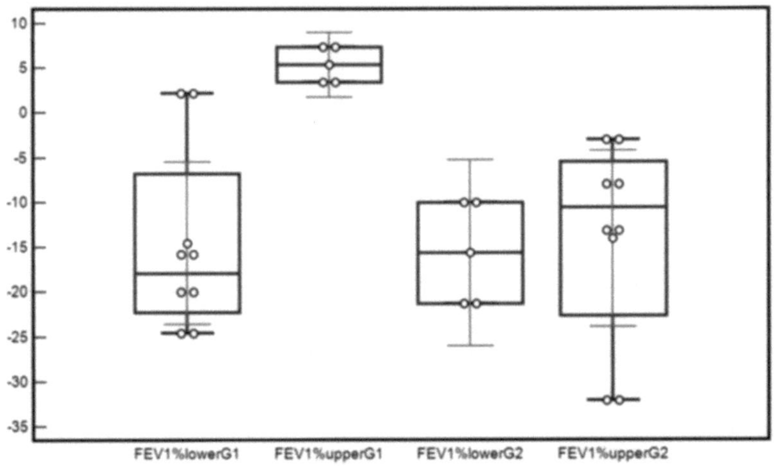

Figure 2. Variations of FEV1% after surgery in the two groups (mean, standard deviation, range), stratified for type of resection (upper Vs lower lobe)

Considering FEV1 as a continuous variable, linear regression analysis showed a significant inverse correlations between preoperative value of FEV1% and FEV1 percentage loss after surgery (B: -0.63, R^2: 0.46 – $p<0.01$), even though linear correlation does not represent effectively the complex physiopathology following lung resection in patients with COPD/emphysema.

Blood gas tests reflected in some way the variations of PFT parameters: in G1 the lower loss in respiratory function resulted in not significant difference in PaO2, PCO2 and pH before and after surgery. Conversely patients in G2 showed a significant PaO2 decrease after surgery. No differences were found between the two groups at time of follow-up.

4.3. Interpretation of results: does LVRS effect act also in octogenarians?

Patients of this series obviously did not accomplish completely the criteria for LVRS and on the other hand apical wedge resection (and not lobectomy) is the recommended surgical option for lung volume reduction. Lobectomy implies removal of functioning lung tissue, together with emphysematous one, and this can explain the significant FVC% loss in G1: this is not observed after LVRS performed in properly selected candidates. However, some physiological effects of LVRS remain and are responsible of the remarkable drop of RV%

and the not significant loss in FEV% after surgery in G1: DLCO showed a gain of +1.5 at follow-up, probably due to more correct redistribution of ventilation and perfusion in lung zones. Patients in G2 having better pulmonary function, had the major impairment (of FEV1% and also DLCO%), because of the resection of a major portion of functioning lung. This results confirmed previous reports [36].

It must be noted that most of these studies report functional results after 1, 3 or 6 months: at this time, the post-thoracotomy pain could be still present in some cases, maybe causing a restrictive pattern and consequently a bias of the results [37]. In our series, all patients received a postero-lateral muscle-sparing thoracotomy, reducing a possible factor conditioning the amount of thoracic pain.

The functional advantage after an upper lobectomy than a lower lobectomy in patients with higher airflow impairment (G1) probably simply reflects predominantly upper lobe emphysema (as usual observed); however the same physiopatologic considerations should be valid in any case of resection of more emphysematous - less functioning lung lobe although no data can be provided supporting this consideration.

It should be kept in mind that PFTs are conditioned by patients collaboration and represent a kind of "surrogate" of effort tolerance which do not necessarily correlate with values measured at a single time. However postoperative global performance status and exercise tolerance seemed to reach a similar level in both mild and moderate COPD patients (G1 and G2), supporting the conclusion that differences in functional status are levelled after a major lung resection.

Although some limitations due retrospective nature of the study, and possible presence of bias such as the preoperative optimization of respiratory reserve through medications and/or physical rehabilitation, we tried to select an homogeneous cohort of patients with strict inclusion criteria in order to establish the pure effect of lobectomy after a long time, enough to allow remodelling processes of lung and thoracic wall until the final steady result. The inadequacy of sample size often did not allow to reach statistical significance in some tests. Lung perfusion scintigraphy was not routinely performed, so we had to use CT-scan estimation method as surrogate to obtain corrected ppoFEV1.

Finally the retrospective nature of the study itself implies that some patients were denied surgery resulting, for example, in unavailability of data for patients with lower preoperative FEV1 and homogeneous pattern of emphysema undergone to lower lobectomy, so the benefit of upper lobectomy could be deducted only on physiological basis.

5. Surgery – RT

Since chemotherapy is not well tolerated by elderly people and yields very disappointing results in local control of disease, radiation therapy (RT) has ever been considered the most feasible and valuable therapeutic option in patients not fitting criteria for operability.

Consequently, literature reports several series of patients treated with RT. In an old report dated 1988, results on 50 patients not candidate to surgery with peripherally located stage I NSCLC were analyzed: the overall response rate was 90%, with 50% complete responses in tumors smaller than 4 cm, resulting in overall survival rates of 56% at 2 years and 16% at 5 years (median survival of 27 months). Complete responders (20/50) showed a remarkable 5-years survival of 42% with 25% of local relapse of disease. On the contrary none of the patients having a tumor greater than 4 cm was alive at 5 years. Results were favorable compared to those of a group of 70 patients surgically resected (median survival of 23 months).

The same positive results were reported several years later in a larger series of 347 patients: curiously, better results were achieved in elderly people (aged > 70), although the difference was not significant, in terms of crude survival and disease-free survival [38]. Other Authors reported worse results of RT compared to surgery, with 5-year survival rate of only 10 to 20% after curative intent radiotherapy [39].

Unfortunately, very few studies report results of surgery and RT in the same Institution, most of them being retrospective and non-randomized.

Yendamuri compared overall survival after surgery (wedge resection) and three dimensional conformation radiation therapy in a retrospective study on 160 patients with early stage lung malignances unable to tolerate lobectomy. Propensity score-matched analysis and cost assessments were performed to compare outcomes with both modalities. Propensity matching was also performed to assure homogeneity between arms in terms of gender, histology, tumor size, performance status, and age The most frequent long term complications encountered were post-thoracotomy pain syndrome and radiation pneumonia with pulmonary fibrosis. . Surgery arm showed a trend to improved outcome towards radiotherapy one (57,1 months Vs 40,9 months), while mean cost of radiation therapy ($32,735) was not statistically significantly different from surgery ($30,411). Propensity matched analysis however failed to confirm a clear benefit of sublobar pulmonary resections, and it could be explained by inadequacy of number of patients and other bias (retrospective – not randomized trial, increased comorbidities of patients treated with 3-D conformal radiation) [40].

In another smaller series of compromised patients (not suitable for lobectomy) retrospectively reviewed (17 treated by sublobar resections, either segmentectomy or wedge resection and 18 by radiation therapy alone) overall 5-years survival rates were 55% after surgery and 14,4% after radiation therapy (p=0.004), without significant more complications due to lung resections. The advantage in long-term survival was maintained even considering only total or partial responders among patients treated with radiation therapy (+18.8%, p=0.008). Even in this series complications reported did not differ between the two treatment modalities (11.8 compared to 11.1). Local recurrence at margins of resection occurred in 4 patients in which tumour diameter was greater than 2 cm. Authors concluded that surgery carries advantage over radiotherapy, especially for smaller lesions measuring less than 2 cm [41].

A prospective analysis of QOL after radical radiotherapy noted benefit on haemoptysis, pain and anorexia, while cough, dyspnea and fatigue were poorly alleviated; also global QOL responded poorly [42].

6. Novel perspective for management of lung cancer in octogenarians

6.1. Diagnosis – Staging

Histological proven diagnosis is significant less frequent in elderly: this may reflect the poor perceived fitness of withstand bronchoscopy, CT guided biopsy and other invasive techniques [43].

Preoperative histopatological confirmation should preferably be obtained in elderly people to avoid unnecessary surgery for benign lesions or, to identify patients with poor prognosis related histology (small-cell carcinoma, large-cell undifferentiated neuroendocrine carcinoma).

Trans-thoracic Ultrasound or CT guided Fine Needle Aspiration was found to have equivalent safety and tolerance to procedure in elderly patients (aged 70 or more), with majority of cases performed as a day-case [44].

In our series of patients, concordance of clinical and pathological staging was a not exciting 63%: the use of sole CT-scan and blind transbronchial/trans-tracheal endoscopic fine needle biopsy has certainly played a role in understaging. The introduction of PET-CT scan in routine assessment for staging purpose in most Institution demonstrated to enhance conventional staging, both for nodal status and distant metastasis, resulting in a 10% of downstaging and 33% upstaging. This changed intent of treatment from palliative to curative in 4% and vice-versa in 22% of cases [45].

Endoscopic UltraSound guided Fine Needle Aspiration (EUS-FNA) performed by bronchoscopy by skilled operators promises to improve sensitivity in metastasis detection of PET positive lymph-nodes not necessarily increased in size (CT-scan nodal assessment is essentially based on dimensional criteria and post-contrast perfusion nodal pattern and is operator-dependent).

A prospective study on 86 with mediastinal adenopathies provided impressive negative and positive predictive value (94% and 100% respectively). This allowed to shift to non-surgical management in 80% of cases [46].

6.2. Image Guided Radiotherapy/Intensity Modulated Radiation Therapy (IGRT/IMRT)

This novel techniques promise to be a milestone in radiation treatment for capacity to delineate tumour contour and correct it for patients positioning, resulting in two theoretical high advantages compared to traditional radiation therapy.

1. Greater precision in irradiating tumour volume with minimal toxicity of neighbouring healthy tissues (→lower incidence of side effects)
2. Possibility to deliver higher dosage with presumed higher efficacy

Unfortunately, despite this convincing rationale, literature lacks of robust studies to confirm promising clinical benefits. To date, there is enough evidence on technical performance, encouraging but not yet conclusive information on safety, very weak evidence in clinical effectiveness and none on cost-effectiveness. The proportion of patients with the clinical indications for IGRT/IMRT inferred by the RER (Regione Emilia Romagna) regional database result in an estimate 10% of all lung cancers (the lowest percentage among several solid tumours considered – brain, prostate, head and neck, pancreatic).

Nonetheless IGT/IMRT are worthy to be seriously considered in future clinical trials, preferably involving a surgery arm.

6.3. Minimally invasive surgery: VATS lobectomy

Videothoracoscopic Assisted Thoracic Surgery has in recent years gained again popularity and has become of routinely use in some Institutions for early stages lung cancers not involving fissures of hilar elements. Octogenarians seem to have the proper characteristics for indication to VATS major resections. Firstly, as stated above, only patients with stage I-II tumours amenable to be resected by standard lobectomy should be operated on; secondly, advantages of VATS compared to thoracotomy (less postoperative pain, lenght of stay, functional impairment) are theoretically able to reduce complications and mortality in such frail patients.

A recent study on 95 octogenarians who received surgery either by VATS (n=58) or standard thoracotomy (n=37) in a single Institution, demonstrated that major cardiopulmonary complications occurred in 13.8% of VATS group and 32.4% of open surgery group (p=0.03). Five-years survival was not affected but study was retrospective, non-randomized and suffers some bias in patients selection (more I stages in VATS group) [47]. However efficacy of VATS has been reported by several other Authors [48, 49]. It has been demonstrated that VATS surgery generates less cytokine production in early postoperative phase and less impairment of postoperative pulmonary function, which ultimately could decrease in-hospital complications, as stated in the text.

Therefore there is enough evidence to support minimally invasive surgery especially in very elderly people.

6.4. Thermal ablation

Thermal ablation has been shown to be effective as local treatment of solid tumours. The main modalities to achieve thermal damage of malignant tissue are radiofrequency (RF), microwave (MW) and cryoablation; all them are applied directly to tumour through different devices positioned percutaneously through an image-guided procedure.

Lung tissue has unique characteristics which maximizes the so called *heat sink* effect: airflow and bloodflow limits in fact the intended tissue damage, that results smaller in vivo versus in vitro experiments, acting as an air/liquid-cooled radiator. Lung has therefore a small thermal conductivity.

In these regards MW has some theoretical advantages over RF ablation, because thermal damage is realized through electromagnetic waves that cause polar water molecules to rotate rapidly; MW is not limited by thermal and electric conductivity of tissue, reaching so larger zones and higher temperatures in lung [50]. Histopathological studies indicates that a margin of 8 mm for adenocarcinomas and 6 mm for squamous cell carcinoma are necessary to cover 95% of microscopic disease [51].

Thermal ablation techniques presents similar limits regarding to:

- The lack of pathological data, especially histological and molecular features of tumour, nodal status and margins of treatment: regarding the last issue, cryoablation is more attractive because the ablated zone correlates with the ice-ball image visualized by CT-scan; this imply nonoptimal planning of adjuvant therapies
- Local control of disease: tumours greater than 3 cm in diameter have a low likelihood of successful ablation with RF; MW ablation has shown promising rates of local control also for tumours until 5 cm; overall local tumour progression rate was reported to be 50% after RF for c-I NSCLC, compared to 28.6% after surgery [52]; some studies indicate that combination of thermal ablation (more effective in the centre of tumour) and external beam radiotherapy (more effective at periphery of the lesion) could remarkably improve local control of disease [53]
- Evaluation of treatment response and monitoring of recurrences is more challenging after thermal ablation, because both residual mass and ablation zone are present: inflammatory response to heat damage may be responsible of initial apparent increase in size of tumour; FDG uptake at PET scan, in addition to CT criteria, is useful to predict completeness of tumour ablation but it should not be performed before 3 months to prevent false positives due to inflammatory response [54]
- Complications: major complication (pneumothorax requiring chest tube drainage, air embolism and pulmonary abscess) are reported in about 8% of procedures, depending on tumour size and pulmonary reserve; minor complications as hemoptysis, fever, pleuritis with effusion, damages to phrenic or intercostals nerves are much more frequent (cumulative incidence: 50%) and may sometimes significantly impair quality of life of patients with poor baseline performance status [50]

Regarding the last point, Tada and coll. reported that pulmonary function significantly decreased after RF, with FEV1 and VC at 1 and 3 months significantly lower than the baseline: predictive factor of major functional loss were severe pleuritis (at 1 and 3 month) and ablation of large volume of marginal parenchyma (at 3 months). Shrinkage of ablated zone during healing process may retract surrounding lung tissue, resulting in a decrease of alveoli compliance [55].

Indications to RF should therefore adequately determined for severely impaired patients as well as indications to surgery.

A recent review based on medically inoperable, early-stage NSCLC patients reports an advantage in 5-years survival and local recurrence rates of patients treated with stereotactic RT versus those treated by RF, at the cost of more disabling and lasting complications (actinic pneumonia, fatigue) [56].

We can conclude that thermal ablation should be part of the armamentarium against lung cancer in a multidisciplinary setting: its undeniable advantages (single session treatment, feasibility in marginal patients, repeatability) make it not only an alternative to surgery (e.g.: multiple small nodules) but primarily a complementary treatment (e.g.: treatment of recurrences after surgery, persistence of local disease after RT).

7. Take home messages

Provided that marginal patients should be evaluated in multi-disciplinary setting and on individual basis, some concepts should be kept in mind in management of octogenarians affected by NSCLC.

- Age above than 80 is neither a contraindication to operative treatment nor a routine indication for lesser resection; even octogenarians, with reduced life expectancy, dead of cancer rather than of comorbidities
- The presence of comorbidities (cardio-respiratory in particular) predict increased operative risk. This support the hypothesis that the potential association between advancing age and operative mortality is a reflection of increased co-morbidity rather than age per se.
- Even healthy octogenarians could have reduced organ function, resulting in low tolerance of postoperative major complications, which are fatal in a considerable percentages of patients.
- Extended resections should be avoided in octogenarians: lesions in early stages and yet not resectable with a standard lobectomy should therefore preferably managed in non-operative way.
- Complete and accurate clinical staging is crucial since pathological stage is the only predictive factor affecting long term survival. Accurate preoperative clinical staging is imperative and in this respect, a more standard use of PET-TC appear to be necessary. In case of doubt, invasive staging with mediastinoscopy should be used in the process of selection of candidates for surgery to avoid unnecessary operative risk in poor prognosis patients.
- Surgery remains to date the benchmark in terms of local control of disease and should therefore be preferred to radiation therapy and thermal ablation until future studies will eventually provide evidences of better risk/benefit ratio. Minimally invasive surgery promises to carry a benefit on postoperative outcome of elderly people

- Lung volume reduction criteria applied to lung surgery could move the limit of operability: in case of poor respiratory reserve, additional considerations should be made before excluding them from surgery, because ppoFEV1% is inaccurate in particular cases. These more compromised patients could benefit of a preoperative pulmonary rehabilitation program: in this way it could be possible to minimize the rate of minor postoperative complications that are probably related to 1st day FEV1% [57]. Lung volumes remodelling in fact takes at least some months to complete and favourable effects are not immediately available.

The critical issue is then to define which octogenarians will have the best chance of avoiding complications and ultimately benefit in terms of long survival after pulmonary resection and which are medically inoperable.

8. Conclusion

Octogenarians with adequate organ function affected by potentially resectable lung cancer are worthy of curative treatments because life expectancy almost always exceed prognosis of disease. Octogenarian should be considered as a patient with higher possibility to have multiple comorbidities and or reduced organ function (even subclinical) and should have access to lung cancer services regardless of age. High accuracy is recommended in clinical staging and functional assessment in order to select healthy patients who could really benefit of lung surgery with acceptable operative risk and with acceptable postoperative QOL. Surgical therapy is nowadays well accepted for healthy octogenarians. In marginal patients, appropriate counselling can support physician to decide on case-by-case basis whether to favour QOL over survival or vice-versa (as usually in the younger patients). Such patients should ideally be enrolled in randomised trials to provide an evidence base.

Author details

Cristian Rapicetta, Massimiliano Paci, Tommaso Ricchetti,
Sara Tenconi and Giorgio Sgarbi
Thoracic Surgery Unit, Arcispedale Santa Maria Nuova – Istituto di Ricerca e Cura a Carattere Scientifico, Reggio Emilia, Italy

Salvatore De Franco
Medical Education – Health Innovation Unit, Arcispedale Santa Maria Nuova – Istituto di Ricerca e Cura a Carattere Scientifico, Reggio Emilia, Italy

9. References

[1] Ginsberg RJ, Hill LD, Eagan RT, et al. Modern thirty-day operative mortality for surgical resections in lung cancer. J Thorac Cardiovasc Surg 1983;86:654-658.

[2] Romano PS, Mark DH. Patients and hospital characteristics related to in-hospital mortality after lung cancer resection. Chest 1992;101:1332-1337.

[3] Smith TJ, Penberthy L, Desch CE, Whittemore M, Newschaffer C, Hillner BE, McClish D, Retchin SM. Differences in initial treatment patterns and outcomes of lung cancer in the elderly. Lung Cancer 1995;13:235-252.

[4] Janssen-Heijnen MLG, Smulders S, Lemmens VEPP, et al. Effect of comorbidity on the treatment and prognosis of elderly patients with non-small cell lung cancer. Thorax 2004;59:602-607.

[5] National Cancer Intitute. SEER statistics review 1973-1997. Bethesda, MD: National Cancer Institute, 2000.

[6] Voltolini L, Rapicetta C, Ligabue T, Luzzi L, Scala V, Gotti G. Short and long-term results of lung resection for cancer in octogenarians. Asian Cardiovasc Thorac Ann 2009;17(2):147-52.

[7] Pagni S, Federico JA, Ponn RB. Pulmonary resection for lung cancer in octagenarians. Ann Thorac Surg 1997;63:785-789.

[8] Port JL, Kent M, Korst RJ, Lee PC, Levin MA, Flieder D, Altorki NK. Surgical resection for lung cancer in the octogenarian. Chest 2004;126:733-738.

[9] Aoki T, Yamato Y, Tsuchida M, Watanabe T, Hayashi J, Hirono T. Pulmonary complications after surgical treatment of lung cancer in octogenarians. Eur J Cardiothorac Surg 2000;18:662-665.

[10] Brock MV, Kim MP, Hooker CM, Alberg AJ, Jordan MM, Roig CM, Xu L, Yang SC. Pulmonary resection in octogenarians with stage I non-small cell lung cancer: a 22 year experience. Ann Thorac Surg 2004;77:271-277.

[11] Harvey JC, Erdman C, Pisch J, Beattie EJ. Surgical treatment of non-small cell lung cancer in patients older than seventy years. J Surg Oncol 1995;60:247-9.

[12] Naunheim KS, Kesler KA, D'Orazio SA, et al. Lung cancer surgery in the octogenarian. Eur J Cardiothorac Surg. 1994;8:453-6.

[13] Mountain CF. Revision in the International System for staging lung cancer. Chest 1997;111:1710-1717.

[14] Sirbu H, Schreiner W, Dalichau H, Busch T. Surgery for non-small cell carcinoma in geriatric patients: 15-year experience. Asian Cardiovasc Thorac Ann. 2005;13(4):330-6.

[15] Sioris T, Salo J, Perhoniemi V, Mattila S. Surgery for lung cancer in the elderly. Scand Cardiovasc J. 1999;33(4):222-7.

[16] Au J, el-Oakley R, Cameron EW. Pneumonectomy for bronchogenic carcinoma in the elderly. Eur J Cardiothorac Surg 1994;8:247-250.

[17] British Thoracic Society, Society of cardiothoracic Surgeons of Great Britain, and Ireland Working Party. Guidelines on the selection of patients with lung cancer for surgery. Thorax 2001;56:89-108.

[18] Thomas P, Sielezneff I, Ragni J, Giudicelli R, Fuentes P. Is lung cancer resection justified in patients aged over 70 years? Eur J Cardiothorac Surg.1993;7:241-245.

[19] Miller DL, Orszulak TA, Pairolero PC, Trastek VF, Schaff HV. Combined operation for lung cancer and cardiac disease. Ann Thorac Surg. 1994 Oct;58(4):989-93.

[20] Dominguez-Ventura A, Allen MS, Cassivi SD, Nichols FC 3rd, Deschamps C, Pairolero PC. Lung cancer in octogenarians: factors affecting morbidity and mortality after pulmonary resection. Ann Thorac Surg 2006;82:1175-9.
[21] Suemitsu R, Yamaguchi M, Takeo S, Ondo K, Ueda H, Yoshino I, Maehara Y. Favorable surgical results for patients with nonsmall cell lung cancer over 80 years old: a multicenter survey. Ann Thorac Cardiovasc Surg. 2008;14(3):154-60.
[22] Fanucchi O, Ambrogi MC, Dini P, Lucchi M, Melfi F, Davini F, Mussi A. Surgical treatment of non-small cell lung cancer in octogenarians. Interact Cardiovasc Thorac Surg. 2011;12(5):749-53.
[23] Brantigan OC. Surgical treatment of pulmonary emphysema. Maryland State Med J 6:409, 1957.
[24] DeMeester SR, et al. Lobectomy combined with volume reduction for patients with lung cancer and advanced emphysema. J Thorac Cardiovasc Surg 1998;115:681,.
[25] DeRose JJ, et al: Lung reduction operation and resection of pulmonary nodules in patients with severe emphysema. Ann Thorac Surg 1998;65:314.
[26] Kearney DJ, Lee TH, Reilly JJ, DeCamp MM, Sugarbaker DJ. Assessment of operative risk in patients undergoing lung resection. Importance of predicted pulmonary function. Chest. 1994;105(3):753-9.
[27] Yoshimoto K, Nomori H. Prediction of pulmonary function after lung lobectomy by subsegments counting, computed tomography, single photon emission computed tomography and computed tomography: a comparative study. Eur J Cardiothorac Surg. 2009;35(3):408-13.
[28] McKenna RJ Jr, Brenner M, Fischel RJ, Singh N, Yoong B, Gelb AF, Osann KE. Patient selection criteria for lung volume reduction surgery. J Thorac Cardiovasc Surg. 1997 Dec;114(6):957-64; discussion 964-7.
[29] Schattenberg T, Muley T, Dienemann H, Pfannschmidt J. Impact on pulmonary function after lobectomy in patients with chronic obstructive pulmonary disease. Thorac Cardiovasc Surg 2007;55: 500-504.
[30] Liao W, Ma G, Fang Y, Wang CM. Influence of chronic obstructive pulmonary disease on postoperative lung function of lung cancer patients and predictive value of lung perfusion scan. Ai Zheng. 2009;28(6):642-6.
[31] Santambrogio L, Nosotti M, Baisi A, Ronzoni G, Bellaviti N, Rosso L. Pulmonary lobectomy for lung cancer: a prospective study to compare patients with forced expiratory volume in 1 second less than 80% of predicted. Eur Cardiothorac Surg 2001; 20:684-687.
[32] Luzzi L, Tenconi S, Voltolini L, Paladini P, Ghiribelli C, Di Bisceglie M, Gotti G. Long term respiratory functional results after pneumonectomy. Eur J Cardiothorac Surg 2008;34(1):164-8.
[33] Rapicetta C, Tenconi S, Voltolini L, Luzzi L. Impact of lobectomy for non-small-cell lung cancer on respiratory function in octogenarian patients with mild to moderate chronic obstructive pulmonary disease. Eur J Cardiothorac Surg. 2011;39(4):555-9.
[34] Goddard PR, Nicholson EM, Laszo G, Watt I. Computed tomography in pulmonary emphysema. Clin Radiol 1982; 33:379-387.

[35] Glaab T, Banik N, Rutscmann OT, Wenker M. National survey of guideline-compliant COPD management among pneumologist and primary care physicians. COPD 2006;3(3):141-8.
[36] Marchand E, Gayan-Ramirez G, De Leyn P, Decramer M. Physiological basis of improvement after lung volume reduction surgery for severe emphysema: where are we? Comment in: Eur Respir J. 1999;13(3):480-1.
[37] Sabanathan S, Eng J, Mearns AJ. Alterations in respiratory mechanics following thoracotomy. J R Coll Surg Edinb. 1990 Jun;35(3):144-50. Review.
[38] Gauden SJ, Tripcony L. The curative treatment by radiation therapy alone of Stage I non-small cell lung cancer in a geriatric population. Lung Cancer. 2001 Apr;32(1):71-9.
[39] Sibley GS, Jamieson TA, Marks LB, Anscher MS, Prosnitz LR. Radiotherapy alone for medically inoperable stage I non-small cell lung cancer: the Duke experience. Int J Radiat Oncol Biol Phys 1998;40:149–54.
[40] Yendamuri S, Komaki R, Correa AM, Allen P et al. Comparison of limited surgery and three-dimensional conformal radiation in high-risk patients with stage I non-small cell lung cancer. J Thorac Oncol 2007; 2: 1022-1028.
[41] Yano T, Yokoyama H, Yoshino I, Tayama K, Asoh H, Hata K, Ichinose Y. Results of limited resection for compromised or poor-risk patients with clinical stage I non-small cell lung carcinoma of the lung. J Am Coll Surg 1995; 181: 33-37.
[42] Langendijk JA, Aaronson NK, de Jong JM, ten Velde GP, Muller MJ, Lamers RJ, Slotman BJ, Wouters EF. Prospective study on quality of life before and after radical radiotherapy in non-small-cell lung cancer. J Clin Oncol. 2001;15;19(8):2123-33.
[43] Booton R, Jones M, Thatcher N. Lung cancer 7: management of lung cancer in elderly patients. Thorax. 2003;58(8):711-20.
[44] Brown TS, Kanthapillai P. Transthoracic needle biopsy for suspected thoracic malignancy in elderly patients using CT guidance. Clin Radiol. 1998;53(2):116-9.
[45] Hicks RJ, Kalff V, MacManus MP, Ware RE, Hogg A, McKenzie AF, Matthews JP, Ball DL. (18)F-FDG PET provides high-impact and powerful prognostic stratification in staging newly diagnosed non-small cell lung cancer. J Nucl Med. 2001;42(11):1596-604.
[46] Wiersema MJ, Vazquez-Sequeiros E, Wiersema LM. Evaluation of mediastinal lymphadenopathy with endoscopic US-guided fine-needle aspiration biopsy. Radiology. 2001;219(1):252-7.
[47] Igai H, Takahashi M, Ohata K, Yamashina A, Matsuoka T, Kameyama K, Nakagawa T et al. Surgical treatment for non-small cell lung cancer in octogenarians: the usefulness of video-assisted thoracic surgery. Interact Cardiovasc Thorac Surg. 2009;9(2):274-6.
[48] Mun M, Kohno T. Video-assisted thoracic surgery for clinical stage I lung cancer in octogenarians. Ann Thorac Surg. 2008;85(2):406-11.
[49] Cattaneo SM, Park BJ, Wilton AS, Seshan VE, Bains MS, Downey RJ, Flores RM, Rizk N, Rusch VW. Use of video-assisted thoracic surgery for lobectomy in the elderly results in fewer complications. Ann Thorac Surg. 2008;85(1):231-5.

[50] Sonntag PD, Hinshaw JL, Lubner MG, Brace CL, Lee FT Jr. Thermal ablation of lung tumors. Surg Oncol Clin N Am. 2011;20(2):369-87.

[51] Ambrogi MC, Fontanini G, Cioni R, Faviana P, Fanucchi O, Mussi A. Biologic effects of radiofrequency thermal ablation on non-small cell lung cancer: results of a pilot study. J Thorac Cardiovasc Surg. 2006 May;131(5):1002-6.

[52] Kim SR, Han HJ, Park SJ, Min KH, Lee MH, Chung CR, Kim MH, Jin GY, Lee YC. Comparison between surgery and radiofrequency ablation for stage I non-small cell lung cancer. Eur J Radiol. 2012 Feb;81(2):395-9. doi:10.1016/j.ejrad.2010.12.091.

[53] Grieco CA, Simon CJ, Mayo-Smith WW et al. Percutaneous image-guided thermal ablation and radiation therapy: outcomes of combined treatment for 41 patients with inoperable stage I/II non-small-cell lung cancer. J Vasc Interv Radiol. 2006;17(7):1117-24.

[54] Deandreis D, Leboulleux S, Dromain C, Auperin A, Coulot J, Lumbroso J, Deschamps F, Rao P, Schlumberger M, de Baère T. Role of FDG PET/CT and chest CT in the follow-up of lung lesions treated with radiofrequency ablation. Radiology. 2011;258(1):270-6.

[55] Tada A, Hiraki T, Iguchi T, Gobara H, Mimura H, Toyooka S, Kiura K, Tsuda T, Mitsuhashi T, Kanazawa S. Influence of Radiofrequency Ablation of Lung Cancer on Pulmonary Function. Cardiovasc Intervent Radiol. 2011 Jul 2. [DOI: 10.1007/s00270-011-0221-z].

[56] Bilal H, Mahmood S et al. Is radiofrequency ablation more effective than stereotactic ablative radiotherapy in patients with early stage medically inoperable non-small cell lung cancer? Interact Cardiovasc Thorac Surg. 2012 May 10. doi: 10.1093/icvts/ivs1.

[57] Varela G, Brunelli A, Rocco G, Novan N, Refai M, Jimenez MF, Salati M et al .Measured FEV1 in the first postoperative day, and not ppoFEV1, is the best predictor of cardio-respiratory morbidity after lung resection. Eur J Cardiothorac Surg 2007;32(5):783-6.

[58] Wu MT, Chang JM, Chiang AA, Lu JY, Hsu HK, Hsu WH, Yang CF. Use of quantitative CT to predict postoperative lung function in patients with lung cancer. Radiology 1994;191:257-262.

[59] Noordijk E, Poest C, Hermans J et al: Radiotherapy as an alternative to surgery in elderly patients with respectable lung cancer. Radiother Oncol 1988; 13:83.

[60] Janssen F, Kunst A. The choice among past trends as a basis for the prediction of future trends in old-age mortality. Popul Stud (Camb). 2007;61(3):315-26.

[61] Korst RJ, Ginsberg RJ, Ailawadi M, Bains MS, Downey RJ Jr, Rusch VW, Stover D. Lobectomy improves ventilatory function in selected patients with severe COPD. Ann Thorac Surg 1998;66:898.

[62] Volpino P et al. Risk of mortality from cardiovascular and respiratory causes in patients with chronic obstructive pulmonary disease submitted to follow-up after lung resection for non-small cell lung cancer. J Cardiovasc Surg (Torino). 2007;48(3):375-83.

[63] Ambrogi MC, Lucchi M, Dini P, Melfi F, Fontanini G, Faviana P, Fanucchi O, Mussi A. Percutaneous radiofrequency ablation of lung tumours: results in the mid-term. Eur J Cardiothorac Surg. 2006;30(1):177-83.

Chapter 5

Risk Prediction and Outcome Analysis

Constance K. Haan

Additional information is available at the end of the chapter

http://dx.doi.org/10.5772/54136

1. Introduction

There are at least three perspectives from which one can think about using risk prediction and outcomes data in cardiothoracic surgery. The first is the perspective of the patient in need of cardiothoracic surgery procedure and care, who wishes to know, "What are my chances?" An engaged patient and family are interested in the patient's survival of the acute condition or event, but also interested in the near- and long-term outlook and quality of life beyond the recovery period.

The second is the perspective of the surgeon, wishing to know, "How am I doing?" This is the essence of the general competency in medical education known as practice-based learning and improvement, which entails review of and reflection on one's practice patterns and using this self-assessment to improve one's practice, particularly assessing against standards of care and specialty practice guidelines. Moreover, it can be argued that as health care is a team sport, rather than a solo act, that perspective should be expanded to reflect the whole interdisciplinary team asking, "How are *we* doing?"

Finally, the societal perspective—including regulators and payers—seeks information that answers whether or not we are delivering care that is safest and of highest quality for the cost and the resources invested.

The Institute of Medicine in *To Err is Human* articulates six key parameters by which quality of care is assessed and which are important to all three perspectives, with those parameters being for care that is safe, timely, effective, efficient, equitable and patient-centered [1]. As decisions are made and care is delivered for each patient as an individual case, the practitioner makes what he or she believes to be the best decisions for care based on the individual patient characteristics and needs and the information available at the time. However, it is the decision-making and care delivery *trends* that are highly informative to all three perspectives described above.

This chapter focuses on the following areas of risk and outcome data use: 1) clinical cardiothoracic databases; 2) risk factors and risk prediction models; 3) application of risk prediction in clinical decision-making and care delivery; 4) process and outcomes data for reporting and improvement; and 5) use of database linkages to determine factors and decisions contributing to outcomes across the continuum of care.

2. Cardiothoracic databases

Surgeons have been interested in monitoring and improving outcomes since Ernest Amory Codman pioneered the study of medical outcomes. He kept "end result cards" on his patients, including long-term outcomes of at least one year, and wrote several papers on the "end result idea" in the early 1900s [2]. The ability to speak knowledgably about risk assessment and clinical outcomes for any clinical specialty requires data gathered on the patients treated by that specialty—whether based on diagnostic category, acute event or performance of a particular procedure or set of procedures. This is of even greater value when one can speak about one's own patient population and performance data, using data that are complete and valid and analyzed in comparison to a large number of patients of comparable condition.

2.1. Administrative databases

Administrative data, such as the data from the Centers for Medicare and Medicaid Services database, are readily available, relatively inexpensive, and provide information on large numbers of patients. However, administrative data are usually collected by coding for billing purposes rather than collection for clinical studies and improvement, so that critical clinical context and variables are unavailable and the differentiation of comorbidities from complications can be problematic [3,4].

The University HealthSystem Consortium (UHC) is an alliance if 101 academic medical centers and nearly 200 of their affiliate hospitals—representing more than 90% of the US nonprofit academic medical centers—which has developed risk-adjusted mortality models based on discharge abstracts and include adjustments for differences in patient severity using the All Patient Refined Diagnosis Related Groups (APR-DRG). The UHC refers to its data and risk model as clinical (versus administrative), because the data are derived from coding of clinical conditions. However, it should be noted that the source of the data sent to UHC by hospitals and healthcare systems is the financial and administrative data from the system, and therefore dependent on coding and demographic information, and drawn from the same data source used to report patient billing data to Medicare and other payers [5].

2.2. Clinical databases

There are numerous notable clinical registries and databases for cardiothoracic surgery patients. Local and regional databases are particularly noteworthy for their ability to draw data from physician groups and hospitals that are traditionally competitive relative to one another, but who agree to contribute data to build valid assessment of quality in cardiac care. Regional databases of note include those of the Northern New England Cardiovascular Disease Study Group (NNE) [6,7]. The New York State Department of Health has been building databases for reporting on adult cardiac surgery and percutaneous coronary interventions since the early 1990s, and subsequently added pediatric congenital cardiac surgery [8,9,10]. The Pennsylvania Health Care Cost Containment Council has databases that include hip and knee replacement, diabetes and health-associated infections, besides cardiac care [11]. Other states have followed, with a statewide approach to quality, such as the State of New Jersey Department of Health and Senior Services Office of Health Care Quality Assessment [12], the Minnesota Cardiac Surgery Database [13], the Michigan Society of Thoracic and Cardiovascular Surgeons Quality Collaborative [14], and the Virginia Cardiac Surgery Quality Initiative [15].

The Veterans Affairs (VA) Cardiac Surgery Database [16,17] has been a leading force in national cardiac databases. The Department of Veterans Affairs has built on the experience in cardiac surgery to develop a database for major surgery outcomes and quality of care, as seen in the National VA Surgical Quality Improvement Program (NSQIP) database [18]. NSQIP has proven so valuable as to now be applied to surgery programs across the country, well beyond the VA medical centers.

The predominant national adult cardiac database in the US, beyond the VA, is the Society of Thoracic Surgeons (STS) National Cardiac Database (NCD) [19,20,21]. Building on the experience with the adult cardiac surgery database, the STS now has three components to the STS National Database—Adult Cardiac, General Thoracic Surgery Database, and Congenital Heart Surgery, with availability of anesthesiology participation in addition to surgeon participation in the Congenital Heart Surgery Database. The STS Congenital Heart Surgery Database has worked collaboratively at the international level on a joint European Association for Cardiothoracic Surgery (EACTS)-STS Congenital Database Committee, particularly on standardization of definitions and naming conventions [22,23,24]. Moreover, the World Society for Pediatric and Congenital Heart Surgery has gathered surgeons from over 50 countries and from all continents except Antarctica to work on pediatric cardiology and pediatric cardiac surgery [25,26,27].

In addition to EACTS, other international registry endeavors in cardiothoracic surgery include the Society for Cardiothoracic Surgery in Great Britain and Ireland [28], the Australian and New Zealand Society of Cardiac and Thoracic Surgeons Database [29], the Japan Cardiovascular Surgery Database Organization [30], and the Chinese coronary artery bypass grafting (CABG) registry [31]. While there are numerous country and international region registries, the STS also now provides the opportunity for international participants to contribute to the Adult Cardiac Surgery Database. The awareness of need for process and outcome data for reporting and improvement has caught fire and driven endeavors around the world. Next, this chapter will explore how the data is analyzed and utilized.

3. Risk prediction—Assessing risk

When outcomes and performance results are first brought up, it seems to be an almost reflexive defense response to say, "My patients are sicker." Thus, it is the risk-adjusted outcomes that essentially level the playing field, comparing like with like to as close a degree as possible. It is therefore of great importance to gather information that is both clinically relevant and comprehensive, to get as complete a picture as possible of the patient factors, over which the surgeon has little control, as well as aspects that can impact both decision-making, care delivery and outcomes of that care.

Further upstream in the continuum of care, a cardiothoracic surgeon depends on clinical judgment to assess the patient's cardiac condition in the context of his/her general health, and then to determine whether there is technically something to offer the patient to improve that cardiac condition. Beyond the ability to do something for the patient, there then follows the consideration of whether surgical intervention is appropriate, given the patient's condition, circumstances and preferences, and when. This is where there is great utility in having access to a reliable, easy-to-use risk prediction scoring system and tool. Granton and Cheng [32] have gathered information describing several of the predictive scoring systems available: the EuroSCORE [33,34], the STS score, the Parsonnet score [35,36], and regional models such as the Cleveland Clinic model and the NNE score. Additionally, the AusSCORE [37] has been developed and studied for Australian patients.

A core set of variables associated with outcomes in cardiothoracic surgery have evolved over time. Accuracy of risk models developed based on administrative data in New York [10] and Pennsylvania [11] have been shown to be substantially improved by addition of a few critical clinical variables—ejection fraction, reoperation, and left main coronary artery obstruction. One may further question how many variables are actually needed to have a robust risk prediction model. Studies from Ontario [38] and the Cooperative CABG Database Project [39] identified six and seven core variables, respectively. In the STS NCD, it has been demonstrated that 78% of the explained variance from the 28-variable model is derived from the eight most important predictors, which are age, surgical acuity, reoperative status, creatinine level, dialysis, shock, chronic lung disease, and ejection fraction [40].

While there are minor variations between the data collection forms for the various databases, the primary differences are derived from the correlation coefficients for the risk factors as calculated from the different patient populations. For purposes of description of data collection, the STS National Databases—Adult Cardiac Surgery [41], General Thoracic Surgery [42], and Congenital Heart Surgery [43]—are used in the section that follows.

3.1. Risk factors

Preoperative risk factors. Preoperative risk factors that are collected relate primarily to the presenting features of the patient. These start with such factors as age, gender, race and ethnicity. Also collected are general resource factors such as referral pattern information via patient zip code and hospital zip code, and the payer type.

The next section after demographic information contains fields for admission, surgery and discharge dates, as well as hours of intensive care unit (ICU) stay. The general health factors are captured by fields for height, weight, smoking status, family history for heart disease, hematocrit, and white blood cell count. The comorbidities recorded include the presence or absence of the following: diabetes, dyslipidemia, renal failure requiring dialysis, hypertension, infectious endocarditis, chronic lung disease, immunosuppressive therapy, peripheral arterial disease, cerebrovascular disease and the form and timing of its effect. In addition, the current renal function is logged as the last creatinine, and for diabetics, the method of diabetes control.

The cardiac presentation section contains fields for the following: previous myocardial infarction and time interval, heart failure, NYHA classification, cardiac presentation on admission, cardiogenic shock, resuscitation, arrhythmia and type, and previous cardiovascular interventions. Preoperative medications are recorded as yes, no or contraindicated/not indicated. Preoperative hemodynamics and catheterization and echocardiographic information are also recorded.

The preoperative risk factors for general thoracic surgery include weight loss over prior three months, steroids, preoperative chemotherapy, pulmonary function tests and results, Zubrod (activity tolerance) score, and clinical staging for lung and esophageal cancer.

For the congenital database, there is the additional information required on date of birth, prematurity, non-cardiac anatomic abnormalities, chromosomal abnormalities and congenital syndromes. The resuscitative preoperative factors captured for the congenital heart surgery patient include cardiopulmonary resuscitation, mechanical circulatory support, and shock. Metabolic risk factors include diabetes mellitus, hypothyroidism, and steroid requirement. Gastrointestinal risk factors relate to presence of colostomy, enterostomy, gastrostomy or esophagostomy, as well as hepatic dysfunction, or necrotizing entero-colitis. Neurological risk factors include neurological deficit, seizures, and stroke or intracranial hemorrhage. Respiratory risk factors include mechanical ventilation, respiratory syncytial virus, single lung, and trachesotomy. Additional factors captured include: coagulation disorder, endocarditis, sepsis, and renal dysfunction.

For congenital heart surgery, there is an additional aspect of risk-adjustment that has been employed and tested. The Risk Adjustment for Congenital Heart Surgery-1 (RACHS-1) was developed by Dr. Kathy Jenkins and investigators from Children's Hospital Boston [44]. The RACHS-1 goal was to adjust for baseline differences in case-mix and risk when comparing mortality prior to discharge from the hospital among patients under 18 years of age undergoing surgery for congenital cardiac disease or defect. It is important to note that the RACHS-1 was not created to predict the risk of death for individual patients, but to be a tool that allows meaningful comparisons across groups of patients [44].

It is worth noting that the available databases do not account for nutritional state, especially for malnourished patients. This is an aspect of general health that significantly impacts wound healing ability and immune system capacity to fight infectious complications.

Cardiac databases do not capture rehabilitation potential, as would be captured by a preoperative activity level and a realistic activity goal following recovery. For patients with a severely limited preoperative functional level, it would generally be unrealistic to expect a normal rate of separation from mechanical ventilation or length of stay. This also speaks to the level of postoperative recovery support required once the patient can be discharged from the hospital. Homelessness or severely limited social network support is also not captured by available databases. While these aspects of patient condition may not negatively impact the ability to heal and recover from a surgical procedure, they do affect the healthcare resources needed to achieve recovery, both in the hospital and following discharge.

Perioperative risk factors. All of the procedural databases include surgeon identification, diagnosis, primary and secondary procedures, operative start and end dates and times (including operating room entry and exit, anesthesia start and end, and skin incision start and stop), antibiotic selection and timing for administration and discontinuation. Operation status—elective, urgent, emergent/salvage, or palliative is recorded. Blood product administration is also captured.

Cardiopulmonary bypass utilization and associated features are recorded, including use of circulatory arrest, aortic occlusion, cardioplegia, and cerebral oximetry. Medication administration and use of intra-aortic balloon pump support are also captured. For coronary artery bypass surgery, the number of anastomoses is recorded for each type of conduit. Valve surgery procedures are captured, by valve, for type of procedure and prosthesis type utilized. Initial extubation date and time is captured to reflect the interval of intubation and ventilator support.

The general thoracic surgery perioperative data also include pathologic staging for cancer and ICU length of stay. The congenital heart surgery data also include capture of procedure location, temperature, cerebral perfusion and oximetry utilized. In addition, pediatric cardiac surgeons have found it important to address the issue of stratification of complexity in surgery for congenital cardiac diseases. The Aristotle Complexity Score was developed by an expert panel, and consists of assignment of an Aristotle Basic Complexity score to a given procedure based on potential for mortality, potential for morbidity, and technical difficulty [44].

Postoperative data collected. Postoperative transfusion and complications are collected for the databases. The complications are reflected by category: reoperation and reason, cardiac, neurologic, renal, pulmonary, infectious, vascular and other (gastrointestinal, urologic, hematologic). The discharge status, interval after surgery, and destination are key components, as well as the discharge medications. If readmission is necessitated, the reason is recorded. Key quality measures are captured for each of the databases.

The congenital heart surgery collection forms include sections for gathering key information for anesthesiology participation in the database—preoperative assessment, anesthetic technique, monitoring, intraoperative and postoperative pharmacology, and anesthesia adverse events. As there are a growing number of patients surviving their congenital heart defects to reach adulthood, the congenital heart surgery database also includes sections for adult cardiac surgery data components.

3.2. Risk models

Ivanov and colleagues studied the predictive accuracy of a statistical model against clinicians' estimates of outcomes after coronary bypass surgery [45]. They found that clinicians, when given the option, preferred to trust their own judgments. Experienced surgeons significantly overestimated the risk of operative mortality compared to their junior colleagues. Overall, the clinicians significantly overestimated the probability of operative mortality (for survivors to a greater degree than non-survivors) and ICU stay greater than 48 hours. Although no predictive model can predict the specific individual who will have an adverse event, statistical models permit reasonably accurate estimates of event rates for subgroups of patients [45].

The risk factors gathered by the database collection form for each patient are entered into the database, and aggregated for analysis and reporting. This can be accomplished by the individual surgeon or group with paper and pencil or an Excel spreadsheet. However, most clinicians are interested in risk-adjusted analysis of performance and outcomes to account for the particular characteristics of the patients and patient population to which care is rendered. Kozower and colleagues described their head-to-head comparison of the ability to predict risk-adjusted mortality by UHC and STS risk models [5]. What they found is that although the UHC model demonstrated better performance in the total study population, the difference was achieved by reflecting postoperative complications, and therefore the predictive discrimination was equivalent to random chance. Thus, it is critical to use a well-constructed and validated clinical risk model that reflects the patient comorbidities and acuity, with high correlation to the endpoints of interest. The next section describes the processes by which a robust clinical risk model is developed and validated.

3.3. Development of a clinical risk model

The study population is key to the quality and performance of the statistical model, and no risk adjustment model is better than the data on which it is based [40]. The population must be adequately defined, and exclusion applied for key missing data elements. The population is then randomly divided into two samples. The first sample of 60% of the population, known as the training sample, is for development of the risk model—used to identify predictor variables and estimate model coefficients [46,47,48]. Data from the other 40%, known as the test sample, is for the validation of the model, to assess model fit, discrimination and calibration.

The endpoints and outcomes of interest then need to be identified and defined. The nine major endpoints of interest for the STS adult cardiac surgery database [46,47,48] are as follows:

1. operative mortality—defined as death during the same hospitalization as surgery regardless of timing, or within 30 days of surgery regardless of venue or site;
2. permanent stroke or cerebrovascular accident—a central neurologic deficit persisting longer than 72 hours;
3. renal failure—an increase of the serum creatinine to more than 2.0 mg/dL and double the most recent preoperative creatinine level, or a new requirement for dialysis;
4. prolonged requirement of mechanical ventilation support(longer than 24 hours);
5. deep sternal wound infection—in most recent database versions recorded for as long as 30 days postoperatively;
6. reoperation for any reason;
7. major morbidity or mortality—a composite defined as the occurrence of any of the above endpoints;
8. prolonged postoperative length of stay—length of stay more than 14 days; and
9. short postoperative length of stay—length of stay less than six days and patient alive at discharge.

The major endpoints for the general thoracic surgery database are selected using similar principles, but with appropriate differences of interest to general thoracic surgeons and their patients. Adverse outcome measure selection is based on clinical judgment, literature review and preliminary data analysis. The postoperative endpoints selected for lung surgery are: mortality (in-hospital mortality regardless of timing or within 30 days of the procedure), tracheostomy, reintubation, initial ventilator support greater than 48 hours, adult respiratory distress syndrome, bronchopleural fistula, pulmonary embolus, pneumonia, bleeding requiring reoperation, and myocardial infarction [49,50]. The selected major outcomes for esophageal surgery consist of the following conditions: bleeding requiring reoperation, anastomotic leak requiring medical or surgical treatment, reintubation, initial ventilation greater than 48 hours, pneumonia, or in-hospital mortality (same hospitalization) regardless of timing [51].

The STS Congenital Database Taskforce and the Joint EACTS-STS Congenital Database Committee have critically reviewed and defined endpoints as well. Operative mortality is again defined as any death, regardless of cause, occurring within 30 days after surgery in or out of the hospital and after 30 days during the same hospitalization subsequent to the operation [22]. Because of the extensive spectrum of congenital heart defects and the wide variety of procedures for same, the complications of interest for the congenital databases are also more extensive and detailed, with significant attention to definitions [23,43].

All candidate variables are considered, and screened for relevance to prediction at population and at individual levels. It is of great value to have expert clinician review as well, to assure clinical relevance of the variables to be included. The validity—on its face, as well as of construct and content—is key to the value of the risk model, and so it needs to make sense to the clinician users.

The definitions for predictor variables and for endpoints must be strictly standardized. Even for an unambiguous endpoint like mortality, the time period and location become important components of the definition. There are important statistical and policy implications of using in-hospital mortality (without time limit) versus 30-day all-cause mortality (without consideration of where it occurs) versus operative mortality as either of the two. The fixed time period is statistically preferable, although more difficult to obtain with completeness and accuracy than in-hospital mortality [40].

The risk model development team has to assess the database for several aspects of variable reporting to determine inclusion or exclusion. The first for consideration is the frequency of missing data for each variable. A second consideration is identification of variables that are collected inconsistently or with questionable reliability, even for clinically unavoidable reasons. Use of derived variables (e.g., body mass index) or redundant variables, such as glomerular filtration rate which is a complex function of variables that are consistently and regularly included, should be assessed for appropriateness of inclusion in the model. Finally, there is consideration of whether to include potentially controversial variables, especially those that raise clinical, statistical or health policy issues. Examples of such variables include race and ethnicity, and preoperative intra-aortic balloon pump. As a confirmatory check, it is helpful to review potential candidate variables against external resources, such as previous versions of a risk model, and other comparable risk models from other groups or organizations.

As described by both Clark and by Shahian and colleagues, there are three principal techniques that have been utilized for construction of cardiac surgery risk models [40,52]. Bayesian models are useful in early database experience as they are robust in the face of missing data. Logistic regression models are the most common statistical technique for risk modeling—utilized by regional and national databases such as those in New York, the VA, and the NNE. Multivariable logistic regression is utilized for the STS national databases. Some use simple, additive scores with weights derived from the logistic regression model. Shahian and colleagues found that comparative studies have generally demonstrated that logistic models offer the best overall performance [40,53,54]. There is interest in the potential advance offered by application of algorithmic models, which are also known as machine-learning techniques, as these models permit complex, nonlinear information processing. However, tests of these models have not yet shown significant improvement over logistic or Bayesian models [40,55,56].

3.4. Risk model validation

Once the multivariable logistic regression is applied, the test sample of the defined population is used to test model performance and to validate the new model against its performance for the development sample and against the old model, if an update. The C-index is assessed for the training or development sample and the test or validation sample, looking for close agreement between the two samples for each endpoint. Alternatively, calibration can be assessed by plots of observed versus expected event proportions within deciles of predicted risk for the various endpoints, such as described by Shahian and colleagues [46,47,48].

For each of the STS risk models—CABG surgery, valve surgery, and combined CABG and valve—there have been multiple iterative refinements and updates to each. Calibration is required after obtaining raw STS risk scores, done annually (in quarterly increments), so that the calibration factors are dynamic, updated quarterly after each data harvest [40]. Jin and colleagues have reported that if the risk models are used without calibration, the risk scores are almost always higher than they should be, overstating risk and understating the observed-to-expected ratio [57].

Numerous types of validity can be used to scrutinize a statistical risk model. One is face validity, where the model is reasonable to experts. A second is content validity, where all important variables have been included. A third type is attributional validity, in which risk adjustment is adequate to insure that differences in outcome are not due to patient characteristics. Finally, there is predictive validity, which provides a measure of how well it performs on a data set other than the one from which it is developed, internal or external [40]. There are two tests applied to test predictive validity. The first, calibration, assesses reliability, or the extent to which the model assigns appropriate risk to the population under consideration, the most common of which is the degree of concordance between deciles of observed and expected risk, or the Hosmer-Lemeshow test [40]. By extension, and as is demonstrated by Tran and colleagues [58] and Zhang and colleagues [59], there is also naturally great interest in comparing the risk models against each other, including extension into intermediate timeframes (e.g., one-year survival). The second test, discrimination, assesses the tradeoff between specificity and sensitivity of the risk model at various probability cut points [40,60].

Following the calculation of the model performance measures, the final regression coefficients can then be estimated from the combined training (development) and test (validation) samples. The algorithm, intercept and coefficients can then be deployed for the risk model, for application for risk prediction for individuals and for population analysis.

4. Application of risk prediction in decision-making and care

4.1. Application at the bedside

Risk prediction tools that are easily accessible and user-friendly are the most valuable for application in the clinic or at the bedside. Tools providing calculations as the data are entered contribute to clinical decision-making in real-time. The STS provides an on-line risk calculator for just such a purpose [61]. It is at the bedside or in the clinic where the counseling is being provided, and the patient's and family's questions and concerns for risk versus benefit and chances for recovery versus adverse outcomes are being actively considered. Data-driven decision-making is extremely helpful, especially as applied to consideration of the patient preferences and expectations for the care plan and procedure being recommended.

When the patient is high-risk for surgery, the data help convey the statistical chances for mortality and adverse outcomes to provide realistic expectations and balance to the hope for a good outcome that can potentially be held out of proportion to the reality of the situation. Sometimes this may even take the form of supporting data-driven decision-making to recommend against a surgical procedure. A surgeon's knowing how to do a procedure does not automatically obligate the surgeon to operate, nor does it make a procedure right for every patient. In other words, it is important to consider when it may be appropriate to say 'no,' but doing so in an objective manner, based on the best available data and evidence.

When the patient condition and/or the cardiac anatomy is complex, and the recommendations by cardiologist and cardiac surgeon are not clearly guided by the evidence in the literature, data provided by the risk prediction tool can help provide input for shared decision-making by clinicians and patient. This is particularly enhanced by data-driven risk prediction for medical and surgical therapy, and for proceduralists from both medical and surgical subspecialties.

4.2. Individual performance trends

The clinician needs an accurate and reliable data source to answer the question, "How am I doing?" Practice guidelines, building on the evidence in the literature, provide recommendations for the standards of care on which proficient and expert clinicians have built consensus. The guidelines, however, do not provide information on the individual practitioner's application of and adherence to the guidelines. It should be noted that following guidelines does not absolve the surgeon of applying good judgment for extenuating patient needs and circumstances. The guidelines and standards should be generally applied, however, and the exceptions and variance should occur rarely. Risk models help to assess the trend in decision-making and practice patterns. This is an important opportunity to allow the data to tell the story about actual practice patterns, as opposed to the good intentions to follow guidelines and apply standard of care. One's perceptions of practice patterns are not always borne out by the data; thus, it is important, even imperative, to regularly evaluate oneself for practice-based learning and improvement.

Individual provider decisions on patient selection for operation are important to assess against appropriateness guidelines. Variance from recommended indications for operation should only be considered as a part of a research study, such as would be employed to assess procedure and timing of surgery for lung cancer.

4.3. Group or hospital performance trends

The trends in patient selection and provider practice patterns are also assessed for the group practice or hospital clinical service—the site of practice—by aggregating the individual provider data within the group or hospital practice. Within a group of providers there may be varying degrees of experience, and providers may be at different points along the lifelong learning curve of evolution from competence to proficiency to expertise and mastery. However, the clinical pathways by which the care is delivered offer an opportunity for setting the expected logistics for delivery of care in the perioperative cardiothoracic surgery patient. The risk-adjusted data provided as feedback to the group help the group to assess the impact of the processes and decision-making strategies commonly employed.

Although hospital and/or provider case volume have long been used as a proxy measure for quality, it is important to note that data show only modest association of hospital procedural volume with CABG outcomes [62]. Thus, volume may not be an adequate quality metric for CABG surgery. Database participation allows for demonstration of where low-volume providers and hospitals achieve high quality outcomes, and where high-volume providers and hospitals do not.

Assessing patient referral and selection trends for the group or hospital against appropriateness guidelines further allow objective data-driven feedback. A new cardiac or thoracic surgery program may be perceived to get good outcomes because it is too conservative in patient selection for surgery—by "cherry-picking" cases to enhance outcomes. Alternatively, a new cardiac or thoracic surgery program may wish to build volume and be or become too liberal in its patient selection for surgery. Database feedback provides valuable perspective against which to weigh public perspective—among the provider and the general community—based on data and the appropriateness guidelines.

5. Performance data for reporting and improvement

5.1. Performance data types

There are two primary types of performance data—process measures and outcome measures. A process measure reflects how an aspect of care is delivered. An outcome measure reflects the impact of care on the patient—or how the patient does as a result of the processes of care.

5.2. Process measures

Process measures may be captured as timed intervals, as exemplified by the time interval between myocardial infarction and operation, time on cardiopulmonary bypass, cross-clamp time, time interval for mechanical ventilation (or time to extubation), length of stay in the ICU and postoperative length of stay. Other process measures are reflected as counts, such as lowest hematocrit on bypass and number of blood products transfused. A third type of process measure is reported as a yes/no response, as in the reporting of use of the internal mammary (or thoracic) artery (IMA) as bypass conduit, use of cardiopulmonary bypass (versus off-pump), or use of recommended medications at discharge, specifically aspirin, beta blockade, and cholesterol-lowering statin therapy.

Preoperative process measures include time from presentation with myocardial infarction to operation, use of intra-aortic balloon pump, preoperative creatinine, and administration of preoperative beta blockade. In general thoracic, preoperative process measures include administration of induction chemotherapy, and urgent versus elective procedure status. Intraoperative process measures in cardiac surgery include use of cardiopulmonary bypass versus off-pump surgery, use of the left IMA as a conduit for bypass, and perioperative transfusion. General thoracic intraoperative process measures include thoracotomy versus video-assisted thoracoscopic surgery, and procedure selection (extent of resection versus wedge resection). These measures are important in the assessment of patient selection and management prior to operation, as related to risk prediction for postoperative outcomes.

Postoperative process measures for cardiac surgery include administration of blood transfusion and discharge medication regimen (antiplatelet med such as aspirin, beta blockade, and statin). Hospital postoperative length of stay, discharge destination and readmission are of increasing importance in assessing care coordination for optimal outcomes.

5.3. Outcome measures

As noted above in relation to development of risk prediction models, it is key to identify endpoints of interest for the database users, providers and patients. Obviously, it is impossible for a database to capture every conceivable outcome, but there is consensus on major adverse events for which the database or registry can provide a robust and valuable resource.

The most familiar outcome measure, of course, is mortality rate. Mortality can be reported as a raw mortality rate—a count of deaths per the patient or case denominator, or as a comparison ratio of the observed mortality rate over the expected or predicted mortality rate. Furthermore, in the section above on risk model endpoints, the various definitions for mortality consideration were reviewed. But why is there so much detail to be worked out around such an unambiguous endpoint of mortality (living versus dead is usually thought of as an easy distinction to determine), and what does it mean to the provider and/or organization? Is the surgery any more successful if the patient gets out of the hospital alive, but dies at home? What is the impact to the patient versus the provider and/or hospital if the patient dies on the 31st day after surgery instead of sooner? And why is it important to capture all-cause mortality versus cardiac or thoracic surgery-specific causes? As an example, all-cause mortality means that death from a bowel obstruction during the same hospitalization as the cardiothoracic procedure would count as in-hospital or operative mortality for the cardiac surgeon. Questions like these are what engage the concerted efforts of the taskforces and expert panels that work to build consensus on the definitions for their databases and the performance reporting from those databases.

Major morbidities, or non-fatal adverse outcomes, commonly reported in cardiac surgery are represented by rates for unplanned reoperation (usually for postoperative hemorrhage), prolonged ventilator support requirement (>24 hours), cerebrovascular accident or new neurologic defect, new renal insufficiency or renal failure, deep sternal wound infection, prolonged length of stay (>7 days). Readmission within 30 days is of growing importance as providers and payers assess quality across the continuum of care, and not just around the in-hospital procedural event.

Major morbidity in general thoracic surgery includes pneumonia, adult respiratory distress syndrome, empyema, sepsis, bronchopleural fistula, pulmonary embolism, ventilator support beyond 48 hours, reintubation, tracheostomy, atrial or ventricular arrhythmias requiring treatment, myocardial infarction, reoperation for bleeding, and central neurologic event.

There is one additional way of thinking about outcomes. This is as a standardized incidence ratio for the composite outcome of any adverse outcome—any mortality or major morbidity. This allows for discussion and counseling that takes into consideration the collective impact of multiple risk factors and comorbidities on successful, uncomplicated recovery and return to quality of life.

5.4. Application of performance measures for reporting quality

Those databases with mandatory participation, such as the New York and Pennsylvania databases and the VA database described previously, provide regular reports, usually on an annual basis. Voluntary databases, such as NNE and STS, also provide regular reports to participants, although on a more frequent interval.

One of the uses of the regular reporting is to provide the individual and group with their own performance results. A second is to place those results in the context of national normative data. This allows the individual and group to assess their practice patterns against not only the guidelines and evidence in the literature, but against other practicing physicians in the specialty as a whole.

Process prevalence and variability can be studied and reported to advance the practice of cardiothoracic surgery. One example is provided by Tabata and colleagues regarding the use of the IMA graft in multivessel CABG surgery [63]. Since use of the IMA graft has been repeatedly shown to be associated with significantly improved short-term and long-term survival in CABG, it is encouraging to see the frequency of IMA use in CABG surgery to be increasing. However Tabata's study shows that many patients do not receive the benefits of IMA grafts, and some hospitals have a very low IMA use rate, which offers a significant opportunity for continued improvement [63].

The STS database, as with other databases such as the NNE, has been the source of data for numerous studies on risk factors and association with outcomes. Studies have been done on relationship to outcomes of gender, race, obesity, diabetes, age, renal function, off-pump CABG, and emergency CABG, as examples [64]. Risk profiles and outcomes can be studied by procedure, as has been done with CABG trends over time as shown by Ferguson and colleagues [65] and ElBardissi and colleagues [66], and with 15-year valve surgery outcome trends as has been done by Lee and colleagues [67]. Risk factors and outcomes, especially mortality, can be studied by region, to assess outcomes in an effort to identify regional best practices and to spread improvements in cardiac surgical outcomes [68].

In addition to providing reports that allow individuals and groups to compare with their peers, regionally and nationally, cardiothoracic surgery databases can also be compared with each other, to compare patient populations and assess the quality of their reports relative to one another. One example of such a study has been provided by Grover and colleagues, comparing the VA and STS cardiac surgery databases [69]. Grover's findings were that, in spite of the major difference in the male proportion of patients between the two databases, risk factors are otherwise very similar. Moreover, both databases have shown a significant reduction in the risk-adjusted operative mortality rate over a decade of provide risk-adjusted performance to their participants, with observed-to-expected death ratios decreasing from 1.05 to 0.9 in the VA system, and 1.5 to 0.9 for the STS participants. This reinforces the conclusion that the availability of data reports for practice-based learning and improvement is thus shown to improve care and outcomes for patients.

As previously noted, procedure volume has long been associated with quality outcomes. Database reports on outcomes have prompted studies of procedure volume in comparison with clinical quality measures—mortality, morbidity, and processes of care [70]. For a voluntary database, critics have expressed concern that not having full participation can potentially skew the data, and thus, the outcomes. In this case the comparison of outcomes against the higher volume in a larger database (e.g., Medicare), can help to reinforce the accuracy of the quality of the data reported [71].

The quality measurements in adult cardiac surgery have been applied to develop a methodology for comprehensive assessment of adult cardiac surgery quality of care, including both individual measures and an overall composite quality score. A Cardiac Surgery Performance Measures Steering Committee and the associated Technical Advisory Panel convened by the National Quality Forum (NQF) selected a set of 21 structure, process, and outcomes measures to assess quality of cardiac surgery care in the US. Incorporating the trend in health care quality assessment for the use of bundled measures and "all-or-none" scoring, the STS Quality Management Taskforce (QMTF) chose eleven individual quality measures grouped within four domains that included all relevant CABG process and outcomes measures endorsed by the NQF. The four domains of STS quality measures are 1) perioperative medical care of preoperative beta blockade, discharge aspirin, discharge beta blockade, and discharge antilipid therapy; 2) operative care of the use of at least one IMA; 3) risk-adjusted operative mortality; and 4) absence of postoperative morbidity, specifically renal insufficiency, deep sternal wound infection, re-exploration for any cause, stroke, and prolonged ventilation/intubation [72]. The STS QMTF has developed and tested a composite measure of cardiac surgery quality that encompasses multiple domains of care, uses Bayesian random-effects analyses, uses all-or-none scoring where appropriate, and avoids subjective weighting of individual measures, to provide validated quality measures useful to various types of users [73]. With the STS composite quality score in use, Shahian and colleagues looked at the association of hospital CABG volume to the STS composite quality score, and found only 1% of composite score variation was explained by volume [70].

5.5. Application of performance measures for improving quality

With the data reports described above, data becomes information provided for self-examination and self-assessment, which in turn can be the starting point for improving quality and outcomes. The individual and group reports have prompted the response of,

"What does this mean?...and what can I do to improve it?" This is the start of the necessary self-examination and self-reflection, followed by system examination, on which to build the quality improvement. When the data is shared with the other members of the interdisciplinary team, it is even more powerful, as it prompts self-assessment and drives buy-in for a collaborative approach to improvement. Carefully designed and disciplined teamwork and reliable implementation of evidence-based protocols applied by an empowered front line helps make improvements, especially decreasing complications and increasing cost savings [74].

6. Database use across the continuum of care

6.1. Linkage of databases

The STS database, as a national voluntary participation database, has seen growing participation, especially over recent years. However, it has still been important to quantify the completeness of the STS database as representative of cardiac surgery care in the US. To that end, the STS linked successfully with the Centers for Medicare and Medicaid Services (CMS) Medicare database and demonstrated high and increasing penetration and completeness of the STS database [75]. In addition, this linkage should facilitate studying long-term outcomes of cardiothoracic surgery. The STS Congenital Heart Surgery database has also performed successful linkage to the Pediatric Health Information System database, an administrative database. This will similarly allow providers to conduct database research that capitalizes on the enhancements provided by linking both types of data to answer important clinical questions [76].

It has been noted repeatedly in this discussion that the surgical databases have focused on short-term outcomes, with mortality being captured as in-hospital or 30 days. But what can we learn about how the patients are doing after 30 days? What data sources may be available to the provider, beyond personal provider or staff follow-up with the patient and/or his/her primary physician? The NNE has linked that database to the National Death Index, to provide long-term survival outcomes [77]. In the interest of more complete and accurate objective data, the STS has linked to the Social Security Death Master File, which allows for verification of "life status." This successful linkage of the STS database to social security data has allowed examination of survival after cardiac operations—CABG, aortic valve replacement and mitral valve operations—with initial reporting on one-year survival [78].

In an important study looking at long-term outcomes, the STS, the American College of Cardiology Foundation, and the Duke Clinical Research Institute are collaborating on a comparative effectiveness study (American College of Cardiology Foundation—Society of Thoracic Surgeons Collaboration on the Comparative Effectiveness of Revascularization Strategies [ASCERT]) of CABG and percutaneous coronary interventions (PCI). This study has developed a long-term mortality (or survival) risk prediction model for CABG and PCI, i.e., considering outcomes across the continuum of care [79]. In another early report on comparative effectiveness of revascularization strategies, Weintraub and colleagues have found that, among older patients with multivessel coronary artery disease not requiring emergency treatment, there was a long-term survival advantage among patients who underwent CABG as compared to patients who underwent PCI [80]. Studies like this will continue to inform providers as they improve shared decision-making and quality, using the data-driven comparative effectiveness research.

6.2. Future opportunities for database improvement

Databases have been firmly established as sources of data for driving learning and improvement. Providers who participate in clinical registries or databases are therefore facilitating their own individual and collective practice-based learning and improvement. The variables captured in these databases will continue to be improved—by building evidence-based consensus on definitions, and by addition of variables needed to more completely represent the patients. In the risk factor discussion above, it was mentioned that there are aspects of patient condition that are not currently captured—including poor nutritional status and homelessness. Also discussed under risk factors was the challenge of capturing rehabilitation potential, relative to anticipated quality of life goal following postoperative recovery. It should be noted that Afilalo and colleagues have proposed using an integrative approach combining frailty, disability, and STS risk scores to better characterize elderly patients referred for cardiac surgery, and especially to identify those at increased risk [81].

While there is benefit in enhancing the databases by adding or refining variables where appropriate, it will remain imperative to exercise excellent quality control of data entered into the database, especially by applying consistent standardized definitions [82]. As the electronic medical record becomes more pervasive in the US and elsewhere, this process may become more streamlined, but it will remain important to conduct appropriate audits for completeness and accuracy of data to decrease variability that would make the data and derived calculations suspect.

In the spirit of Dr. Codman, who in 1917 called for hospitals to release and compare outcomes data [2], the STS has initiated voluntary public reporting of database participant performance [83]. The rationale is to provide transparency and promote accountability. With implementation, will follow the continued need for appropriate auditing and reporting of composite measures using credible data and methodologies, thus decreasing the likelihood of other entities developing measures from inferior methodologies which use unadjusted or inadequately adjusted administrative data [83,84].

7. Conclusion

A complete and accurate database is essential in order to provide vital information to patients, to providers, and to society. The patient needs valid and accurate prediction derived from data on procedural risk to aid in decision-making and to set realistic expectations for outcomes of care. The provider needs a valid and accurate risk prediction tool with which to appropriately counsel patients, families and colleagues. The provider needs valid and trusted reports on process and outcome measures in order to carry out appropriate and necessary assessment of self and system by which to improve. The public needs to see that the providers and the profession are measuring and monitoring, and using data for improvement of decision-making and care delivery, to ensure safe, timely, effective care. Cardiothoracic surgeons have been leaders in database development and testing, but even stronger leaders in applying the data to improve practice and outcomes for patients. This is a critical role and responsibility, but also an opportunity to make an invaluable contribution to our patients.

Author details

Constance K. Haan
University of Florida College of Medicine-Jacksonville, Jacksonville, FL, USA

8. References

[1] Committee on Quality of Heath Care in American, Institute of Medicine. To err is human: building a safer health system. Washington: National Academies Press; 1999.
[2] Codman EA. A study in hospital efficiency. Oakbrook Terrace, IL: Joint Commission on Accreditation of Healthcare Organization; 1996. [Originally published in Boston in 1917.]
[3] Iezzoni LI. The risks of risk adjustment. JAMA. 1997;278:1600-7.
[4] Hannan EL, Racz MJ, Jollis JG, Peterson ED. Using Medicare claims data to assess provider quality for CABG surgeyr: does it work well enough? Health Serv Res. 1997;31:659-78.
[5] Kozower BD, Aiulawadi G, Jones DR, Pates RD, Lau CL, Kron IL, Stukenborg GJ. Predicted risk of mortality models: surgeons need to understand limitations of the University HealthSystem Consortium models. J Am Coll Surg. 2009;209:551-6.
[6] O'Connor GT, Plume SK, Olmstead EM, Coffin LH, Morton JR, Maloney CT, Nowicki ER, Tryzelaar JF, Hernandez F, Adrian L, Casey KJ, Soule DN, Marrin CAS, Nugent WC, Charlesworth D, Clough R, Katz S, Leavitt BJ, Wennberg JE. A regional prospective study of in-hospital mortality associated with coronary artery bypass grafting. The Northern New England Cardiovascular Disease Study Group. JAMA. 1991;266:803-9.
[7] O'Connor GT, Plume SK, Olmstead EM, Morton JR, Maloney CT, Nugent WC, Hernandez F Jr, Clough R, Leavitt BJ, Coffin LH, Marrin CAS, Wennberg D, Birkmeyer JD, Charlesworth DC, Malenka DJ, Quinton HB, Kasper JF, for the Northern New England Cardiovascular Disease Study Group. A regional intervention to improve the hospital mortality associated with coronary artery bypass graft surgery. JAMA. 1996;275:841-6.
[8] Hannan EL, Kilburn H Jr, Racz M, Shields E, Chassin MR. Improving the outcomes of coronary artery bypass surgery in New York State. JAMA. 1994;271:761-6.
[9] Hannan EL, Siu AL, Kumar D. The decline in coronary artery bypass graft surgery mortality in New York State. JAMA. 1995;273(3):209-13.

[10] New York State Department of Health. Cardiovascular disease data and statistics [Internet]. 2012 [cited 2012 Apr 7]. Available from: http://www.health.ny.gov/statistics/diseases/cardiovascular/
[11] Pennsylvania Health Care Cost Containment Council. Public reports—cardiac care [Internet]. 2012 [cited 2012 Apr 7]. Available from: http://www.phc4.org/reports/cabg/
[12] State of New Jersey Department of Health and Senior Services. Office of Health Care Quality Assessment—Cardiac surgery [Internet]. 2012 [cited 2012 Apr 16]. Available from: http://www.state.nj.us/health/healthcarequality/cardiacsurgery.shtml
[13] Arom KV, Petersen RJ, Orszulak TA, Bolman RM 3rd, Wickstrom PH, Joyce LD, Spooner TH, Tell BL, Janey PA. Establishing and using a local/regional cardiac surgery database. Ann Thorac Surg. 1997 Nov;64(5):1245-9.
[14] Blue Cross and Blue Shield of Michigan. Michigan Society of Thoracic and Cardiovascular Surgeons quality collaborative [Internet]. 2012 [cited 2012 Apr 7]. Available from: https://www.bcbsm.com/provider/value_partnerships/cqi/society-of-thoracic-cardiovascular-surgeons-quality-collaborative.shtml
[15] Virginia Cardiac Surgery Quality Initiative. The Virginia cardiac surgery quality initiative [Internet]. 2012 [cited 2012 Apr 15]. Available from: http://www.vcsqi.org/about_us.php
[16] Hammermeister KE, Johnson R, Marshall G, Grover FL. Continuous assessment and improvement in quality of care. Ann Surg. 1994;219(3):281-90.
[17] Grover FL, Shroyer ALW, Hammermeister KE. Calculating risk and outcome: the Veterans Affairs Database. Ann Thorac Surg. 1996;62:S6-11.
[18] Khuri SF, Daley J, Henderson W, Hur K, Demakis J, Aust JB, Chong V, Fabri PJ, Gibbs JO, Grover F, Hammermeister K, Irvin G 3rd, McDonald G, Passaro E Jr, Phillips L, Scamman F, Spencer J, Stremple JF. The Department of Veterans Affairs' NSQIP: the first national, validated, outcome-based, risk-adjusted, and peer-controlled program for the measurement and enhancement of the quality of surgical care. National VA Surgical Quality Improvement Program. Ann Surg. 1998 Oct;228(4):491-507.
[19] Edwards FH, Clark RE, Schwartz M. Coronary artery bypass grafting: The Society of Thoracic Surgeons National Database experience. Ann Thorac Surg. 1994 Jan;57:12-9.
[20] Edwards FH, Clark RE, Schwartz M. Practical considerations in the management of large multiinstitutional databases. Ann Thorac Surg. 1994 Dec;58:1841-4.
[21] The Society of Thoracic Surgeons. STS National Database [Internet]. 2012 [cited 2012 Apr 7]. Available from: http://www.sts.org/national-database
[22] Jacobs JP, Mavroudis C, Jacobs ML, Maruszewski B, Tchervenkov CI, Lacour-Gayet FG, Clarke DR, Yeh T Jr, Walters HL, Kurosawa H, Stellin G, Ebels T, Elliott MJ. What is operative mortality? Defining death in a surgical registry database: a report of the STS Congenital Database Taskforce and the Joint EACTS-STS Congenital Database Committee. Ann Thorac Surg. 2006;81:1937-41.
[23] Jacobs JP, Jacobs ML, Mavroudis C, Maruszewski B, Tchervenkov CI, Lacour-Gayet FG, Clarke DR, Yeh T Jr, Walters HL, Kurosawa H, Stellin G, Ebels T, Elliott MJ, Vener DF, Barach P, Benavidez OJ, Bacha EA. What is operative morbidity? Defining complications in a surgical registry database. Ann Thorac Surg. 2007;84:1416-21.

[24] Franklin RCG, Jacobs JP, Krogmann ON, Beland MJ, Aiello VD, Colan SD, Elliott MJ, Gaynor JW, Kurosawa H, Maruszewski B, Stellin G, Tchervenkov CI, Walters HL III, Weinberg P, Anderson RH. Nomenclature for congenital and paediatric cardiac disease: historical perspective and The International Pediatric and Congenital Cardiac Code. Cardiol Young. 2008;18(Suppl 2):70-80.

[25] Jacobs JP, Maruszewski B, Kurosawa H, Jacobs ML, Mavroudis C, Lacour-Gayet FG, Tchervenkov CI, Walters H 3rd, Stellin G, Ebels T, Tsang VT, Elliott MJ, Murakami A, Sano S, Mayer JE Jr, Edwards FH, Quintessenza JA. Congenital heart surgery databases around the world: do we need a global database? Semin Thorac Cardiovasc Surg Pediatr Card Annu. 2010;13(1):3-19.

[26] Sandoval N, Kreutzer C, Jatene M, DiSessa T, Novick W, Jacobs JP, Bernier PL, Tchervenkov CI. Pediatric cardiovascular surgery in South America: current status and regional differences. World J Pediatr Congenital Heart Surg. 2010;1:321-7.

[27] Tchervenkov CI, Jacobs JP, Bernier PL, Stellin G, Kurosawa H, Mavroudis C, Jonas RA, Cicek SM, Al-Halees Z, Elliott MJ, Jatene MB, Kinsely RH, Kreutzer C, Leon-Wyss J, Liu J, Maruszewski B, Nunn GR, Ramirez-Marroquin S, Sandoval N, Sano S, Sarris GE, Sharma R, Shoeb A, Spray TL, Ungerleider RM, Yangni-Angate H, Ziemer G. The improvements of care for paediatric and congenital cardiac disease across the world: a challenge for the World Society for Pediatric and Congenital Heart Surgery. Cardiol Young. 2008;(Suppl 2):63-9.

[28] Society for Cardiothoracic Surgery in Great Britain & Ireland. UK cardiac surgery is safe no matter what day of the week: an analysis of the SCTS database [Internet]. 2012 [posted 2012 Apr 2; cited 2012 Apr 7]. Available from: http://www.scts.org/modules/news/newsstory.aspx?n=24

[29] The Australian and New Zealand Society of Cardiac and Thoracic Surgeons. Cardiac surgery database [Internet]. 2012 [cited 2012 Apr 7]. Available from: http://www.anzscts.org/ascts-surgical-database/

[30] Motomura N, Miyata H, Tsukihara H, Okada M, Takamoto S, and Japan Cardiovascular Surgery Database Organization. Ann Thorac Surg. 2008;86:1866-72.

[31] Li Y, Zheng Z, Hu S. The Chinese coronary artery bypass grafting registry study: analysis of the national multicentre database of 9248 patients. Heart. 2009;95:1140-4.

[32] Granton J, Cheng D. Risk stratification models for cardiac surgery. Semin Cardiothorac Vasc Anesth. 2008;12:167-74.

[33] Qadir I, Salick MM, Perveen S, Sharif H. Mortality from isolated coronary bypass surgery: a comparison of the Society of Thoracic Surgeons and the EuroSCORE risk prediction algorithms. Interact Cardiovasc Thorac Surg. 2012;14(3):258-62.

[34] Nashef SAM, Roques F, Hammill BG, Peterson ED, Michel P, Grover FL, Wyse RKH, Ferguson TB. Eur J Cardiothorac Surg. 2002;22:101-5.

[35] Parsonnet V, Bernstein AD, Gera M. Clinical usefulness of risk-stratified outcome analysis in cardiac surgery in New Jersey. Ann Thorac Surg. 1996;61:S8-11.

[36] Parsonnet V, Dean D, Bernstein AD. A method of uniform stratification of risk for evaluating the results of surgery in acquired adult heart disease. Circulation. 1989;79:I3-12.

[37] Reid C, Billah B, Dinh D, Smith J, Skillington P, Yii M, Seevanayagam S, Mohajeri M, Shardey G. An Australian risk prediction model for 30-day mortality after isolated coronary artery bypass: the AusSCORE. J Thorac Cardiovasc Surg. 2009;138:904-10.

[38] Tu JV, Sykora K, Naylor CD. Assessing the outcomes of coronary artery bypass graft surgery: how many risk factors are enough? Steering Committee of the Cardiac Care Network of Ontario. J Am Coll Cardiol. 1997;30:1317-23.

[39] Jones RH, Hannan EL, Hammnermeister KE, DeLong ER, O'Connor GT, Leupker RV, Parsonnet V, Prior DB. Identification of preoperative variables needed for risk adjustment of short-term mortality after coronary artery bypass graft surgery. The Working Group Panel on the Cooperative CABG Database Project. J Am Coll Cardiol. 1996;28:1478-87.

[40] Shahian DM, Blackstone EH, Edwards FH, Grover FL, Grunkemeier GL, Naftel DC, Nashef SAM, Nugent WC, Peterson ED. Cardiac surgery risk models: a position article. Ann Thorac Surg. 2004;78:1868-77.

[41] The Society of Thoracic Surgeons. Adult cardiac surgery database data collection form version 2.73 [Internet]. 2011 [posted 2011 Jan 14; cited 2012 Apr 15]. Available from: http://www.sts.org/sites/default/files/documents/STSAdultCVDataCollectionForm2_73.pdf

[42] The Society of Thoracic Surgeons. General thoracic surgery database major procedure data collection form version 2.2 [Internet]. 2012 [posted 2012 Feb 10; cited 2012 Apr 7]. Available from:
http://www.sts.org/sites/default/files/documents/STSThoracicNonAnnotatedDataCollectionFormV2_2_MajorProc_1.2012_0.pdf

[43] The Society of Thoracic Surgeons. Congenital heart surgery database data collection from version 3.0 [Internet]. 2012 [posted 2009 Sep 16; cited 2012 Apr 7]. Available from: http://www.sts.org/sites/default/files/documents/pdf/ndb/CongenitalDataCollectionForm3_0_NonAnnotated_20090916.pdf

[44] Jacobs ML, Jacobs JP, Jenkins KJ, Gauvreau K, Clarke DR, Lacour-Gayet F. Stratification of complexity: the Risk Adjustment for Congenital Heart Surgery-1 method and the Aristotle Complexity Score—past, present, and future. Cardiol Young. 2008;18(Suppl2):163-8.

[45] Ivanov J, Borger MA, David TE, Cohen G, Walton N, Naylor CD. Predictive accuracy study: comparing a statistical model to clinicians' estimates of outcomes after coronary bypass surgery. Ann Thorac Surg. 2000;70:162-8.

[46] Shahian DM, O'Brien SM, Filardo G, Ferraris VA, Haan CK, Rich JB, Normand SLT, DeLong ER, Shewan CM, Dokholyan RS, Peterson ED, Edwards FH, Anderson RP. The Society of Thoracic Surgeons 2008 cardiac surgery risk models: part 1 coronary artery bypass grafting surgery. Ann Thorac Surg. 2009;88:2-22.

[47] O'Brien SM, Shahian DM, Filardo G, Ferraris VA, Haan CK, Rich JB, Normand SLT, DeLong ER, Shewan CM, Dokholyan RS, Peterson ED, Edwards FH, Anderson RP. The Society of Thoracic Surgeons 2008 cardiac surgery risk models: part 2 isolated valve surgery. Ann Thorac Surg. 2009;88:23-42.

[48] Shahian DM, O'Brien SM, Filardo G, Ferraris VA, Haan CK, Rich JB, Normand SLT, DeLong ER, Shewan CM, Dokholyan RS, Peterson ED, Edwards FH, Anderson RP. The

Society of Thoracic Surgeons 2008 cardiac surgery risk models: part 3 valve plus coronary artery bypass grafting surgery. Ann Thorac Surg. 2009;88:43-62.
[49] Kozower BD, Sheng S, O'Brien SM, Liptay MJ, Lau CL, Jones DR, Shahian DM, Wright CD. STS database risk models: predictors of mortality and major morbidity for lung cancer resection. Ann Thorac Surg. 2010;90:875-83.
[50] Shapiro M, Swanson SJ, Wright CD, Chin C, Sheng S, Wisnivesky J, Weiser TS. Predictors of major morbidity and mortality after pneumonectomy utilizing the Society of Thoracic Surgeons General Thoracic Surgery Database. Ann Thorac Surg. 2010;90:927-35.
[51] Wright CD, Kucharczuk JC, O'Brien SM, Grab JD, Allen MS. Predictors of major morbidity and mortality after esophagectomy for esophageal cancer: a Society of Thoracic Surgeons General Thoracic Surgery Database risk adjustment model. J Thorac Cardiovasc Surg. 2009;137(3):587-96.
[52] Clark RE. Calculating risk and outcome: the Society of Thoracic Surgeons Database. Ann Thorac Surg. 1996;62:S2-5.
[53] O'Brien SM, Dunson DB. Bayesian multivariate logistic regression. Biometrics. 2004;60:739-46.
[54] Marshall G, Grover FL, Henderson WG, Hammermeister KE. Assessment of predictive models for binary outcomes: an empirical approach using operative death from cardiac surgery. Stat Med. 1994;13:1501-11.
[55] Lippman RP, Shahian DM. Coronary artery bypass risk prediction using neural networks. Ann Thorac Surg. 1997;63:1635-43.
[56] Orr RK. Use of a probabilistic neural network to estimate the risk of mortality after cardiac surgery. Med Decis Making. 1997;17:178-85.
[57] Jin R, Furnary AP, Fine SC, Blackstone EH, Grunkemeier GL. Using Society of Thoracic Surgeons risk models for risk-adjusting cardiac surgery results. Ann Thorac Surg. 2010;89:677-82.
[58] Tran HA, Roy SK, Hebsur S, Barnett SD, Schlauch KA, Hunt SL, Holmes SD, Ad N. Performance of four risk algorithms in predicting intermediate survival in patients undergoing aortic valve replacement. Innovations. 2010;5(6):407-12.
[59] Zhang C, Xu J, GE Y, Wei Y, Yang Y, Liu F, Shi Y. Validation of four different risk stratification models in patients undergoing heart valve surgery in a single center in China. Chin Med J. 2011;124(15):2254-9.
[60] O'Brien SM. Cutpoint selection for categorizing a continuous predictor. Biometrics. 2004;60:504-9.
[61] The Society of Thoracic Surgeons. STS National Database risk calculator [Internet]. 2012 [cited 2012 Apr 15]. Available from: http://sts.org/quality-research-patient-safety/quality/risk-calculator-and-models
[62] Peterson ED, Coombs LP, DeLong ER, Haan CK, Ferguson TB. Procedural volume as a marker of quality for CABG surgery. JAMA. 2004;291(2):195-201.
[63] Tabata M, Grab JD, Khalpey Z, Edwards FH, O'Brien SM, Cohn LH, Bolman RM III. Prevalence and variability of internal mammary artery graft use in contemporary multivessel coronary artery bypass graft surgery. Analysis of the Society of Thoracic Surgeons National Cardiac Database. Circulation. 2009;120:935-40.

[64] Caceres M, Braud RL, Garrett HE Jr. A short history of the Society of Thoracic Surgeons National Cardiac Database: perceptions of a practicing surgeon. Ann Thorac Surg. 2010;89:332-9.

[65] Ferguson TB Jr, Hammill BG, Peterson ED, DeLong ER, Grover FL, for the STS National Database Committee. A decade of change—risk profiles and outcomes for isolated coronary artery bypass grafting procedures, 1990-1999: a report from the STS National Database Committee and the Duke Clinical Research Institute. Ann Thorac Surg. 2002;73:480-90.

[66] ElBardissi AW, Aranki SF, Sheng S, O'Brien SM, Greenberg CC, Gammie JS. Trends in isolated coronary artery bypass grafting: an analysis of the Society of Thoracic Surgeons adult cardiac surgery database. J Thorac Cardiovasc Surg. 2012;143:273-81.

[67] Lee R, Li S, Rankin JS, O'Brien SM, Gammie JS, Peterson ED, McCarthy PM, Edwards FH, for the Society of Thoracic Surgeons Adult Cardiac Surgical Database. Fifteen-year outcome trends for valve surgery in North America. Ann Thorac Surg. 2011;91:677-84.

[68] Quin JA, Sheng S, O'Brien SM, Welke KF, Grover FL, Shroyer AL. Regional variation in patient risk factors and mortality after coronary artery bypass grafting. Ann Thorac Surg. 2011;92:1277-83.

[69] Grover FL, Shroyer ALW, Hammermeister K, Edwards FH, Ferguson TB Jr, Dziuban SW Jr, Cleveland JC Jr, Clark RE, McDonald G. A decade's experience with quality improvement in cardiac surgery using the Veterans Affairs and Society of Thoracic Surgeons National Databases. Ann Surg. 2001;234(4):464-74.

[70] Shahian DM, O'Brien SM, Normand SLT, Peterson ED, Edwards FH. Association of hospital coronary artery bypass volume with processes of care, mortality, morbidity, and the Society of Thoracic Surgeons composite quality score. J Thorac Cardiovasc Surg. 2010;139:273-82.

[71] Welke KF, Peterson ED, Vaughan-Sarrazin MS, O'Brien SM, Rosenthal GE, Shook GJ, Dokholyan, Haan CK, Ferguson TB Jr. Comparison of cardiac surgery volumes and mortality rates between the Society of Thoracic Surgeons and Medicare databases from 1993 through 2001. Ann Thorac Surg. 2007;84:1538-46.

[72] Shahian DM, Edwards FH, Ferraris VA, Haan CK, Rich JB, Normand SLT, DeLong ER, O'Brien SM, Shewan CM, Dokholyan RS, Peterson ED. Quality measurement in adult cardiac surgery: part 1—conceptual framework and measure selection. Ann Thorac Surg. 2007;83:3-12.

[73] O'Brien SM, Shahian DM, DeLong ER, Normand SLT, Edwards FH, Ferraris VA, Haan CK, Rich JB, Shewan CM, Dokholyan RS, Anderson RP, Peterson ED. Quality measurement in adult cardiac surgery: part 2—statistical considerations in composite measure scoring and provider rating. Ann Thorac Surg. 2007;83:13-26.

[74] Culig MH, Kunkle RF, Frndak DC, Grunden N, Maher TD Jr, Magovern GJ Jr. Improving patient care in cardiac surgery using Toyota production system based methodology. Ann Thorac Surg. 2011;91:394-400.

[75] Jacobs JP, Edwards FH, Shahian DM, Haan CK, Puskas JD, Morales DLS, Gammie JS, Sanchez JA, Brennan JM, O'Brien SM, Dokholyan RS, Hammill BG, Curtis LH, Peterson ED, Badhwar V, George KM, Mayer JE Jr, Chitwood WR Jr, Murray GF, Grover FL. Successful linking of the Society of Thoracic Surgeons Adult Cardiac Surgery Database

to Centers for Medicare and Medicaid Services Medicare data. Ann Thorac Surg. 2010;90:1150-7.

[76] Pasquali SK, Jacobs JP, Shook GJ, O'Brien SM, Hall M, Jacobs ML, Welke KF, Gaynor JW, Peterson ED, Shah SS, Li JS. Linking clinical registry data with administrative data using indirect identifiers: implementation and validation in the congenital heart surgery population. Am Heart J. 2010;160(6):1099-1104.

[77] Malenka DJ, Leavitt BJ, Hearne MJ, Robb JF, Baribeau YR, Ryan TJ, Helm RE, Kellett MA, Dauerman HL, Dacey LJ, Silver MT, VerLee PN, Weldner PW, Hettleman BD, Olmstead EM, Piper WD, O'Connor GT. Comparing long-term survival of patients with multivessel coronary disease after CABG or PCI: analysis of BARI-like patients in northern New England. Circulation. 2005;112:I371-6.

[78] Jacobs JP, Edwards FH, Shahian DM, Prager RL, Wright CD, Puskas JD, Morales DLS, Gammie JS, Sanchez JA, Haan CK, Badhwar V, George KM, O'Brien SM, Dokholyan RS, Sheng S, Peterson ED, Shewan CM, Feehan KM, Han JM, Jacobs ML, Williams WG, Mayer JE Jr, Chitwood WR Jr, Murray GF, Grover FL. Successful linking of the Society of Thoracic Surgeons database to social security data to examine survival after cardiac operations. Ann Thorac Surg. 2011;92:32-9.

[79] Shahian DM, O'Brien SM, Sheng S, Grover FL, Mayer JE, Jacobs JP, Weiss JM, Delong ER, Peterson ED, Weintraub WS, Grau-Sepulveda MV, Klein LW, Shaw RE, Garratt KN, Moussa ID, Shewan CM, Dangas GD, Edwards FH. Predictors of long-term survival after coronary artery bypass grafting surgery: results from the Society of Thoracic Surgeons Adult Cardiac Surgery Database (the ASCERT study). Circulation. 2012 Mar 27;125(12):1491-500. Epub 2012 Feb 23.

[80] Weintraub WS, Grau-Sepulveda MV, Weiss JM, O'Brien SM, Peterson ED, Kolm P, Zhang Z, Klein LW, Shaw RE, McKay C, Ritzenthaler LL, Popma JJ, Messenger JC, Shahian DM, Grover FL, Mayer JE, Shewan CM, Garratt KN, Moussa ID, Dangas GD, Edwards FH. Comparative effectiveness of revascularization strategies. N Engl J Med. 2012 Mar 27 [Epub ahead of print] Available from: http://www.nejm.org/doi/pdf/10.1056/NEJMoa1110717

[81] Afilalo J, Mottillo AJ, Eisenberg MJ, Alexander KP, Noiseux N, Perrault LP, Morin JF, Langlois Y, Ohayon SM, Monette J, Boivin JF, Shahian DM, Bergman H. Addition of frailty and disability to cardiac surgery risk scores identifies elderly patients at high risk of mortality or major morbidity. Circ Cardiovasc Qual Outcomes. 2012;5(2):222-8.

[82] Brown ML, Lenoch JR, Schaff HV. Variability in data: the Society of Thoracic Surgeons National Adult Cardiac Surgery Database. J Thorac Cardiovasc Surg. 2010;140:267-73.

[83] Shahian DM, Edwards FH, Jacobs JP, Prager RL, Normand SLT, Shewan CM, O'Brien SM, Peterson ED, Grover FL. Public reporting of cardiac surgery performance: part 1 history, rationale, consequences. Ann Thorac Surg. 2011;92:2-11.

[84] Shahian DM, Edwards FH, Jacobs JP, Prager RL, Normand SLT, Shewan CM, O'Brien SM, Peterson ED, Grover FL. Public reporting of cardiac surgery performance: part 2 implementation. Ann Thorac Surg. 2011;92:12-23.

Chapter 6

Robot Assisted Thoracic Surgery (RATS)

Naohiro Kajiwara, Masatoshi Kakihana, Jitsuo Usuda, Tatsuo Ohira,
Norihiko Kawate and Norihiko Ikeda

Additional information is available at the end of the chapter

http://dx.doi.org/10.5772/53896

1. Introduction

Robotic surgery using the da Vinci® Surgical System (dVS; Intuitive Surgical, Inc., Sunnyvale, CA, U.S.A) has been approved in many countries for cardiovascular surgery, urology, and gynecology. However, unlike mediastinal tumors, which can be located in many different sites, in other organs treated with the dVS (heart, bladder, prostate, and uterus), the targets are generally found in similar locations. Moreover, the anatomical structures surrounding mediastinal tumors are vital (heart, aorta, lungs, pulmonary vessels, esophagus, and vertebrae), and it is crucial to pay careful attention in performing operations. Video-assisted thoracic surgery (VATS) is less invasive than standard thoracotomy, but there is the problem of postoperative pain caused by the inevitable leverage of instruments on the chest wall during the procedure, and the difficulty of manipulation in the mediastinum. The most crucial aspect is the limited movement of long rigid instruments (stick surgery). The instrument arms used in the dVS inflict less stress on the chest wall than conventional VATS, especially when highly skilled techniques are needed to operate on lesions in difficult-to-access areas [1].

Recently, Ruckert and his colleagues reported a comparison of robotic and nonrobotic thoracoscopic thymectomy [2]. After a follow-up of 42 months, they reported the cumulative complete remission rates of myasthenia gravis for robotic and nonrobotic thymectomy were 39% and 20%, respectively. Their conclusions reveal an improved outcome for myasthenia gravis after robotic thoracoscopic thymectomy compared with thoracoscopic thymectomy. In November 2011, Park and his colleagues reported robotic lobectomy for non–small cell lung cancer (NSCLC) concern with long-term oncologic results [3]. This report is the first concerning outcome about long term prognosis of lung cancer the robotic surgery in a total of 325 consecutive patients underwent robotic lobectomy for early-stage NSCLC at 3 institutions. They reported that overall 5-year survival was 80% and by pathologic stage, 91% for stage IA, 88% for stage IB and 49% for all patients with stage II disease. They concluded robotic lobectomy for early-stage NSCLC can be performed with low morbidity and mortality and long-term stage-specific survival is acceptable and consistent with previous results for VATS and thoracotomy. These data are very important, and these two reports support the scientific basis of robotic surgery. Thus, robotic surgery has gradually produced improved clinical outcomes, making it attractive for many surgeons. In the near future, robotic surgery may replace conventional VATS.

In this chapter, we set out to establish a procedure for resection of a variety of targets located in various thoracic areas difficult to reach by the VATS technique using robotic assisted thoracic surgery (RATS).

2. The da Vinci® surgical system

The dVS consists of a surgeon's console connected to the body of the dVS, a manipulator unit with 3-4 instrument arms, including a central arm to guide the endoscope camera, to which the surgeon's movements are transmitted, shown in Figure 1.

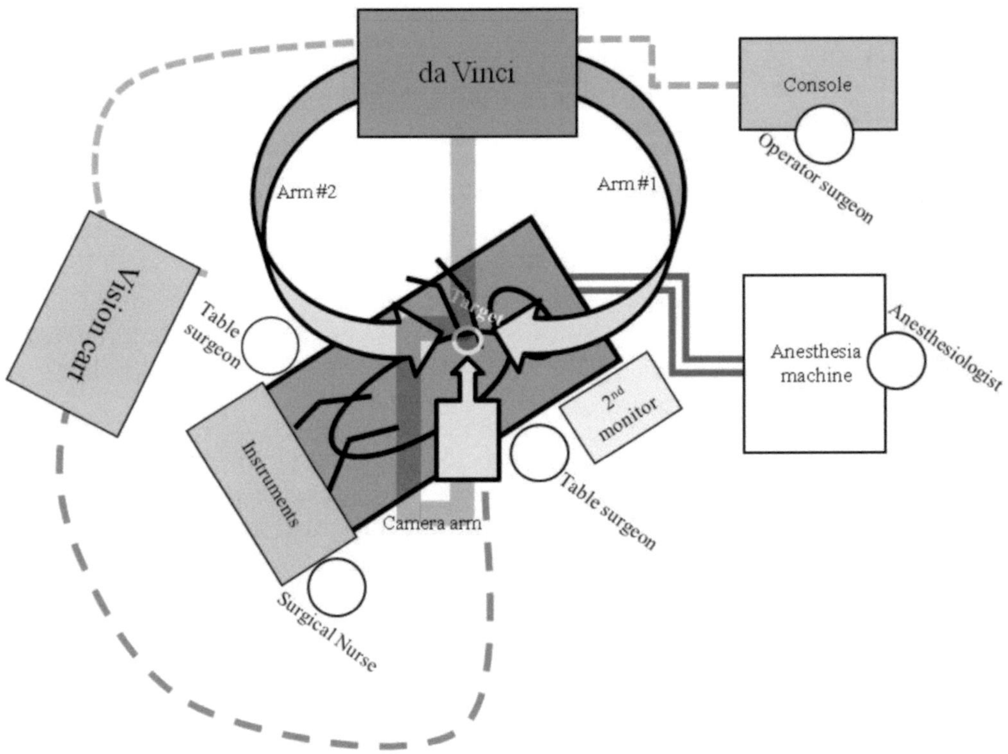

Fig.1-a

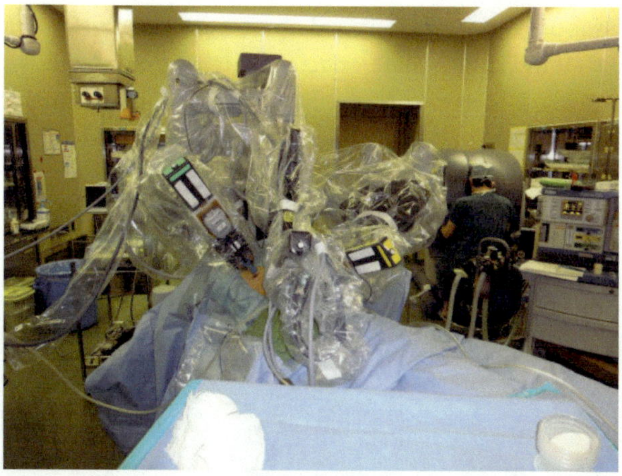

Fig. 1-b

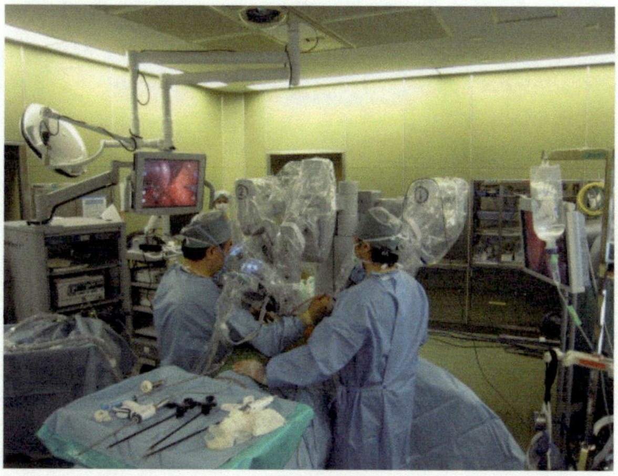

Fig.1-c

Figure 1. Positioning of all units for RATS

Appropriate positioning of all units for RATS is essential (Figure 1-a). The operating surgeon sits at the console (Figure 1-b) and there are two operating table surgeons (Figure 1-c), an anesthesiologist and a surgical nurse. The roles of table surgeons include setting and adjustment of the arms of the dVS, changing of instruments, surgical assistance using VATS devices and, most importantly, conversion to open thoracotomy if necessary, e.g. in cases of massive hemorrage,, during robotic surgery.

Accurate setup of the dVS is crucial to the success of thoracic operations, and this varies according to the location of the target in the mediastinum [4].

The flexible joint movements of robotic surgery enables dissection of targets located in sites that are difficult to access in the thoracic space, such as the upper, lower, anterior and posterior mediastinum. Dissection of various type mediastinal tumors with this system enables an accurate, smooth, and safe surgical operation, because the range of motion of the robotic arms and wrists within small spaces is extremely extensive. The EndoWrist® operative arm of the dVS is capable of replicating minute human wrist-like movements within the thoracic cavity (shown in Figure 2). Moreover the EndoWrist® system has motion scaling that eliminates physiological vibrations of the hands of the human surgeon.

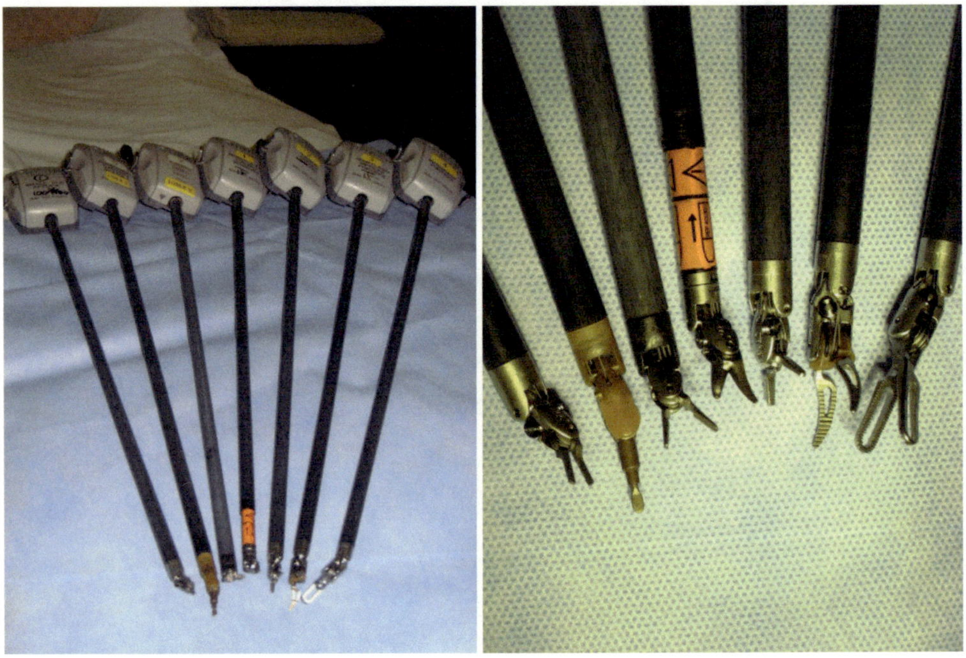

Figure 2. Instruments device

Figure 2 shows some of the accessory arms which are useful for general thoracic surgery (from left side; small clip applier, permanent cautery spatula, DeBakey forceps, monopolar curved scissors, large needle driver, Maryland bipolar forceps, ProGrasp forceps; usually attached the monopolar curved scissors on arm 1; as the right hand in thoracic procedure, and Maryland bipolar forceps or Cadiere forceps on arm 2; as the left hand in thoracic procedure).

The endoscope of the dVS system provides a 3-dimensional high-resolution binocular view of the surgical field, and is capable of a 12-fold enlarged view. The operation with the system enables accurate and simple safe surgery, because the range of motion of the robot arms within small spaces such as the thorax is extremely extensive. The crucial factors for successful dVS surgical procedures in thoracic surgery are selection of the appropriate placement and angle of the dVS ports, selected in relation to the individual target and patient position, which varies according to the target location.

2.1. Robot assisted thoracic surgery (RATS)

2.1.1. RATS set up

Care in selecting the pre-setting according to target location is the most important stage for robotic surgery in such lesions. Adjustments to the position of the instrument arms are also necessary, depending on the level of the target lesion.

Typical positioning of the instrument arm ports shown in Figure 3 is important. The camera port is placed approximately 20 cm from the target through the disposable 12-mm trocar. Instrument arm ports are placed at least 10 cm away from the camera port or the other Intuitive instrument arm ports. Assistant port (s) consisting of disposable 5–12 mm trocars are placed at least 5 cm away from any camera or instrument arm ports.

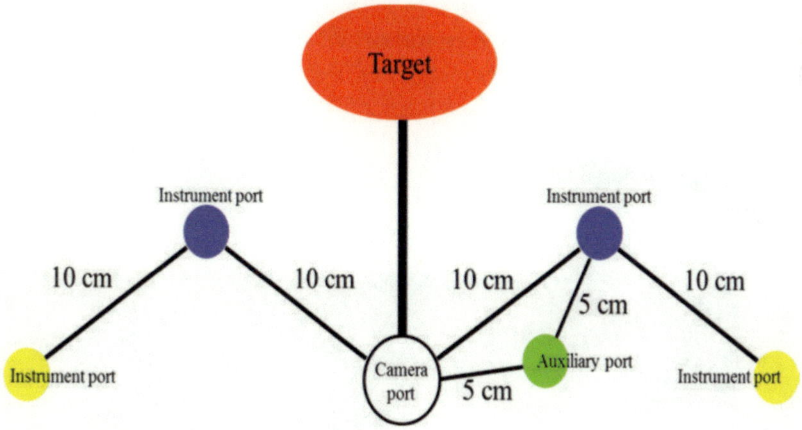

Figure 3. Positioning of Instrument Arm Port

- In the instrument-port procedure, the first port is positioned for the 3-dimensional camera placed in the 6-7th intercostal space on the mid-axillary line as shown in Figure 4.
- Another two ports for arms #1 (right hand in the thoracic procedure) and #2 (left hand in the thoracic procedure) are made. Arm port #1 is usually placed in the 6- 8th intercostal space on the mid-posterior axillary line, and arm port #2 is often placed in the 4–6th intercostals spaces on the anterior axillary line for left-sided anterior tumors, as shown in Figure 4.
- The 4th port is used as an accessory port for other devices such as those for vessel sealing and clipping, continuous suction, and washing. It is placed at least 5 cm apart from the other ports to prevent clashing of instrument arms. This accessory port is usually placed at the additional 1-2 cm incision made in the anterior axillary line in the 7-8th intercostal space.
- The settings of the dVS for thoracic surgery are generally classified into four patterns. The placement of arm-ports for typically lobectomy and thymectomy are classified in the pattern of Figure 4, and as for posterior targets, the approach shown in Figure 5 is recommended [5].

- For targets located in the opposite side of the thoracic cavity, the system and instrument ports positions are reversed, and areas for arms #1 and #2 should be changed correspondingly.
- The patient position on the operating table is also extremely important for the dVS procedure. A semi-lateral prone position is appropriate for resection of posterior targets, to avoid contacting the lung anteriorly under gravity. The lower limbs of the patient are also flexed downward so that the pelvis does not disturb the movement of the instrument arms [5].
- In urgent conversion to open thoracotomy cases, it is important to mark a line on the skin between the instrument-ports of arm #1 and arm #2.
- To widen the narrow working space, CO_2 inflation into the thoracic space (high-flow; 8–10 mm Hg) is carried out during the dVS procedure.

As Figures (4-6) show, target level is very important to decide the direction of approach of the dVS. Such this idea is a very crucial procedure to lose a perioperative blind spot in thoracic space.

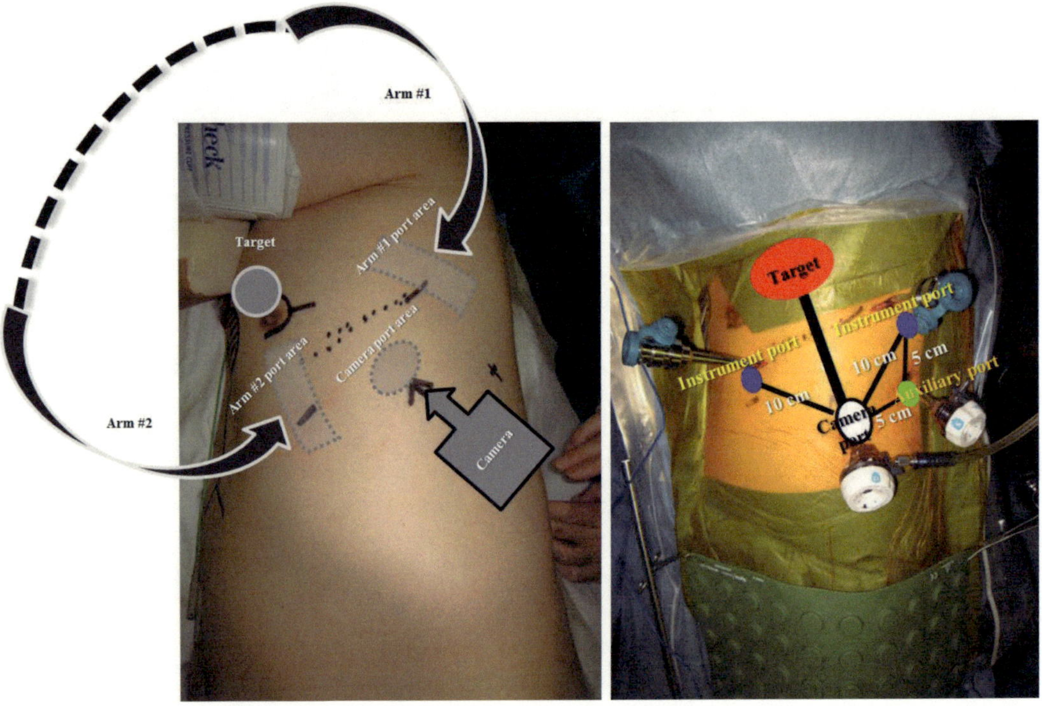

Figure 4. Appropriate parts replacement for thymectomy and lobectomy

The camera port is placed approximately 20 cm from the target through a disposable 12-mm trocar. Instrument arm ports are placed a minimum of 10 cm away from the camera port or the other Intuitive instrument arm ports. The assistant port, containing disposable 5- to 12-mm trocars, are placed at least 5 cm away from any camera or Intuitive instrument arm ports. Instrument arms are very useful in general thoracic surgery, especially the monopolar curved scissors, the Maryland bipolar forceps, Cadiere forceps and the DeBakey forceps and the permanent cautery spatula.

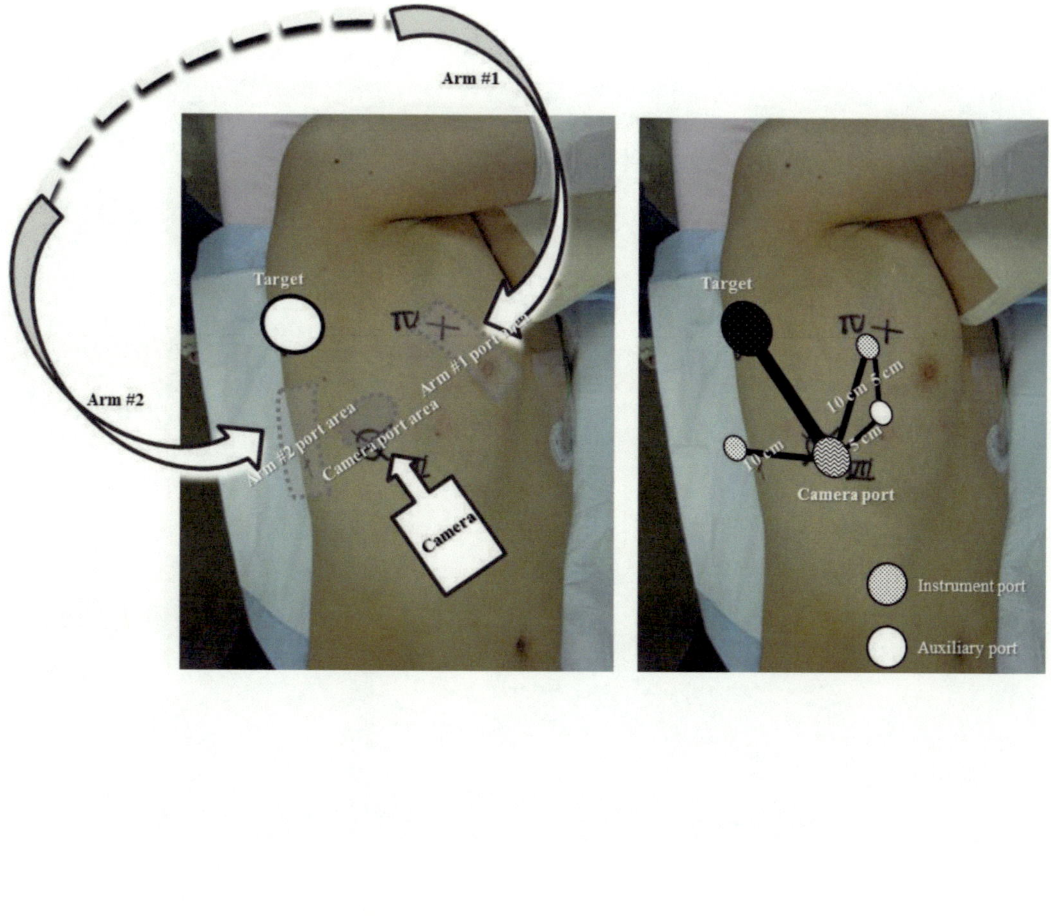

Figure 5. Appropriate placement of instrument ports for posterior tumors

Figure 5 shows the pattern of the location for right posterior-upper target with appropriate placement of instrument arm ports. The 3-D camera port is placed in the area of 6th intercostal in anterior-mid axillary line. Arm #1 is placed in the 3-4th intercostal in anterior axillary line. Arm #2 is placed in the 8-9th intercostal in the mid-posterior axillary line. The accessory port is placed in the 5th intercostal space in the anterior axillary line.

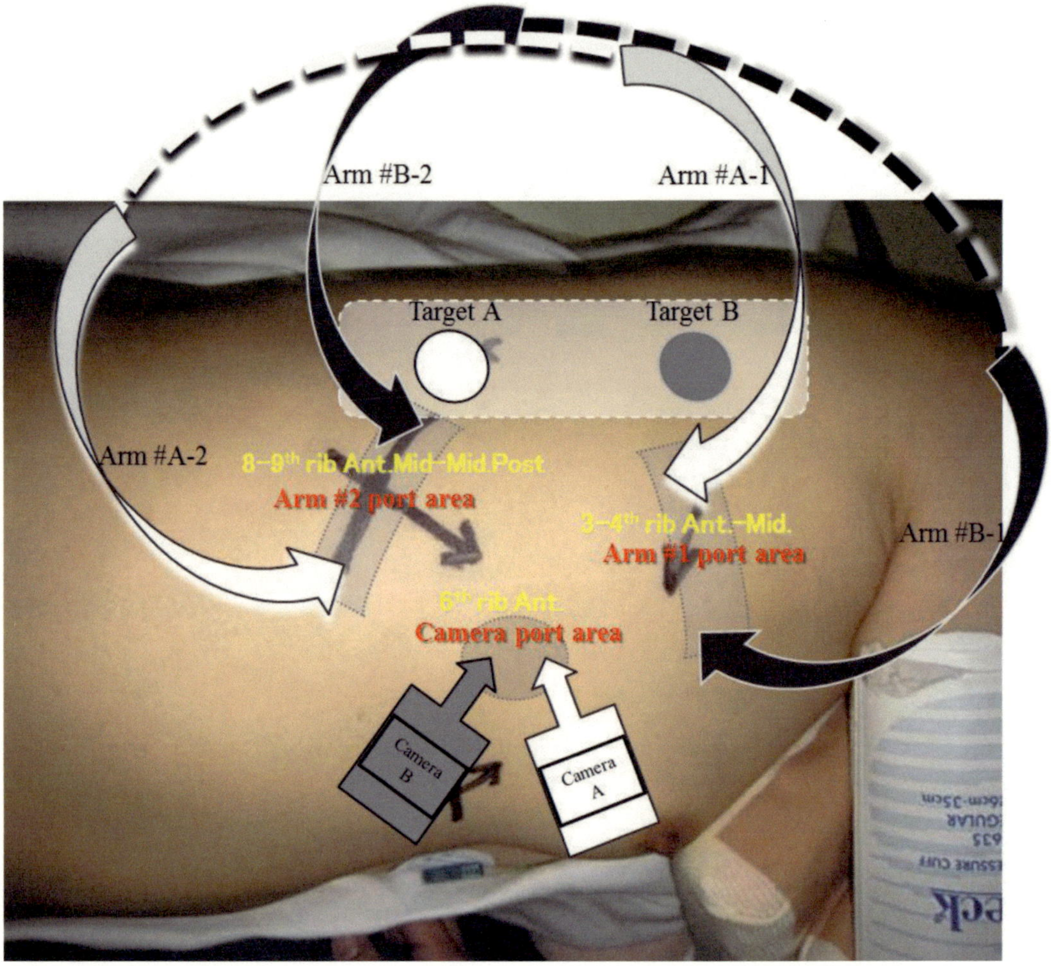

Figure 6. Appropriate placement of instrument arm ports for the right posterior targets location

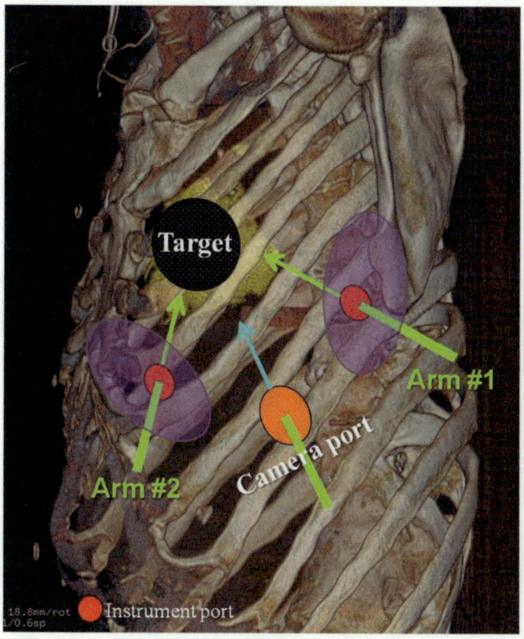

Fig. 7-a

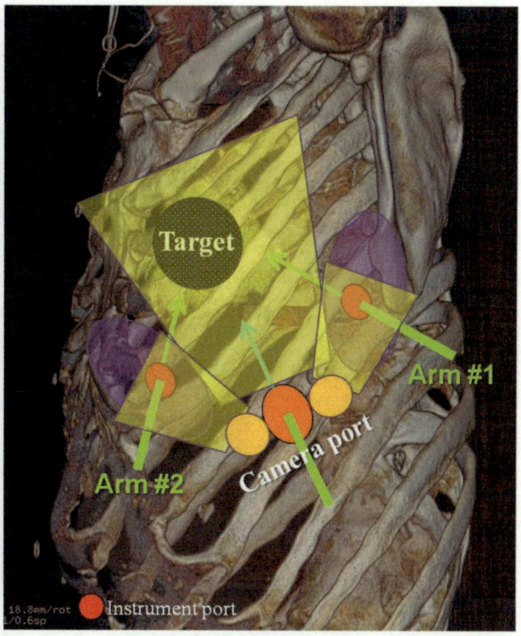

Fig. 7-b

Figure 7. Pitfalls of RATS

Target level is important to decide the direction of approach of the dVS. Instrument arm ports for a right posterior target: the camera port is placed in the 6th intercostal space area on the anterior axillary line; arm #1 (A and B) is placed in the 3rd–4th intercostal space in the anterior axillary line; arm #2 (A and B) is placed in the 8–9th intercostal space in the mid-axillary line; an accessory port is placed in the 5th intercostal space in the anterior axillary line. For a left-sided target, both arms (#1 and #2) should be interchanged.

2.1.2. Pitfalls of RATS

Arms of the dVS can be difficult to change position intraoperatively unlike in VATS so that preoperative fixation is important as described previously. That is the reason why the primary positioning of each unit and setting of instrument arms of the dVS is an essential step for the RATS procedure. The most important point regarding safety is to ensure a setting that eliminates or minimizes any blind spots of the console-operator, depending on target localization.

In clinical cases, trouble due to inappropriate manipulation in the blind spots (Figure 7-a; violet areas) in thoracic procedures seem empirically to depend on lack of function in that the tentacle of the arm tip against the organ is not transmitted to the console-operator. If the instruments give damage to lung in blind area, the operator sitting in the console could not know how to avoid this accident except for confirming with their own eyes.

In insertion of devices into the thoracic cavity and also in replacing them, it is essential during the process to confirm the exact position of the arm tip while watching the movement of the arms in the thoracic cavity closely by camera surveillance. Furthermore, table surgeons occasionally need to confirm the intrathoracic space with another sub-monitor or wide-view camera for safe manipulations during operation shown in Figure 7-b. These pitfalls are also crucial points for procedures in the abdominal space, and steps to avoid them can lead to the minimization of accidents.

Violet areas, which areas show the intrathoracic instrument port, are sometimes blind-spot from central camera view.

3. Future developments

RATS is generally better for the treatment of targets located in difficult to access areas than conventional VATS. However, the positioning of all units and the location of arm ports need suitable directional setting, which depends on the target location.

Several support safety developments are expected in the near future.

These ideas include following;

- instruments with tactile sensor tips,
- wide-angle view combined with the 3D main camera to eliminate blind spots,
- installing several supplementary cameras for total coverage of blind areas,

- devices uses in conventional VATS, i.e., stapler, vessel sealing system, soft coagulation device.

Reduction in size and weight, and a more economical price is always a problem for the dVS.

In addition to reduction in size, the manipulation of several arms through a single thoracic incision has become possible. Furthermore, surgeons should be able to perform detailed treatment within the thoracic space even in areas difficult to reach and very tiny spaces in which to perform manipulation. In this way possibilities will continue to improve. Moreover the speed of such improvements might begin to increase exponentially.

That this is technology for the patient entirely is something that a surgeon must never forget, and it means that primarily we must think first about safety for patients.

Author details

Naohiro Kajiwara*, Masatoshi Kakihana, Jitsuo Usuda, Tatsuo Ohira,
Norihiko Kawate and Norihiko Ikeda
Department of Surgery, Tokyo Medical University, Japan

Naohiro Kajiwara* and Norihiko Kawate
Department of Health Science and Social Welfare, Waseda University School of Human Sciences, Japan

Acknowledgement

The authors are grateful to Prof. J. Patrick Barron, Chairman of the Department of International Medical Communications of Tokyo Medical University for reviewing the English manuscript.

4. References

[1] Kajiwara N, Taira M, Yoshida K et al. (2011). Early experience using the da Vinci® surgical system for the treatment of mediastinal tumors. Gen Thorac Cardiovasc Surg. 59: 693–698

[2] Rückert JC, Swierzy M, Ismail M. (2011). Comparison of robotic and nonrobotic thoracoscopic thymectomy. A cohort study. J Thorac Cardiovasc Surg. 141(3): 673-7.

[3] Park BJ, Melfi F, Mussi A, Maisonneuve P, Spaggiari L, Da Silva RK, Veronesi G. (2012). Robotic lobectomy for non–small cell lung cancer (NSCLC): Long-term oncologic results. J Thorac Cardiovasc Surg. 143(2): 383-9.

[4] Kajiwara N, Kakihana M, Kawate N et al. (2011). Appropriate set-up of the da Vinci® surgical system in relation to the location of anterior and middle mediastinal tumors. Interact Cardiovasc Thorac Surg. 12: 112–116

* Corresponding Author

[5] Kajiwara N, Kakihana M, Usuda J et al. (2012). Extended indications for robotic surgery for posterior mediastinal tumors. Asian Cardiovascular & Thoracic Annals. 20(3): 308 - 313

Chapter 7

Valved Conduits Right Ventricle to Pulmonary Artery for Complex Congenital Heart Defects

Antonio F. Corno

Additional information is available at the end of the chapter

http://dx.doi.org/10.5772/51081

1. Introduction

The surgical implantation of a valved conduit to establish the continuity between the right ventricle and the pulmonary artery made possible the repair of a huge variety of complex congenital heart defects.

Diagnoses included tetralogy of Fallot, pulmonary atresia with ventricular septal defect, truncus arteriosus, transposition with ventricular septal defect and pulmonary stenosis or atresia, and various forms of double outlet right ventricle, ventricular septal defect, with or without pulmonary stenosis (1-7).

Right ventricle to pulmonary artery valved conduits have also been used in the pulmonary autograft replacement (Ross procedure) (8,9).

Various types of prosthetic and biological valved conduit have been used through the last decades, generally with satisfactory early hemodynamic performance, but most have been abandoned because of unsatisfactory long-term results.

Since any type of valved conduit utilized for clinical application present with some problem or complication in the long-term observations, the search for the ideal conduit is still ongoing.

For the decision making process among the various valved conduits currently available for surgical implantation, several options have been to taken into consideration regarding the type of conduit.

2. Types of biological valved conduits

2.1. Dacron valved conduits

Prosthetic Dacron conduits with incorporated a biological valve, porcine, bovine, or constructed with heterologous pericardium, have been used in the early period of this type of surgery (4-7,10).

The main advantage of this type of conduits was the off the shelf availability in a complete range of sizes, which made their use very attractive and practical.

The medium term results of Dacron valved conduits were complicated by failure of the conduits due to two main reasons (5-7,10-18):

a. the rapid development of thick pseudointima, causing conduit obstruction;
b. the rapid calcification of the glutaraldehyde preserved porcine valves, particularly in young children.

The combination of pseudointima formation and valve calcification resulted in conduit obstruction substantially reducing the freedom for conduit replacement, even in children where large size conduit had been implanted.

In favor of this type of valved conduits remained the slow and easy to detect progression of conduit stenosis, allowing timely plan of conduit replacement, facilitated by the easy shelling out of the covering pseudoadventitia, with a relatively low risk operation.

More recently aceptable long-term results have been reported with Dacron porcine valved conduits used for the right ventricular outflow tract reconstruction, particularly in patients with limited pulmonary vascular bed and high pulmonary artery pressures (19). Even in this reported positive experience the main limit of these conduits remained their rigidity, reducing the suitability for neonates and small infants.

2.2. Aortic and pulmonary homografts

After the first report of Rastelli on 1965 (1), Ross on 1966 introduced the use of the aortic valve with aortic root and ascending aorta to obtain the continuity between right ventricle and pulmonary artery with a biological valved conduit (2).

The homografts introduced by Ross were harvested from human cadavers, generally within 24-48 after death; after dissection they were treated for few days with antibiotic solution and then stored for up to 4 weeks at 4°C in either a balanced salt solution or in a special tissue culture medium (2).

Two changes were subsequently introduced in the homografts preparation:

a. homografts were sterilized by high-power irradiation
b. homografts were freeze dried

The combination of the two above techniques resulted in cells death, with severe damage to the collagen of the homografts, and particularly to the valve leaflets, resulting in conduit valve stenosis. As a result the use of frozen conduit with the above preparation has been abandoned, and few hospital in Europe continued to use fresh, antibiotic sterilized conduit (20,21).

Unfortunately became evident from clinical studies that homografts stored at 4°C were gradually losing cellular viability and tissue integrity; because of these reasons the fresh homografts had to be discarded 4 to 6 weeks after preparation because not suitable for clinical utilization.

The consequence was a homograft shortage, particularly for the smaller sizes, required for implantation in small children, due to the limited number of donors.

Major progress in the utilization of homografts has been the introduction of cryopreservation technology in the preparation, particularly with the controlled freezing to the temperature of liquid nitrogen (-196°C). This method allowed a large scale introduction of homografts in the clinical practice, despite issues related to the cellular viability of donor cells in the maintenance of the homografts durability (22-26).

The results provided by homografts on medium and long-term clinical observations were quite good, and nowadays these results are still used as comparison with any other type of biological valved conduit introduced in clinical practice (27-28).

Nevertheless the utilization of homografts present with the following issues:

a. the choice between aortic and pulmonary homografts
   The arterial wall of pulmonary homografts is thinner (60% thickness) than the wall of aortic homografts, and the elastin concentration is less.
   Because of this combination rapid dilatation of pulmonary homografts has been reported when implanted in children with pulmonary hypertension, and therefore were exposed to systemic pressure (22,23).

b. the rapid outgrowth of the conduit when implanted in infants and small children
   Longitudinal growth can result in lengthening and narrowing. Severe degree of calcification, due to he accelerated calcium metabolism in children, can reduce the size of the homograft lumen, and also the valve leaflets can rigid and stenotic, and also calcified (29-31). This can oblige to an early conduit replacement, even if very long-term observations have been reported, up to 21 years (32).

c. the reduced availability
   Homografts are not always available worldwide, particularly in the small sizes frequently requested for implantation in infants and small children. The technique of bicuspidalization of adult size homografts has been utilized in order to produce homografts of small size, with decent results even recently reported at long-term follow-up (33).

d. the immunitary reaction
   In most children where an homograft gas been implanted, humoral antibodies developed against human leukocyte antigen specific to the transplanted tissue. Host

antigen recognition and antibody development may be linked to early tissue calcification and structural valved deterioration with valved conduit failure (34-36).

2.3. Bovine jugular vein

The bovine jugular vein (Contegra®, Medtronic Inc., Minneapolis, MN), containing a trileaflet valve, was introduced into clinical practice as an alternative to the use of homografts in 1999 and has provided encouraging results in several reported clinical series, with follow-up reaching more than 10 years (37-45).

Recognized advantages of the bovine jugular vein are:

a. structural continuity between the wall of the jugular vein of the conduit and the valve leaflets, which provides optimal hemodynamics because of the ideal effective orifice area
b. unlimited "off-the-shelf" availability in sizes from 12 to 22 mm diameter, representing a good alternative to the homograft shortage, particularly in the smaller sizes
c. availability of a long length at both inflow and outflow that obviates the need for either proximal or distal augmentation; this facilitates conduit tailoring and positioning which helps to avoid potential distortion and sternal compression
d. exceptional reports of antigenic reaction, due to glutaraldehyde fixation

In contrast to the good clinical results obtained in several institutions (37-45), a disturbing sequence of publications reported stenosis at the level of the distal anastomosis of the conduit, with proximal conduit dilatation, aneurysm or pseudo-aneurysm, in between 6 and 50% of patients (39,40,42,46-54).

The problem of conduit dilatation related to obstruction at the distal anastomosis has been reported as a specific complication of the bovine jugular vein (46-54).

The following mechanisms were recognized as potential causes of distal stenosis:

a. presence of hypoplasia and/or distal stenosis of pulmonary artery branches
b. discrepancy in size between conduit and pulmonary artery
c. surgical technique
d. local immunologic/inflammatory reaction
e. local peel formation
f. thrombosis
g. a combination of two or more of the above (55).

The impact of the surgical technique has previously been studied using Computational Fluid Dynamics comparing two types of distal anastomosis: the conventional end-to-end *"circular"* anastomosis versus the oblique *"elliptical"* anastomosis with the incision extended on to the anterior aspect of the left pulmonary artery and the distal end of the conduit obliquely tailored.

The study confirmed a larger cross sectional area in the *"elliptical"* compared to the *"circular"* type of anastomosis along with more homogeneous velocity, pressure and shear stress distribution (55).

These results suggested that the "elliptical" anastomosis might reduce the incidence and degree of distal stenosis, particularly for smaller conduits.

We have therefore adopted this technique for the distal anastomosis, and in addition careful rinsing (5 minutes X 3 in different saline solutions) of the bovine jugular vein before implantation to clear the glutaraldehyde to reduce the inflammatory reaction, and avoidance of oversized conduits to reduce the discrepancy between conduit and distal pulmonary artery size (45).

Using this protocol the distal conduit stenosis has became a rare observation in our experience even with the smaller conduits (45).

Early calcification of biological valved conduits is frequently reported with homografts, particularly the smaller size conduits implanted in infants or small children in the first few years of life (30,37).

In our experience early conduit calcification causing hemodynamic consequences was never observed, confirming our own previous observations and those of other researchers (39,40,42,45).

We speculate that rinsing the glutaraldehyde off before bovine jugular vein implantation reduces the calcium deposition and then prophylactic antiplatelet treatment (Aspirine 5 mg/kg/day), started immediately after surgery and continued at least for one year, may play a role.

2.5. Tissue engineered decellularized allografts

The most recently introduced biological valved conduits are the decellularized valved conduits.

The principle for the preparation is the decellularization process applied to allografts tissue to reduce the antigenicity. The mechanism of decellularization result in the removal of all native cells from the collagen tissue of the extracellular matrix, with only the collagen and elastin remaining within a structural integrity maintained. The removal of the cellular material should reduce or eliminate the immunologic response and leave the functional vascular matrix available for autogenous remodeling. The progressive migration of the recipient-specific cells into the matrix nay eventually make the graft indistinguishable from other endogenous tissues (56-61).

Different techniques have been used for decellularization, as well as they have been applied to either fresh or cryopreserved valve matrix.

The clinical reports so far were limited to a relatively short follow-up, and therefore longer periods of observation are required before considering this type of conduits as a reliable alternative to the conventional biological valved conduits.

3. Size of the biological valved conduits

The significantly higher incidence (29.4% versus 3.1%, $P<0.0005$) of conduit failure observed with smaller (12 and 14mm) compared to larger (16 to 22mm) bovine jugular vein conduits was directly correlated to the age and body weight at implantation, and was due to the patient outgrowing the conduit (45).

This is a recurrent problem observed with any type of biological valved conduit implanted in small patients, when a difficult balance has to be reached between the need to limit the size of the ventriculotomy, the space available in the mediastinum (particularly in heart defects with anterior aorta), and the instinct to implant the largest possible conduit to avoid early reoperation (30,37,45,62,63).

It has been reported that implantation of oversized pulmonary valved conduits doesn't improve the durability even in infants at high risk of somatic outgrowth (30,37,64).

Since it has been demonstrated that sizing the valved conduit with a Z-score between +1 and +3 minimizes both the post-operative peak pressure gradient through the conduit and the progression of conduit valve regurgitation (64), it is reasonable to implant a biological valved conduit with a Z-score between +1 and +3 in all patients under 2 years of age.

With this regard the choice of relative small size valved conduit is limited by the reduced availability of homografts in small sizes.

4. Conclusions

The ideal biological valved conduit to establish right ventricle to pulmonary artery continuity for the surgical treatment of complex congenital heart defects doesn't exist yet.

Particularly when the operation has to be performed in infants and small children, at least one reoperation has to be planned to replace the original conduit with a larger size conduit.

Alternative surgical options are taken in consideration, like the use of a non-valved conduit implantation to delay the conduit failure due to progressive stenosis and dysfunction of the conduit valve (65-70).

The data available in the literature show that, on a midterm basis, the use of non valved conduit may decrease the need for re-operation for right ventricular outflow tract stenosis and may promote an adequate growth of the pulmonary arteries in selected congenital heart defects, like truncus arteriosus (65-70).

In infants and smaller children where a valved conduit is required, the choice of homografts is limited by the reduced availability of small sizes, and therefore other types of biological valved conduits are utilized more frequently. Because of this reason, the surgeons still preferring the homografts have used the technique of bicuspidalization of adult size homografts to produce homografts of small size (33).

In older children and young adults, since the availability of homografts is extremely variable from country to country, at the moment there is the possibility of deciding among various alternative options, with biological valved conduits available off the shelves in all range of sizes.

At the end the choice regarding type and size of conduit depends upon the mismatch between the congenital heart defect of the specific patient, the local availability of conduits, and the personal experience of the individual surgeon.

Author details

Antonio F. Corno
Pediatric Cardiac Surgery, Prince Salman Heart Center, King Fahad Medical City, Riyadh, Kingdom of Saudi Arabia

5. References

[1] Rastelli GC, Ongley PA, Davis GD, Kirklin JW, Surgical repair for pulmonary valve atresia with coronary-pulmonary artery fistula: report of a case, Mayo Clin Proc 1965;40:521-7

[2] Ross DN, Somerville J, Correction of pulmonary atresia with a homograft aortic valve, Lancet 1966;2:1446-7

[3] Weldon CS, Rowe RD, Gott V, Clinical experience with the use of aortic valve homografts for reconstruction of the pulmonary artery, pulmonary valve, and outflow portion of the right ventricle, Circulation 1968;37(suppl IV):II51-61

[4] Bowman FO, Hancock WD, Malm JR, A valve containing Dacron prosthesis, Arch Surg 1974;107:724-8

[5] Carpentier A, Lemaigre G, Robert L, Carpentier S, Dubost C, Biological factors affecting long-term results of valvular heterografts, J Thorac Cardiovasc Surg 1969;58:467-83

[6] Marcelletti C, Corno AF, Losekoot TG, Olthof H, Schuller JL, Bulterijs AHK, Becker AE, Extracardiac conduits: indications, techniques and early results, G Ital Cardiol 1980;10:1041-54

[7] Corno AF, Giamberti A, Giannico S, Marino B, Picardo S, Ballerini L, Marcelletti C, Long term results after extracardiac valved conduits implanted for complex congenital heart disease, J Card Surg 1988;3:495-500

[8] Ross DN, Replacement of aortic and mitral valve with a pulmonary autograft Lancet 1967;2:956-7

[9] Corno AF, Hurni M, Griffin H, Jeanrenaud X, von Segesser LK, Glutaraldehyde-fixed bovine jugular vein as a substitute for the pulmonary valve in the Ross operation, J Thorac Cardiovasc Surg 2001;122:493-4

[10] Norwood WI, Freed MD, Rocchini AP, Bernhard WF, Castaneda AR, Experience with valved conduits for repair of congenital cardiac lesions, Ann Thorac Surg;1977:223-32

[11] Bailey WW, Kirklin JW, Bargeron LM, Pacifico AD, Kouchoukos NT, Late results with synthetic valved external conduits from venous ventricle to pulmonary arteries Circulation 1976;56:73-9

[12] Alfieri O, Blackstone EH, Kirklin JW, Pacifico AD, Bargeron LM, Surgical treatment of tetralogy of Fallot with pulmonary atresia, J Thorac Cardiovasc Surg 1978;76:321-35

[13] Geha AS, Laks H, Stansel HC, Late failure of porcine valve heterografts in children, J Thorac Cardiovasc Surg 1979;78:351-64

[14] Hellberg K, Ruschewski W, de Vivie ER, Early stenosis and calcification of glutaraldehyde-preserved porcine xenografts in children, Thorac Cardiovasc Surg 1981;29:369-74

[15] Williams DB, Danielson GK, McGoon DC, Puga FJ, Mair DD, Edwards WD, Porcine heterograft valve replacement in children, J Thorac Cardiovasc Surg 1982;84:446-50

[16] Edwards WD, Agarwal KC, Feldt RH, Danielson GK, Puga FJ, Surgical pathology of obstructed, right-sided, porcine-valved extracardiac conduits, Arch Pathol Lab Med 1983;107:400-5

[17] Jonas RA, Freed MD, Mayer JE Jr, Castaneda AR, Long-term follow-up of patients with synthetic right heart conduits, Circulation 1985;72(Suppl-III):II77-83

[18] Kloevekorn WP, Meisner H, Paek SU, Sebening F, Long-term results after right ventricular outflow tract reconstruction with porcine bioprosthetic conduits, J Card Surg 1991;6(Suppl-IV):624-6

[19] Belli E, Salihoğlu E, Leobon B, Roubertie F, Ly M, Roussin R, Serraf A, The performance of Hancock porcine-valved Dacron conduit for right ventricular outflow tract reconstruction, Ann Thorac Surg 2010;89:152-7

[20] Saravalli OA, Somerville J, Jefferson KE, Calcification of aortic homografts used for reconstruction of the right ventricular outflow tract, J Thorac Cardiovasc Surg 1980;80:909-20

[21] Ciaravella JM, McGoon DC, Danielson GK, Wallace RB, Mair DD, Ilstrup DM, Experience with the extracardiac conduit, J Thorac Cardiovasc Surg 1979;78:920-30

[22] Allen MD, Shoji Y, Fujimura Y, Growth and cell viability of aortic versus pulmonic homografts in the systemic circulation, Circulation 1991;84 (Suppl I):III 94-9

[23] Kadoba K, Armiger LC, Sawatari K, Jonas RA, Mechanical durability of pulmonary allograft conduits at systemic pressure: angiographic and histological study in lambs, J Thorac Cardiovasc Surg 1993;105:132-41

[24] O'Brien MF, Stafford EG, Gardner MAH, Pohlner PG, McGiffin DC, The viable cryopreserved allograft aortic valve, J Card Surg 1987;2;153-67

[25] Yankah AC, Wottge HU, Muller-Rucholz W, Prognostic importance of viability and a study of a second set allograft valve: an experimental study, J Card Surg 1988;3:263-70

[26] Mitchell RN, Jonas RA, Schoen FJ, Pathology of explanted cryopreserved allograft heart valves: comparison with aortic valves from orthotopic heart transplants, J Thorac Cardiovasc Surg 1998;115:118-27

[27] Forbess JM, Shah AS, St Louis JD, Jaggers JJ, Ungerleider RM, Cryopreserved homografts in the pulmonary position: determinants of durability, Ann Thorac Surg 2001;71:54-60
[28] Dearani JA, Danielson GK, Puga FJ, Schaff HV, Warnes CW, Driscoll DJ, Late follow-up of 1095 patients undergoing operation for congenital heart disease utilizing pulmonary ventricle to pulmonary artery conduits, Ann Thorac Surg 2003;75:399-411
[29] Bielefeld MR, Bishop DA, Campbell DN, Mitchell MB, Grover FL, Clarke DR, Reoperative homograft right ventricular outflow tract reconstruction, Ann Thorac Surg 2001;71:482-8
[30] Wells WJ, Arroyo H, Bremner RM, Wood J, Starnes VA, Homograt conduit failure in infants is not due to somatic outgrowth, J Thorac Cardiovasc Surg 2002;124:88-96
[31] Brown JW, Ruzmetov M, Rodefeld MD, Vijay P, Turrentine MW, Right ventricular outflow tract reconstruction with an allograft conduit in non-Ross patients: risk factors for homograft dysfunction and failure, Ann Thorac Surg 2005;80:655-64
[32] Corno AF, Can you top this?, J Thorac Cardiovasc Surg 1998;116:670-1
[33] Bramer S, Mokhles MM, Takkenberg JJ, Bogers AJ, Long-term outcome of right ventricular outflow tract reconstruction with bicuspidalized homografts, Eur J Cardiothorac Surg 2011;40:1392-5
[34] Yankah AC, Alexi-Meskhishvili V, Weng Y, Schorn K, Lange PE, Hetzer R Accelerated degeneration of allografts in the first two years of life, Ann Thorac Surg 1995;60:S71-7
[35] Rajani B, Mee RB, Ratliff NB, Evidence for rejection of homograft cardiac valves in infants, J Thorac Cardiovasc Surg 1998;115:111-7
[36] Konuma T, Devaney EJ, Bove EL, Gelehrter S, Hirsch JC, Tavakkol Z, Ohye RG, Performance of CryoValve SG decellularized pulmonary allografts compared with standard cryopreserved allografts, Ann Thorac Surg 2009;88:849-55
[37] Karamlou T, Blackstone EH, Hawkins JA, Jacobs ML, Kanter KR, Brown JW, Mavroudis C, Caldarone CA, Williams WG, McCrindle BW, Can pulmonary conduit dysfunction and failure be reduced in infants and children less than age 2 years at initial implantation? J Thorac Cardiovasc Surg 2006;132:829-38
[38] Bove T, Demanet H, Wauthy P, Goldstein JP, Dessy H, Viart P, Deville A, Deuvaert FE, Early results of valved bovine jugular vein conduit versus bicuspid homograft for right ventricular outflow tract reconstruction, Ann Thorac Surg 2002;74:536-41
[39] Breymann T, Blanz U, Woitalik MA, Daenen W, Hetzer R, Sarris G, Stellin G, Planché C, Tsang V, Weissmann N, Boethig D, European Contegra multicentre study: 7-year results after 165 valved bovine jugular vein graft implantation, Thorac Cardiovasc Surg 2009;57:257-69
[40] Brown JW, Ruzmetov M, Rodefeld MD, Vijay P, Darragh RK, Valved bovine jugular vein conduits for right ventricular outflow tract reconstruction in children: an attractive alternative to pulmonary homograft, Ann Thorac Surg 2006;82:909-16
[41] Carrel T, Berdat P, Pavlovic M, Pfammatter JP, The bovine jugular vein: a totally integrated valved conduit to repair the right ventricular outflow, J Heart Valve Dis 2002;11:552-6

[42] Corno AF, Qanadli SD, Sekarski N, Artemisia S, Hurni M, Tozzi P, von Segesser LK, Bovine valved xenograft in pulmonary position: medium-term follow-up with excellent hemodynamics and freedom from calcifications, Ann Thorac Surg 2004;78:1382-8

[43] Hickey ED, McCrindle BW, Blackstone EH, Yeh T, Pigula F, Clarke D, Tchervenkov CI, Hawkins J, Jugular venous conduit (Contegra) matches allograft performance in infant truncus arteriosus repair, Eur J Cardiothorac Surg 2008;33:890-8

[44] Raja SG, Rasool F, Yousuffudin S, Danton MD, MacArthur KJ, Pollock JC, Current status of the Contegra conduit for pediatric right ventricular outflow tract reconstruction, J Heart Valve Dis 2005;14:616-22

[45] Prior N, Alphonso N, Arnold P, Peart I, Thorburn K, Venugopal P, Corno AF, Bovine jugular vein valved conduit: up to 10 years follow-up, J Thorac Cardiovasc Surg 2011;141:983-746.

[46] Bautista-Hernandez V, Kaza AK, Benavidez OJ, Pigula FA True aneurismal dilatation of a Contegra conduit after right ventricular outflow tract reconstruction: a novel mechanism of conduit failure, Ann Thorac Surg 2008;86:1976-7

[47] Boethig D, Thies WR, Hecker H, Breymann T, Mid term course after pediatric right ventricular outflow tract reconstruction: a comparison of homografts, porcine xenografts and Contegra, Eur J Cardiothorac Surg 2005;27:58-66

[48] Boudjemline Y, Bonnet D, Agnoletti G, Vouhé P, Aneurysm of the right ventricular outflow following bovine valved venous conduit insertion, Eur J Cardiothorac Surg 2003;23:122-4

[49] Göber V, Berdat P, Pavlovic M, Pfammatter JP, Carrel TP, Adverse mid-term outcome following RVOT reconstruction using the Contegra valved bovine jugular vein, Ann Thorac Surg 2005;79:625-31

[50] Kadner A, Dave H, Stallmach T, Turina M, Prêtre R, Formation of a stenotic fibrotic membrane at the distal anastomosis of bovine jugular vein grafts (Contegra) after right ventricular outflow tract reconstruction, J Thorac Cardiovasc Surg 2004;127:285-6

[51] Meyns B, van Garsse L, Boshoff D, Eyskens B, Mertens L, Gewillig M, Fieuws S, Verbeken E, Daenen W, The Contegra conduit in the right ventricular outflow tract induces supravalvular stenosis, J Thorac Cardiovasc Surg 2004;128:834-40

[52] Morales DL, Braud BE, Gunter KS, Carberry KE, Arrington KA, Heinle JS, McKenzie ED, Fraser CD, Encouraging results for the Contegra conduit in the problematic right ventricle-to-pulmonary artery connection, J Thorac Cardiovasc Surg 2006;132:665-71

[53] Rastan AJ, Walther T, Daehnert I, Hambsch J, Mohr FW, Janousek J, Kostelka M, Bovine jugular vein conduit for right ventricular outflow tract reconstruction: evaluation of risk factors for mid-term outcome, Ann Thorac Surg 2006;82:1308-15

[54] Shebani SO, McGuirk S, Baghai M, Stickley J, De Giovanni JV, Bu'lock FA, Barron DJ, Brawn WJ, Right ventricular outflow tract reconstruction using Contegra valved conduit: natural history and conduit performance under pressure, Eur J Cardiothorac Surg 2006;29:397-405

[55] Corno AF, Mickaily-Huber ES, Comparative computational fluid dynamic study of two distal Contegra conduit anastomoses, Int Cardiovasc Thorac Surg 2008;7:1-5
[56] Dohmen PM, Ozaki S, Verbeken E, Yperman J, Flameng W, Konertz W, Tissue engineering of a pulmonary xenograft heart valve Asian Cardiovasc Thorac Surg 2002;10:25-30
[57] Konertz W, Dohmen PM, Liu J, Hemodynamic characteristics of the Matrix P decellularized xenograft for pulmonary valve replacement during the Ross operation, J Heart Valve Dis 2005;14:78-81
[58] Bechtel M, Muller-Steinhardt M, Schmidtke C, Brunswik A, Stierle U, Sievers HH, Evaluation of the decellularized pulmonary valve homograft (Synergraft), J Heart Valve Dis 2003;12:734-40
[59] Leyh RG, Wilhelmi M, Rebe P, Fischer S, Kofidis T, Haverich A, Mertsching H, In vivo repopulation of xenogenic and allogenic acellular valve matrix conduits in the pulmonary circulation, Ann Thorac Surg 2003;75:1457-63
[60] Burch PT, Kaza AK, Lambert LM, Holubkov R, Shaddy RE, Hawkins JA, Clinical performance of decellularized cryopreserved valved allografts compared with standard allografts in the right ventricular outflow tract Ann Thorac Surg 2010;90:1301-6
[61] Ruzmetov M, Shah JJ, Geiss DM, Fortuna RS Decellularized versus standard cryopreserved valve allografts for right ventricular outflow tract reconstruction: a single-institution comparison. J Thorac Cardiovasc Surg 2012;143:543-9
[62] Brown JW, Ruzmetov M, Rodefeld MD, Vijay P, Darragh RK, Valved bovine jugular vein conduits for right ventricular outflow tract reconstruction in children: an attractive alternative to pulmonary homograft Ann Thorac Surg 2006;82:909-16
[63] Boethig D, Thies WR, Hecker H, Breymann T, Mid term course after pediatric right ventricular outflow tract reconstruction: a comparison of homografts, porcine xenografts and Contegra Eur J Cardiothorac Surg 2005;27:58-66
[64] Karamlou T, Ungerleider RM, Alsoufi B, Burch G, Silberbach M, Reller M, Shen I Oversizing pulmonary homograft conduits does not significantly decreases allograft failure in children Eur J Cardiothorac Surg 2005;27:548-53
[65] Derby CD, Kolcz J, Gidding S, Pizarro C Outcomes following non-valved autologous reconstruction of the right ventricular outflow tract in neonates and infants Eur J Cardiothorac Surg 2008;34:726-31
[66] Nemoto S, Ozawa H, Sasaki T, Katsumata T, Kishi K, Okumura K, Mori Y Repair of persistent truncus arteriosus without a conduit: sleeve resection of the pulmonary trunk from the aorta and direct right ventricle-pulmonary artery anastomosis Eur J Cardiothorac Surg 2011;40:563-8
[67] Vouhé PR Common arterial trunk repair without extracardiac conduit: technically feasible, potentially advantageous (Editorial comment) Eur J Cardiothorac Surg 2011;40:569-70
[68] Lecompte Y, Neveux JY, Leca F, Zannini L, Tran Viet T, Duboys Y, Jarreau MM Reconstruction of the pulmonary outflow tract without prosthetic conduit J Thorac Cardiovasc Surg 1982;84:727-33

[69] Danton MHD, Barron DJ, Stumper O, Wright JG, DeGiovanni J, Silove ED, Brawn WJ Repair of truncus arteriosus: a considered approach to right ventricular outflow tract reconstruction Eur J Cardiothorac Surg 2001;20:95-104

[70] Raisky O, Ben Ali W, Bajolle F, Marini D, Metton O, Bonnet D, Sidi D, Vouhé PR Common arterial trunk repair: with conduit or without? Eur J Cardiothorac Surg 2009;36:675-82

Chapter 8

Surgical Management of the Aortic Root

B. Goslin and R. Hooker

Additional information is available at the end of the chapter

http://dx.doi.org/10.5772/51831

1. Introduction

The surgical management of aortic root pathology is complicated and challenging. The dynamic structure of the root serves the purpose of being the outflow tract of the left ventricle, a conduit to coronary perfusion, and path for blood flow to the end-organs. The anatomy of the aortic root is the basis of what leads to complex problems needing surgical correction including aortic valve repair, aneurismal disease of the sinuses and root, dissection of the ascending aorta, in addition to other surgically correctable disorders. The anatomy, pathology, pathophysiology, and imaging, as well as the surgical management of the aortic root will be discussed.

2. Anatomy

The aortic root is proximally defined as the left ventricular outflow tract and distally defined as the ascending aorta at the sinotubular junction. (Figure 1) Critical structures of the root include; the aortic valve, sinuses of Valsalva, coronary ostia, and transition at the sinotubular junction into the ascending aorta.[1]

The leaflets of the aortic valve form a transient barrier between the left ventricular outflow tract and the lumen of the proximal aorta. Leaflets are individually suspended around the aortic annulus. [2] There is debate between surgeons and anatomists regarding the anatomy of the fibrous annulus. [1,2] Surgeons grossly perceive the annulus to be a circumferential fibrous structure while anatomists have identified individual histologic hinge points for each of the leaflets. All three leaflets have a rigid border (lunules) which lie adjacent to one another when the aortic valve is in the closed position.[1,3] The lunules of each triangular shaped leaflet convalesce at the apex of the leaflet to form the nodule of Arantius. While the leaflets are able to form a uniform barrier in the closed position along the commissures, they have separate dimensions which affect the flow dynamics and coronary perfusion during systole.[3] The superior side of each leaflet is basket-shaped (open to the aortic lumen) and forms a raphe when closed. Each leaflet is named based upon the respective coronary artery and therefore they are termed the left, right, and non-coronary leaflets. The left coronary leaflet has a larger surface area than the right and non-coronary in the normal valve.[1]

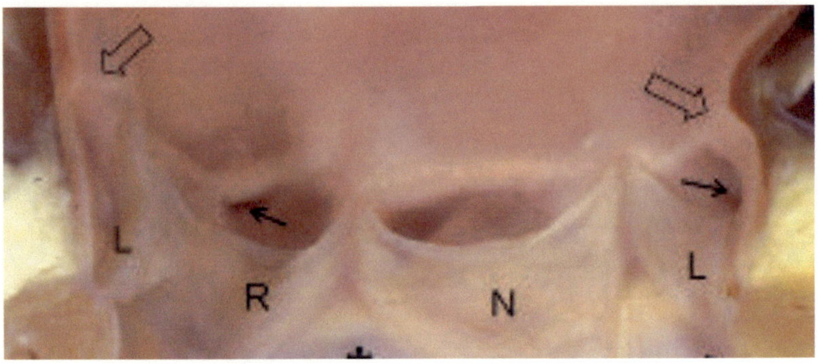

Figure 1. Sectioned aortic root. Hollow arrows signify the sinotubular junction. L, R, and N correspond to the left, right and non-coronary sinuses. Solid black arrows identify the right and left coronary ostia that are located adjacent to their respective sinuses.[1]

In the space immediately superior to the leaflets are the sinuses of Valsalva. The most superior border of each sinus forms the sinotubular junction, a fibrous ridge on the luminal surface.[1,2] In vivo studies have shown that the sinuses not only collect blood during diastole, but dynamically dilate to potentate flow to the coronary ostia.[4] During systole the leaflets project superiorly into the sinus allowing blood to pass into the aortic lumen.[1] Diameters of the sinotubular junction and aortic annulus as well as dimensions of the sinuses of Valsalva are critical in patients needing aortic root surgery, especially in cases of aortic root replacement. Each of these variables is dependent on individual patient characteristics such as age, body surface area, weight, height, and an individual's fitness.[5,6]

The most critical function of the aortic root is to perfuse the coronaries. Typically there are two coronary ostia that perfuse the left and right coronary arteries, respectively. Multiple ostia for both coronaries, however, is not rare and knowledge of ostia anatomical variation is crucial during an aortic root reconstruction and coronary angioplasty.[7,8] In a study by Pejkovic et al, ostia were located 2-10mm inferior to the sinotubular junction in 90% of cases. Additionally, separate conal ostia from the right sinus of Valsalva were found in 33% of cases. The pathologic significance of left and right coronary arteries originating from only one ostia (from either the left or right sinus of Valsalva) has a noted correlation with sudden death at a young age. This anomaly is exceedingly rare.[8]

Histologically, the aortic root is a significant point of transition with regard to supportive tissue. Proximally, collagenous fibers help support the annulus of the aortic valve. The majority of proximal root support, however, is composed of myocardial fibers with a superficial layer of endocardium. More distally, the sinuses of Valsalva has dense elastic fibers interspersed with regions of woven collagen forming the ridge of the sinotubular junction. In regard to the lining of the aortic root lumen, the leaflets are the transition point of for which endocardium lines the inferior surface of each leaflet while endothelium lines the superior surface.[2]

3. Pathology of the aortic root

3.1. Aortic valve disorders

3.1.1. Congenital

Bicuspid aortic valves are present in approximately 0.5-2% of the population.[9] Rather than a simple failure of fusion of two cusps, embryology studies with animals portray a complex interaction between intracellular pathways and between individual stem cells.[9] Multiple formations of bicuspid valves have been described in addition to variable surface sizes (Figures 2 and 3). The most common bicuspid formation is anterior-posterior in nature with the left and right coronary ostia sharing the raphe of anterior sinus of Valsalva.[12] Bicuspid aortic valves, and the associated aortopathy, can lead to valvular stenosis and regurgitation, as well as ascending aneurysms and dissections. One-fourth of patients with bicuspid valves will have normal valvular function and, in one natural history study, required no medical or surgical intervention at 20 years of follow-up.[13,14]

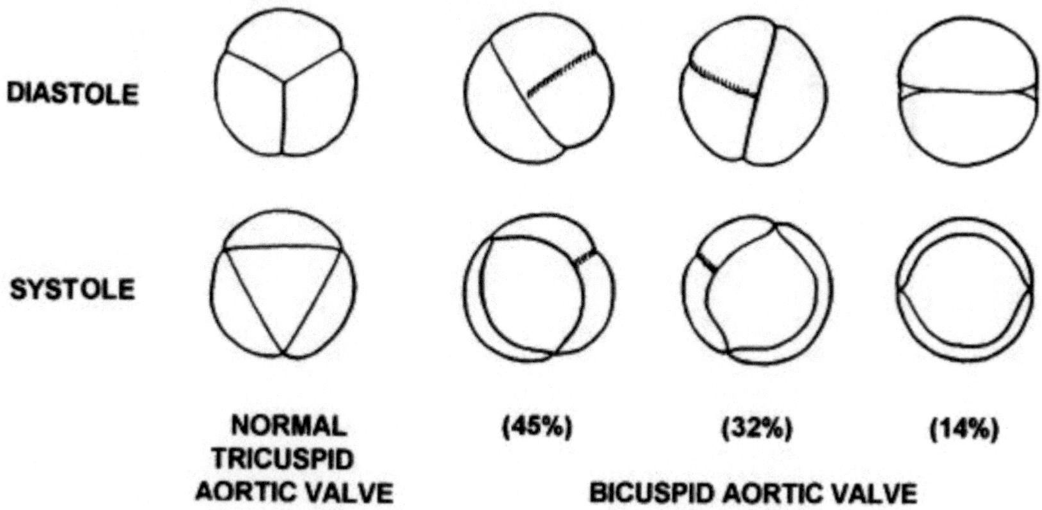

Figure 2. A normal valve in the open and closed compared to a bicuspid valve. Fusion of two leaflets is noted in the closed bicuspid valve positions. The relative frequency of each morphological abnormal leaflet fusion is depicted.[10]

Unicuspid and quadricuspid valves also exist but are less common. Unicuspid valves occur in approximately 1 of 10,000 individuals and patients seem to have similar valve and aortic pathology as compared to patients with bicuspid valves.[15,16] The prevalence of unicuspid aortic valves are so rare that the risk of aortic root disease can not be quantified by clinical studies; only case reports and summaries exist. Likewise, quadracusp valves are rare occurring in 1-10 patients per 100,000. It usually leads to insufficiency at an early age. [17] Anecdotally, authors recommend stress testing prior to undergoing valve replacement. [17]

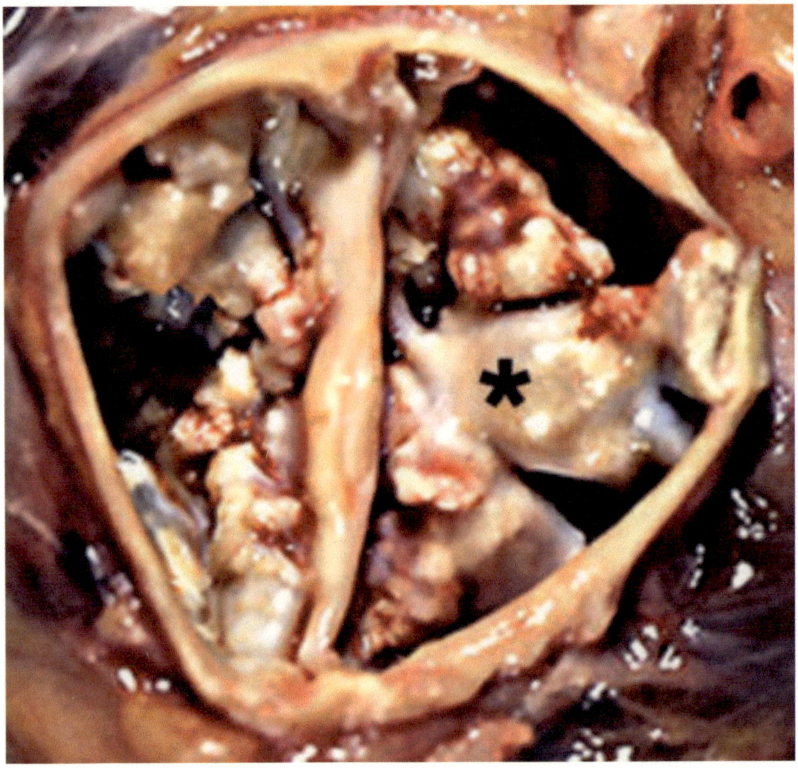

Figure 3. Congenital bicuspid valve as seen from the root position, in vivo. Bulkly calcifications cover the lumenal surface of the valve. One such macrocalcification is identified by an askerisk.[11]

3.1.2. Aquired

The most common acquired condition of the aortic valve is calcific valvular disease.[18] This typically leads to aortic stenosis but can also cause a mixed pathology of both stenosis and regurgitation. During 2009 in the United States alone, over 40,000 patients underwent aortic valve replacement (AVR) with or without coronary artery bypass grafting.[19] Isolated infection of the leaflets typically leads to regurgitation. Usually both of these conditions are not considered "root" problems as they can be treated with surgical replacement of the aortic valve, however they can evolve into root problems when calcium deposition in the aortic wall becomes severe or the infection forms a root abscess, as will be discussed.

3.1.3. Aneurismal disease of the root

Since the ascending aorta begins at the level of the sinotubular junction it is frequently involved with any aneurismal root pathology. Hence, any discussion of root pathology often involves the ascending aorta as well. The ascending aorta is considered to be aneurysmal if the diameter is greater than 3.5cm.[20] The aortic root, however, is not considered aneurismal until it is greater than 4cm.[21] Aneurysms of the root and ascending aorta have multiple etiologies including genetic, inflammatory, acquired and infectious. Disorders that cause degenerative changes in the root wall are most common. Aortic root aneurysms are common, accounting for roughly 70% of all thoracic aneurysms.[22] The risk of fatal complications of these aneurysms strongly correlates with aneurysm size. In one natural history study, the risk of death, dissection, or rupture in patients with aneurysms >6 cm had an incidence of 15% per year.[14] Reports on growth of the aorta are variable with some reports showing little growth while others report growth of up to 0.2 cm/year in patients with aortic stenosis and a bicuspid valve.[14]

3.1.4. Genetic

Marfan's Syndrome, Loeys-Dietz syndrome, Ehlers-Danlos syndrome as well as others are known genetic causes of aneurismal dilatation.[23,24,25] These disorders cause deficits in the formation of the aortic wall during embryogenesis and lead to flow abnormalities. This eventually can result in aneurysm formation.

Marfan's syndrome is a well-characterized, autosomal-dominant disorder that causes cystic necrosis within the media layer of the aortic wall. These patients have mutations in a single fibrillin gene, FBN1. Prevalence of Marfan's ranges from 1 in 10,000 to 20,000 people.[26] Although aortic root problems have the most dramatic sequelae in patients, other systems are adversely affected by this single gene mutation including the lungs, bones, muscles, and the central nervous system. Aortic dissection and subsequent rupture is the most common cause of sudden death in Marfan patients.[27] Patients with Marfan's associated aortic root dilatation are recommended to undergo surgical repair if the diameter of the aorta is >4.5cm.[23] Diagnosis of the disorder at a young age is crucial to prevent catastrophic aortic complications, yet 24% have the initial operation in an emergency setting.[28]

Loeys-Dietz Syndrome is an autosomal-dominant disorder that became known for having an association with aortic root aneurysms. The disorder was first discovered in 2005.[29] The baseline aortic diameter in these individuals are small, yet have a tendency to dissect or become aneurismal at a young age. When ascending aneurysms are identified in these patients, one group of authors recommended fixation when the size reached 4.2 cm.[23]

Ehlers-Danlos Syndrome is an autosomal-dominant disorder with many subtypes and each subtype typically leads to specific end-organ pathology. Vascular type (Type 4) Ehlers-Danlos Syndrome is prone to cause dissection without aneurysm formation.[29,30] Surgical results in these patients have been poor.[30]

Patients with a bicuspid aortic valve are predisposed to root aneurysms because of the associated aortopathy. An exact inheritance pattern for bicuspid disease has not been determined, rather, it's believed that most cases of bicuspid valves are due to multiple genes that interact causing abnormal root structure.[31] Researchers believe that pooling the genetic and histologic changes identified in bicuspid valve patients ultimately leads to aortic root dilatation. Root enlargement is described at a younger age in patients with bicuspid valves and therefore the risk of root disease is higher in these patients.[32] The development of root pathology in patients with bicuspid valves is described later in the chapter.

3.1.5. *Inflammatory*

A variety of inflammatory disorders affect aortic compliance leading to aneurysm formation and dissection, prompting the need for surgical repair.

Giant cell arteritis (GCA) causes inflammation of the endothelium typically involving the temporal arteries leading to malaise, frequent temporal headaches, fevers, and jaw claudication. Infrequently patients will have complete visual loss. The gold standard of diagnosis remains temporal artery biopsy. The temporal artery is found to be involved in approximately 50% of specimens while the proximal aorta and immediate branches have less frequent involvement, 10-15%.[33] In a study of autopsy specimens, 4 in 1000 specimens had giant cell arteritis while 1.5 per 1000 were found to have dissection.[34]

Takayasus's arteritis is a form of large vessel vasculitis characterized by granulomatous inflammation in the aortic wall leading to intimal fibrosis and narrowing. Early symptoms are non-specific including malaise, fevers and rigors while late phase symptoms are ischemic in nature consisting of syncope, angina, and visual disturbance.[35] In rare cases, rupture of the aorta and proximal branches is caused by aneurismal disease of the vessels. Survival with rupture of a lesion due to Takayasu's disease is exceedingly rare. The mainstay of treatment is systemic corticosteroids.[36] In cases of aneurysm formation, surgical intervention should be delayed until the acute inflammatory phase has resolved.[37,38]

Other inflammatory disorders account for a minority of aortic root pathology. Reiter's syndrome is an autoimmune inflammatory disease that is characterized by reactive arthritis. There are rare cases of ascending aneurysms and severe aortic regurgitation in patient's with longstanding inflammatory responses in severe cases of Reiter's.[39] Ankylosing spondylitis is an inflammatory disease that has a strong association with HLA-B27 and is characterized by joint pain involving the axial skeleton. Nearly 20% of patients with ankylosing spondylitis required aortic valve replacement in one case control study.[40]

3.1.6. *Infectious*

Infections of the aortic valve that are uncontrolled can lead to spread to contiguous structures, i.e. spread to the aortic wall causing dehiscense and formation of root abscesses. Left unchecked, the infection can erode further leading to involvement of the mitral and tricuspid valves as well as fistulization to atria and right ventricle.

Syphilis once had a significant impact on the cardiovascular morbidity of the United States population. The need for surgery in the management of cardiovascular complications of syphilis in the past fifty years has been exceedingly rare. Patients in need of surgery because of these complications are usually not diagnosed until after fixation. When surgical correction is required, ascending aortic involvement is diffuse, starting at the sinotubular junction proximally and extending distal to the arch. Grossly and histologically the aortic wall is comparable to those patients with GCA or ankylosing spondylitis.[41]

3.1.7. *Calcific atherosclerosis*

Calcific atherosclerosis of the coronaries is well characterized in the literature. However, within the past decade implications of a heavily calcified aortic root have also become evident, especially in association with calcific aortic stenosis. This may make aortic valve replacement complicated and necessitate root replacement. Severe calcification of the aorta can also extend distally. Cardiac surgeons are aware of the consequences of negligent cross-clamping. Significant aortic calcification as assessed by an intraoperative ultrasound in patients undergoing cardiac surgery is an independent predictor of poor neurologic outcome and all-cause mortality.[42-44].

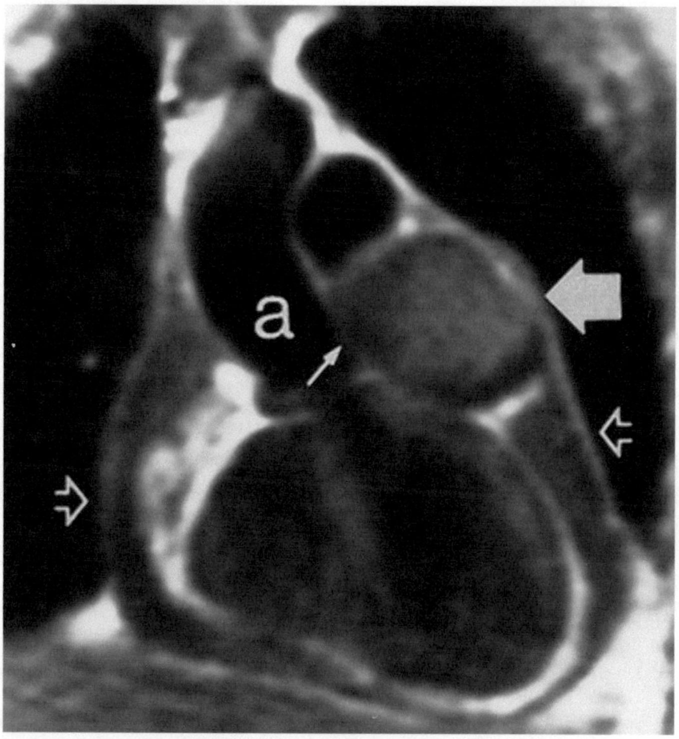

Figure 4. A large sinus of Valsalva aneurysm highlighted by the large bold arrow. A small solid arrow within the aortic lumen identifies the inflow tract to the aneurysm. A small pericardial effusion is associated with the aneurysm (hollow arrows).[41]

3.1.8. *Sinuses of Valsalva aneurysms*

Aneurismal disease of the sinuses of Valsalva occurs between the aortic valve annulus and the sinotubular junction (Figure 5). Relative to the spectrum of other aortic root pathology, sinus of Valsalva aneurysms are very rare. Studies of large patient series show that the rate of these aneurysms found in all cardiac operations is roughly 0.5%, and more so in Eastern populations. Most have extended adjacent to the left ventricle by the time of surgery.[45,46] The sinus most commonly involved is the right coronary, followed by the non-coronary and left coronary sinus.[47] Indications for surgery include rupture, infection, and flow impedance of the coronary ostia. The goal of surgery, regardless of the specific technique, is to close the defect of the wall, resect the fistula if present, and resect the aneurysm sac.[50]

3.1.9. Aortic root trauma

Traumatic injury to the aortic root requiring operative management is rare, yet one needs to be aware of the injury pattern and understand indications for operative repair. Blunt thoracic aortic traumatic injury usually occurs at the level of the ligmentum arteriousum just distal to the branch point of the left subclavian artery.[49] A minority of injuries, <10%, occur at the level of the ascending aorta.[49] When aortic injuries are identified, surgery can often be delayed until other traumatic injuries are corrected according to Mattox et al.[50]

Those patients who are at highest suspicion of aortic injury need CT angiography. The sensitivity of CT is typically high enough to use for screening, however, the assessment of the aortic root is currently regarded as inadequate.[51] Well designed studies in the last two decades sought to provide evidence that transesophageal echocardiogram (TEE) was a reasonable screening test, however, it was no better than CT with regard to all thoracic injuries.[52-54] When sensitivity, cost utilization, and quality of life on follow-up are given equal consideration, it is advocated that chest radiograph and aortography continue to be the best diagnostic tools to assess for proximal aortic and root injury.[55]

Patients with root injuries often have other major injuries requiring management prior to the root and aorta.[56] When surgical repair is indicated it is frequently for contained rupture of the aortic wall. Because the injury is often distal to the sinotubular junction, surgical fixation is feasible.[57] Injuries to the aortic valve leaflets, sinuses, and coronary ostia have also been reported, but only in case reports due to the lack of prevalence.[58,59]

4. Pathophysiology and presentation of aortic root disease

4.1. Aortic stenosis

The etiology can be divided into three separate categories including postinflammatory scarring, senile calcific stenosis, and calcific stenosis of the congenitally deformed valve.[60] Rheumatic fever accounts for less than 10% of all cause aortic stenosis and continues to decline in modern society but is still very common in underdeveloped countries. Regardless of the etiology of aortic stenosis, all have the potential to progress to left heart failure if left untreated.

Grossly, calcific disease of the aortic valve is a heaped up mass of calcium that usually projects into the sinuses.[61] Only recently is this process of calcium deposition being understood as an active regulatory process rather than degenerative. Calcium deposition on the valves is the result of a complex interaction between interstitial cells via paracrine signals.[62]

Valvular sclerosis eventually leads to a pressure gradient between the left ventricular outflow tract and aortic lumen. The left ventricle attempts to compensate and overcome this pressure gradient to maintain perfusion by concentric hypertrophy of the myocardium.[62] Clinically this corresponds to the three hallmarks of aortic stenosis including angina, congestive heart failure (CHF), and syncope. Symptom severity directly correlates with prognosis, as 50% of patients with CHF will die in 2 years without intervention.[63]

4.2. Aortic regurgitation

Regurgitation of flow into the left ventricle occurs during the diastolic phase. Causes of this reverse flow are numerous, however, the predominant causes of include calcific stenosis and a dilated aortic root.[61] Calcific stenosis leads to stiff leaflets that stay in a fixed open position, even in the diastolic phase, and this allows for reflux into the left ventricle.[61] Aortic root disease causing valvular regurgitation is due to tension on and retraction of the cusps. [14]

The Starling principle demonstrates the stretch of the myocardium is increased due to volume expansion from the regurgitant blood.[64] Cardiac contractility is increased due to an added volume at end diastole. This creates a vicious cycle of increased output due to contractility, yet there is also gradually increasing regurgitant flow as left ventricular output increases. Chronically, the forces of volume and pressure overload in addition to increased contractility lead to eccentric hypertrophy. Hypertrophy leads to increased myocardial wall tension causing to fibrosis and ischemia.[65] Chronic reflux of flow back into the left ventricle causes a combination of pressure and volume overload.[65]

Signs and symptoms are not noted until the patient develops congestive heart failure. Patients without significant predisposing factors (Marfan's or bicuspid valve) however may have progressive regurgitation for decades without symptoms.[66] The first symptoms to develop are disguised as primarily pulmonary complaints such as exertional and nocturnal dyspnea. Some patients complain of vague thoracic pain or headaches. Angina is a late finding that signifies end stage left ventricular function.[67]

4.3. Type A dissection

A dissection occurs when there is a tear of the intima and a tunneled pathway is made between the media and adventitia parallel to the lumen of the blood vessel. This dissection flap that is created diverts blood flow through true and false lumens with the false lumen created by the dissection.[68] Type A dissections are located in the ascending aorta and are known for having a high mortality.[69] With respect to the aortic root, patients with dissection can have dilated sinuses, aortic regurgitation, and acute pericardial tamponade and therefore repairing the dissection may also include root replacement or modification.

A number of factors predispose certain populations to getting Type A dissection including genetic and aquired diseases.[70] Once the dissection flap is made, the false lumen diameter expands and there is elongation of the false lumen. It is hypothesized that the false lumen enlarges and true lumen collapses over time for two reasons. First, the relative over-abundance of elastin within the wall of the true lumen causes it to be more compliant and compressible. Second, the pressure within the false lumen is higher causing the dissection flap to collapse the true lumen.[70]

Symptomatically, Type A dissection is characterized by what is often described by patients as being "ripping" or "tearing" chest pain. Because dissections are known to travel retrograde, patients may have profound hypotension if the dissection involves the pericardium or aortic valve. Pericardial tamponade complicates approximately 20% of Type A dissections.[71]

4.4. Ascending aorta & root aneurysms

The majority of patients with ascending aneurysms have inherent tissue abnormalities that result in a weak aortic wall. The most well described disorders associated with proximal aortic aneurysms of patients with a bicuspid valve and Marfan's. Both abnormalities cause cystic medial necrosis by replacement of normal elastic mesenchymal cells with mucoid degenerated cells.

Patients with Marfan's and those with bicuspid aortic valves also have degenerative changes in the media.[72] The aortic roots have variable amounts of elastin and larger baseline aortic root diameters than the general population.[73-75] The underlying genetic association has yet to be determined.

5. Imaging of the aortic root

Imaging modalities most readily available for assessment of aortic root pathology include, echocardiography, both, transthoracic (TTE) and transesophageal (TEE), computed tomography (CT), angiography, and magnetic resonance imaging (MR). Each has advantages and disadvantages when analyzing abnormalities and planning for surgical repair.

Echocardiography can assess aortic root and valve anatomy and function however, it does not give good views of the distal aorta. Echo is also very useful for imaging other heart valves and ventricular size and function, all important for operative planning. While TTE is known to give accurate measurements of aortic root structures, it is not able to adequately detect dissection locations or extent of dissection with accuracy.[76] TEE, has proven to be safe and effective in the pre and post-operative assessment of patients with aortic dissection.[77,78]

Computed tomography is an attractive means of assessing the ascending aorta when pathology such as dissection, aneurysm formation, ulceration, and intramural hematoma are suspected. Arterial wall enhancement with contrast is necessary for this technology to be utilized and patients with renal dysfunction or contrast allergy may have a contraindication. Low volume contrast studies have recently been used safely in patients with renal dysfunction.[80] Most series report the sensitivity for Type A dissection to be >90%.[81] Due to the varying degrees of signal enhancement, CT is able to distinguish between the false and true lumens in addition to the presence of thrombosis or communication of the false lumen. Similarly, the assessment of ascending aneurysms is accurate because of CT's ability to determine size, relative assessment of flow, and the aneurysms relationship to surrounding vital structures.[80] With regard to valve pathology, multidetector CT is able to provide an accurate depiction of aortic annulus size, valve calcification, and degree of stenosis as compared to preoperative TEE and MR.[82] CT scans may be used to image the coronary arteries, heart and other thoracic structures. Indeed, heart surgery has been done safely without coronary angiogram in patients with normal coronaries on CT angiogram.[83,84]

	Sensitivity	Specificity
Echo (TEE)	95-99%	92-97%
Helical CT	96-100%	87-99%
MRI	95-99%	95-100%

Table 1. Result of meta-analysis by Shiga et al describing the sensitivities and specificities of TEE, CT, and MRI for detecting thoracic aortic dissection.[79]

Use of MR angiography is typically an adjunct form of imaging used with echocardiography in patients with complex anatomy. At some institutions MR angiography is replacing CT as the primary imaging modality for assessment of diseases involving the thoracic aorta due to its decreased risk of radiation exposure. MR angiography (CE MR) provides improved diagnostic accuracy of thoracic vascular pathology when compared to other imaging. It has demonstrated a higher sensitivity and specificity than other forms of MR imaging and echocardiography.[85] Emergency use of MR is limited. Steady state free procession MR is a newer technology that allows for better visualization of structures by decreasing surrounding interference without the use of contrast.[83] This method has demonstrated success in the accurate visualization of diseases such as aneurysm, intramural hematoma, dissection, and ulceration of the native aorta as well as assessment of postoperative graft placement.[88] It is particularly attractive for patients who have a contrast allergy.

Coronary angiography remains the gold standard for evaluation of the coronary arteries. Aortography can demonstrate aortic insufficiency and enlargement of the aorta, although we use CT and echo as it is much more accurate and less invasive. Venticulography may also be done, however with severe aortic stenosis it may be difficult to cross the valve and may not be indicated because the risk of emboli.[87] Right and left heart pressures may also be obtained at the time of catherization.

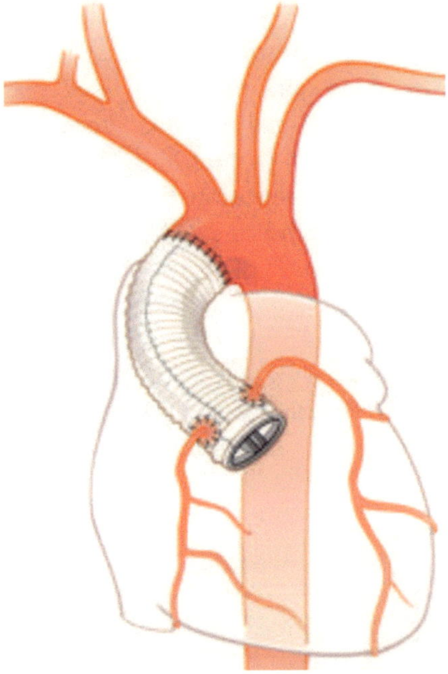

Figure 5. A graphic depiction of the modified-Bentall Procedure. A synthetic graft is identified in the native root position with implantation of both coronary arteries.[83]

6. Surgery of the aortic root

In 1968, Bentall and Bono published the case of a patient with an ascending aortic aneurysm that involved the root and included coronary involvement.[88] In their case, a composite aortic graft was sewn to the annulus with a mechanical Starr valve. The coronaries were attached via an inclusion technique into the wall of the new prosthetic aortic root. Currently, the Kouchoukos modification with direct coronary button modification is the standard for root replacement today. Typically, the aortic valve tissue is removed, all abnormal aortic tissue in the sinuses and the ascending aorta is removed, and buttons of the right and left coronary artery are created. The root is then replaced with one of the following: a valved-conduit (either mechanical or biologic), a stentless valve as a root, a homograft, or a pulmonary autograft. There is a proximal suture line at the level of the left ventricular outflow tract, a distal suture line where the pathology of the aorta usually ends, and suture lines for reimplantation of both the coronary buttons. (Figure 5)

6.1. Biologic options for aortic root surgery

For patients who need aortic root surgery there is the option of using synthetic material (usually Dacron) versus a biologic prosthesis. Biologics are manufactured and treated in the form of xenografts or homografts. The major benefit with a biologic valve is that therapeutic anticoagulation is not required. In July of 1992 the FDA approved the use the first xenograft in the United States, the Medtronic Freestyle. This graft allows similar flow and velocity measurements in addition to peri-operative morbidity and mortality to synthetic grafts.[90] In a prospective, randomized trial comparing homografts to Freestyle grafts, long-term survival was found to be the same for the groups. The main indication for root replacement was aortic valve disease associated with pathologic changes in the root. Homografts were found to have a higher likelihood to need a second operation and a higher rate of root degeneration and calcification.[91] Homographs are commonly indicated in patients with a history of endocarditis. The major factor that deters the use of biologics is long-term degeneration of the biologic material when compared synthetic grafts.

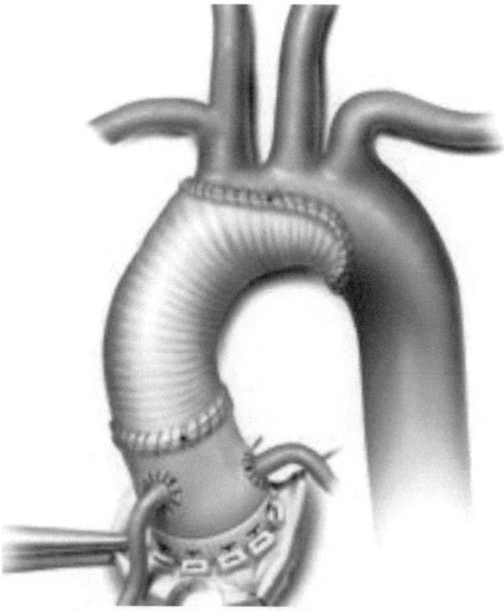

Figure 6. Hemi arch replacement with aortic root replacement using a porcine bioroot. Vertical mattress sutures are noted at the annular anastomosis. Both coronaries are reimplanted with their native peri-aortic tissue.[116]

6.2. Composite versus valve sparing root replacement

The question of to replace the aortic root with a composite graft or to perform a valve-sparing operation is dependent on multiple patient characteristics as well as the surgeon preference. Over the last decade surgeons have debated which technique provides the best peri-operative and long-term results. The major concern with complete root replacement is lifelong therapeutic anticoagulation. The etiology of the aortic root disease, as well as individual patient preferences, must be taken into account so the correct procedure is performed for each patient.

Patients who present with an ascending aneurysm or dissection involving the root have a variety of options for surgical reconstruction. Specific criteria are taken into account including the patient age and if there are early signs of co-morbid aortic valve pathology that may require replacement in the future. Patients with connective tissue disorders, bicuspid valves, or history of valve infection may be best served with Bentall-type replacement rather than valve-sparing reconstruction.

Previous studies have attempted to stratify patients into composite replacement versus a valve-sparing techniques with a heterogenous group of patients. One major study retrospectively examined patients who received root replacement at a single institution. Patients were therefore not prospectively stratified with respect to age, genetic basis of root replacement (patients with Marfan's or bicuspid valves), or additional comorbidities.[92]

Zehr et al reviewed the results at their institution comparing total replacement with valve-sparing techniques, an experience over a 30-year period that served to answer the question of which procedure had improved outcomes.[92] All patients in the study electively underwent a Bentall procedure or valve-sparing (Yacoub or David-type technique). Roughly 75% of the total 208 patients underwent composite root replacement while the remaining patients had valve-sparing operations. They concluded that patients undergoing a Bentall-type procedure have less risk of needing a second operation for aortic valve disease. There was no difference between long-term survival of the two groups which was 93%, 72%, and 59% at five, ten, and twenty years, respectively. However, 37% of the valve-sparing group needed reoperation due to additional valvular or aortic pathology in the follow-up period. Most procedures for reoperation in the valve-sparing patients were due to the need of aortic valve replacement for regurgitation or stenosis. The authors concluded that both types of procedures offered durable results in the peri-operative and long-term periods. This study tells us that, while both procedures are reasonable options, benefits are difficult to determine without patient specific treatment characteristics.

Other studies are published since the Zehr series that have attempted to give credence to either technique for more concentrated patient populations.[93-95] The results from previous large retrospective and prospective studies will be discussed at depth in the upcoming paragraphs. We will review the results of major studies and discuss aortic root reconstructive techniques stratified by disease etiology.

6.3. Aortic root surgery for patients with bicuspid valves- General recommendations and analysis of surgical outcomes

There is strong consensus that patients with bicuspid valves and aortic root enlargement should be considered for replacement when the aneurysm is > 5.0cm or there is an increase in size of >0.5cm per year.[96,97] In 2007, guidelines were published by the European Society of Cardiology regarding replacement of the aortic root with respect to the aortic diameter, recommending replacement when the root diameter is >5.5cm.[98] Subsequently in 2008, the American Heart Association/American College of Cardiology guidelines found class IB evidence that root replacement should be considered when the diameter is >5cm or dilatation progresses at a rate >5mm per year.[99]

While the latest guidelines are straightforward, some controversy still exists with regard to the surgical management of patients who require aortic valve replacement (AVR) of a degenerated bicuspid valve yet who do not have aneurismal change of the ascending aorta or root. It is advocated by some institutions that patients who need aortic valve replacement should also undergo simultaneous replacement of the root and proximal ascending aorta.[100,101] McKellar et al examined outcomes at the Mayo Clinic in patients who had AVR without ascending aorta replacement. These patients did not have signs of root pathology at the time of operation. Analysis showed that patients who did not have aortic valve replacement had a low risk of having subsequent aortic root pathology on follow-up.[102] The most feared complication in the interim, Type A dissection, was very low in follow-up (1%) in patients with a normal size ascending aorta. Interestingly, the risk of aortic complications was the same for patients with and without aortic enlargement at the time of surgery. Median follow-up time was fifteen years. Mortality of aortic root replacement is low at 2-4%,[103] while in specific institutions AVR mortality rates are less than 1%, especially in low-moderate risk populations.[104] Thus we would advocate aortic valve replacement alone and close follow up of the remaining aorta with CT or MR.

Choice of valve in aortic root replacement is also somewhat controversial. Data out of the Mayo Clinic has shown better long-term survival with mechanical aortic valve replacement.[92,105] Patient preference enters into the decision process as patients do not want to take Coumadin. Younger patients who choose a bioprosthesis may face reoperation. Re-operative mortality on a stentless valve has been reported over 10%.[106] Although homograft root replacement has traditionally been used for infectious reasons, it also has a high mortality when it is redone, primarily due to severe calcification of the walls.[107] Lastly, with regard to biologic roots made with a valve inside a tube graft, very little data exists regarding re-operative surgery. Intuitively it would seem to be a safer procedure, as surgery would involve replacing the valve inside the graft and leaving the graft alone. The Ross procedure has been abandoned for bicuspid valves as progression of aneurysmal dilatation over time leads to autograft dysfunction in a significant number of patients.[108]

Valve-sparing aortic root replacement in bicuspid aortic valve situations has been performed. Many fewer cases have been done than with a tricuspid valve. Results are not as good as with a tricuspid valve but nevertheless some have reported good long-term follow-up.[99]

Mortality in most series for root replacement is approximately 2-4% without comparison of independent risk stratification.[109,110] The risks for serious bleeding and stroke are 3.2% and 3.2%, respectively. Long-term survival is variable depending on the age and comorbidities of the patients undergoing replacement. Survival at 1, 3 and 5 years in a study by Ancheck et al was 84.7%, 78.3%, and 72.5%, respectively. The key to survival seems to be recognizing signs of aortic pathology related to the congenital disease and preventing morbidity and mortality of dissection and aneurysm with early root replacement. Van Putte et al. examined their long-term data of root replacement over a 25-year period with over 500 patients. Survival at 5, 10, and 25 years was 87%, 73%, and 29%, respectively. Peri-operative complication rates for myocardial infarction and stroke were 4.0 and 4.2%, respectively. Peri-operative rate for take back to the operating room for bleeding was 19%.[111] In sum, the results of root replacement are safe and are standing the test of time.

When aneurismal change is present, the root replacement may extend distally to include the remainder of the ascending aorta, aortic arch, and descending aorta. The most common operation in combination with the root replacement is hemi-arch replacement. Other operations combined with root replacement include aortic arch replacement and occasionally a frozen elephant trunk procedure. (Figures 6-8) With these more extensive procedures, mortality and morbidity understandably increases. Peri-operative mortality of the hemi arch and total arch procedures is 6.7% and 6.9%, respectively, with comparable morbidity.[115] With the elephant trunk procedure, the latest and best survival data are from Italy.[116] In 2010, Bartolomeo et al published their series of 67 patients who underwent the frozen elephant trunk over a two year period. Peri-operative mortality was 13.4%. Severe neurologic deficit occurred in 17%, although most patients had adequate outcomes with a 2 year survival 70%.[116]

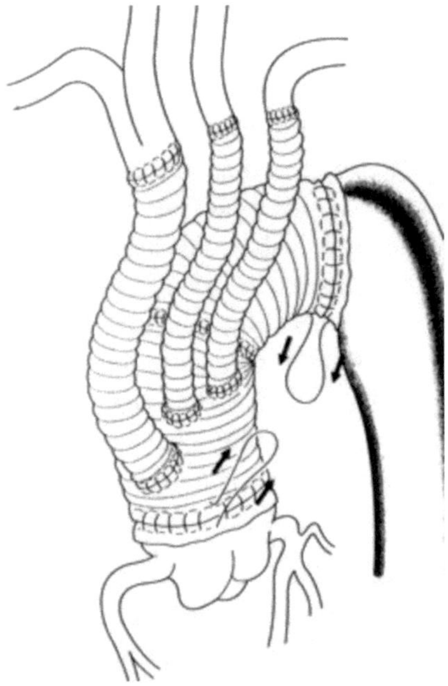

Figure 7. Aortic arch replacement via implantation and proximal grafting of the brachiocephalic, left carotid, and left subclavian arteries. Although not depicted in this image, root reconstruction via modified-Bentall technique can be performed during the same operation.[107]

6.4. Valve sparing aortic root replacement in patients with aneurysms

Aortic root reconstruction without valve replacement has come into popularity with cardiac surgeons because not all aortic root disease is accompanied with aortic valve dysfunction. Yacoub, in 1983,[117] and David, in 1991,[118] separately devised procedures that spare the native aortic valve, or so named, valve-sparing aortic root replacement. The Yacoub procedure is a "remodeling" procedure where the aortic graft is surgically attached to the aortic wall at the level of the commissures.[119] (Figure 9) A modification of the Yacoub procedure is the David, or "reimplantation" procedure. During the reimplantation procedure, the graft is fixed at a level proximal to the annulus, to the tissue of the left ventricular outflow tract[120](Figure 10). Since the origin of the David procedure, there have been multiple modifications to the technique with the latest emphasizing restoration of the sinuses of Valsalva by the creation of neosinuses.[121] Special grafts with sinuses (Gelweave) are also available.

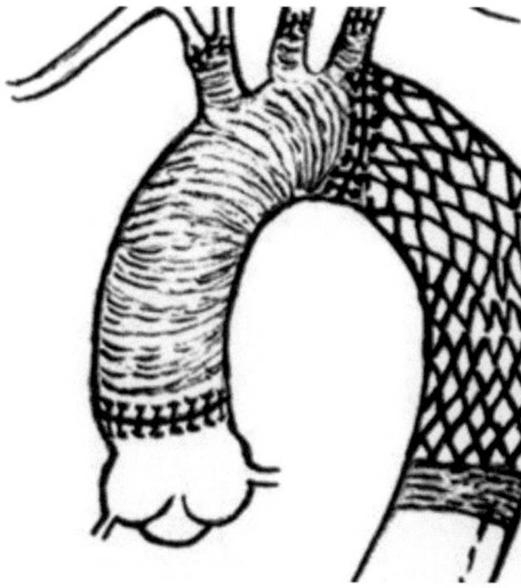

Figure 8. Frozen elephant trunk procedure in which a stent graft is deployed distally in the descending thoracic aorta. Debranching and anastomosis of the proximal arch branches, distal aortic arch, and proximal aorta are then carried out with a Dacron graft.[118]

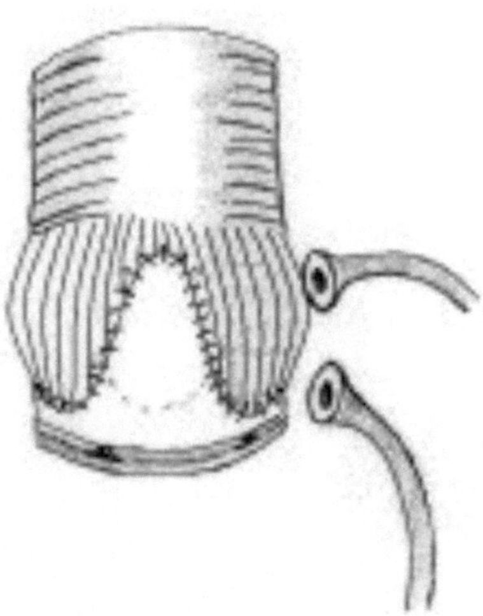

Figure 9. Yacoub procedure. Root replacement by remodeling consists of placing subannular U-stitches, a scalloped Dacron graft attached above the commissural ring, and finally coronary ostia are reimplanted into the graft material.[113]

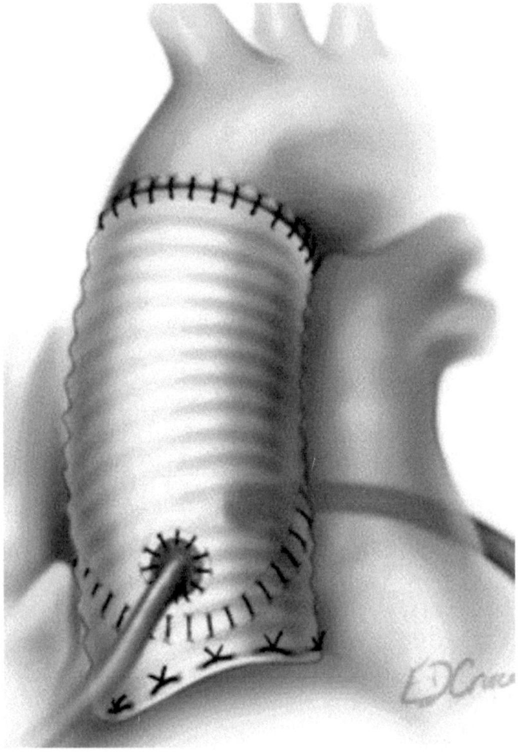

Figure 10. Modified David procedure where the graft is fixed to the level just proximal to the aortic annulus at the left ventricular outflow tract.[114]

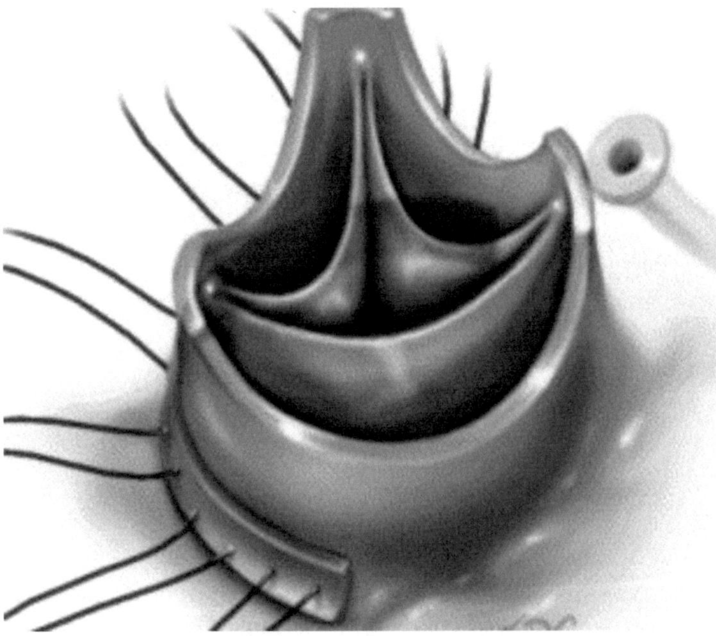

Figure 11. Trimming of the aortic root during modified David Procedure.[121]

The surgical technique involves resecting all aortic tissue except for a 5mm rim of aorta just above the valve and creating buttons of the coronaries (Figure 11). Dissection is carried proximally below the level of the annulus. Great care must be taken during this portion of the procedure to avoid the RVOT and left atrium. Sutures are then placed from inside the LVOT to outside through the graft for the proximal suture line. The graft is seated and the leaflets are inside the graft. After securing the proximal suture line, the valve leaflets are carefully positioned inside the graft to allow coaptation in the same plane for all three leaflets. The leaflets are then sutured inside the graft by running a suture along the small piece of aortic wall and attaching it to the graft. The coronaries are reimplanted and the distal suture line is performed where appropriate. Echo confirms (Figure 12) good coapatation of the leaflets and no aortic insufficiency.

Indications for a valve-sparing procedure are ascending and root aneurysms (>5cm or 4.5cm for patients with Marfan's) with normal aortic leaflets. Typically from sinotubular dilatation there is central aortic insufficiency which is easily corrected by this procedure. Asymmetric regurgitation may require leaflet repair. This is an excellent operation for patients with Marfan's, as it obviates the need for long-term anticoagulation. Recently it has been used in patients with acute Type A aortic dissection who require a root replacement.

Multiple studies are published since the advent of the David procedure that have attempted to give credence to the valve-sparing technique.[93-95] Long-term results of this have been excellent. A meta-analysis summarized the results and conclusions of 16 studies describing complete root replacement and valve-sparing techniques. Ten-year survival for patients undergoing valve-sparing techniques ranged from 82-97% in a heterogeneous group of patients.

Subpopulations that have undergone valve-sparing technique include the elderly and those patients with Marfan's. One study in older patients (>60 years old) demonstrated less favorable, yet still good results.[123] The peri-operative mortality of 63 patients undergoing valve-sparing replacement was 1.4% with an overall 51 month survival of 84%. Immediate post-operative and long-term results for Marfan's patients are also excellent. Volguina et al analyzed the short-term results of 105 patients with Marfan's who underwent valve-sparing technique.[124] There were no inpatient mortalities and significant morbidity included 8% requiring re-exploration of the mediastinum while only 13% had a peri-operative arrhythmia. David et al analyzed the long-term results of their 103 person cohort.[125] Fifteen year survival was 87% and 89% of those alive at fifteen years and patients were free of clinically significant aortic regurgitation.

6.5. Aortic root replacement in patients with acute type A aortic dissection

Patients who have an acute type A aortic dissection are a surgical emergency. Typically the ascending aorta is replaced with an open distal anastomosis such as a hemiarch with antegrade cerebral perfusion. The proximal anastomosis is then done at the sinotubular junction after removing all thrombus between the layers and gluing them together.

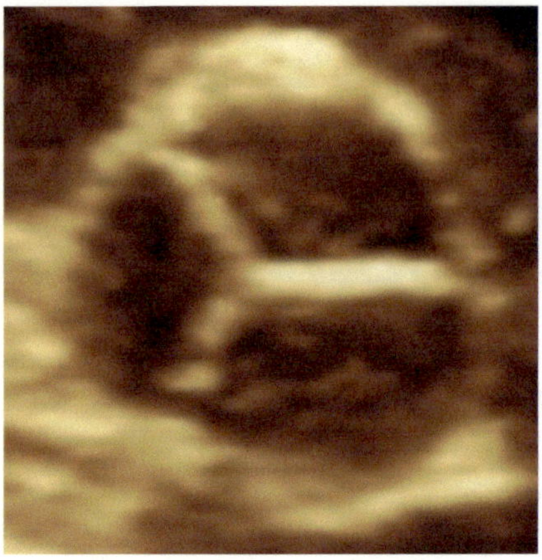

Figure 12. Echo demonstrating coaptation of aortic valve leaflets.[122]

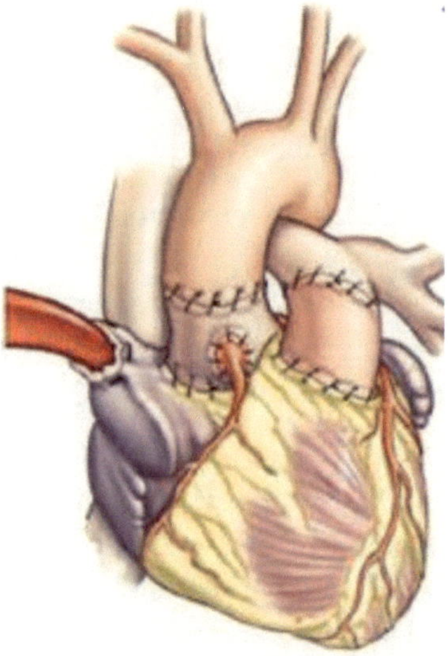

Figure 13. Ross Procedure after reconstruction. The pulmonary allograft is implanted into the left ventricular outflow tract and the coronaries are reimplanted into the autograft. A synthetic valve/root component is then used for the new pulmonary artery and valve.

Approximately 31% of patients will require aortic root replacement as the dissection extends down into the sinuses and around the coronaries.[126] As mentioned earlier, if the valve leaflets are normal then a valve-sparing root replacement is an option. The downside is an extended length of time during this critical operation, however with the proximal suture line below the annulus it may prevent bleeding. This is a major problem in patients with dissection. Because root replacement must be done in a significant proportion of Type A dissections there is incentive to understand outcomes in composite grafts versus stentless grafts. Lai et al examined their experience with Type A dissection patients who had AI and were stratified by root replacement with composite graft and separate valve graft.[127] Composite grafts had slightly improved survival at long-term follow-up then did patients with a separate valve graft. International Registry of Acute Aortic Dissection data should be used to examine this relationship in the future.

6.6. Aortic root replacement for infected endocarditis

Endocarditis is a dangerous condition of the aortic valve that can rapidly spread beyond the leaflets into the tissue around the aortic root. This typically leads to an aortic root abscess. This can further erode into contiguous structures such as the mitral valve, left atrium, right atrium, tricuspid valve, and right ventricle. Surgical principle mandates debridement of all infected tissue. Other valves and chambers must be repaired, prior to the root replacement. In the past it was felt that homograft root replacement was the ideal operation. Indeed the graft was felt to be more resistant to infection and the homograft had the anterior leaflet still attached, which often aided in mitral valve involvement. Recently, the availably and quality of homografts has become less. Results of root replacement with material other than homograft are not substantially different. Jassar et al reviewed the results of root replacement at their institution in patients with active endocarditis.[128] Patients had root replacement with synthetic grafts, biologics, or homografts. There was no significant difference with regard to in hospital mortality or survival with a mean follow-up of 32 months. Five-year survival for the cohort was also similar between groups, ranging from 58-62%.[128] Long-term survival was analyzed in patients receiving homograft roots for endocarditis and results are quite promising.[129] Thirty day survival was 83% while 10-year survival was 47%. One year reoperation rate due to deterioration of the graft was 8.6%. We therefore advocate root replacement in this situation based on factors such as age and patient preference. The Ross procedure is also an option for root replacement in this condition. Excellent long term results have been reported and theoretically the pulmonary autograft may be more resistant to infection.[130]

6.7. Aortic root replacement for a calcific aortic root

Patients who have severe aortic stenosis and a very calcified root may require aortic root replacement because of the difficulty inserting the valve from the distribution of calcium in the root. This can be a very dangerous operation because of the calcium extending into the coronary arteries. Indeed ligation of the coronaries may be required with the addition of bypass grafting. [131]

6.8. Surgery for sinus of valsalva aneurysms- general recommendations and analysis of surgical outcomes

Although sinus of Valsalva aneurysms are rare, they frequently require prompt surgical repair to prevent life threatening complications. A majority of patients present with rupture of the aneurysm into a cardiac chamber, typically the right atrium or ventricle. Eastern cultures have a notable increased incidence when compared to Western cultures. The first aneurysms were treated successfully in the 1950s. A clear distinction in outcome can be seen in patients who have infected versus non-infected aneurysms.[132] Root replacement is infrequently required for this condition, however when it is, the standard considerations about which type of valve to implant are used.

The largest series of patients was compiled by the Texas Heart Institute where the outcomes of 129 patients were analyzed over a 40-year period. Aortic root replacement was only necessary in 12% of patients, while the remaining patients were able to be treated with simple plication or a patch procedure.[132] Peri-operative mortality was 4% and complications included valve malfunction, endocarditis, and recurrence of the aneurysm in 3.9%, 2.6%, and 1.8%, respectively. Other recent retrospective trials have been published.[133,134] Again the vast majority of patients (>90%) were able to attain fixation with either direct closure or patch techniques. Approach for fixation was usually obtained through the chamber that rupture of the aneurysm occurred. Patients who had repair in the last decade demonstrated fewer days in the hospital and fewer peri-operative complications which included wound infection and arrhythmias. Over 90% of patients were alive after 5 years. The factor of highest prognostic significance with regard to long-term survival is time of onset and severity of aortic regurgitation.[135] Unfortunately there was no sub-analysis describing the results in those patients with root replacement.

6.9. The Ross procedure: indications and outcomes

The Ross procedure involves root replacement with the patients pulmonary valve harvested en-bloc as a cylinder from RVOT to distal pulmonary artery (Figure 13). The pulmonary valve is typically replaced with a porcine xenograft or homograft. Drawbacks of this operation include its complexity and it also involves double valve replacement for single valve pathology. Surgical results with the Ross procedure have been excellent except in the cases of bicuspid aortic valve.[136] In bicuspid cases the root undergoes dilatation, possibly from the same underlying abnormality that involved the native aorta of which the cause is not known.

While the procedure is technically very challenging, the peri-operative outcomes are adequate, yet long-term results are still debated.[137,138] One group out of Germany described their outcomes of 203 patients who were at least 10 years out from surgery with a mean follow-up of 12.3 years. Over 90% of patients did not need reoperation on either valve at 10 years of follow-up. They concluded that the Ross operation was safe, as long-term survival did not differ from the general population. Slight increases in the size of the aortic valve annulus and rate of insufficiency was observed.[137] In contrast, a meta-analysis was published in 2009 which summarized the results of Ross procedure outcomes and included 17 studies.[138] They concluded that the peri-operative and short-term outcomes is acceptable, however, there is significant graft durability limitation that is observed after the first decade, especially in younger patients. They concluded that further research to accomplish extended graft function would be helpful to limit possibility of long-term reoperation. It is now well established that patients with a bicuspid aortic valve should not have the Ross operation.

6.10. Reoperation of the aortic root

Structural failure of the root, pseudoaneurysms, or infection may necessitate redo aortic root replacement. This is an operation that typically carries a high risk of mortality and morbidity. Some special considerations when this very difficult operation is undertaken include: calcified homografts or stentless valves, coronary artery length, and infection.

In patients with a very calcified neo-aortic wall it is often extremely difficult to dissect out the wall and redo the root as it becomes very adherent to the adjacent structures and pulmonary artery and coronaries can be injured. Replacing just the aortic valve within the calcified root is an option. With the advent of trans aortic valve implantation (TAVI), this may be an excellent option in high risk patients. El-Hamamsy et al compared the Freestyle graft with homograft aortic root replacement in a prospective, randomized trial.[139] One-hundred sixty-six patients with an average age of 65 years had a mean follow-up of 7.6 years. Significant conclusions were made from this data including an improved age of survival (80 vs. 77 years), lower rate of reoperation (100% vs. 90%), and echocardiographically patients had less signs of valvular deterioration (86% vs. 30%) in the FreeStyle group.

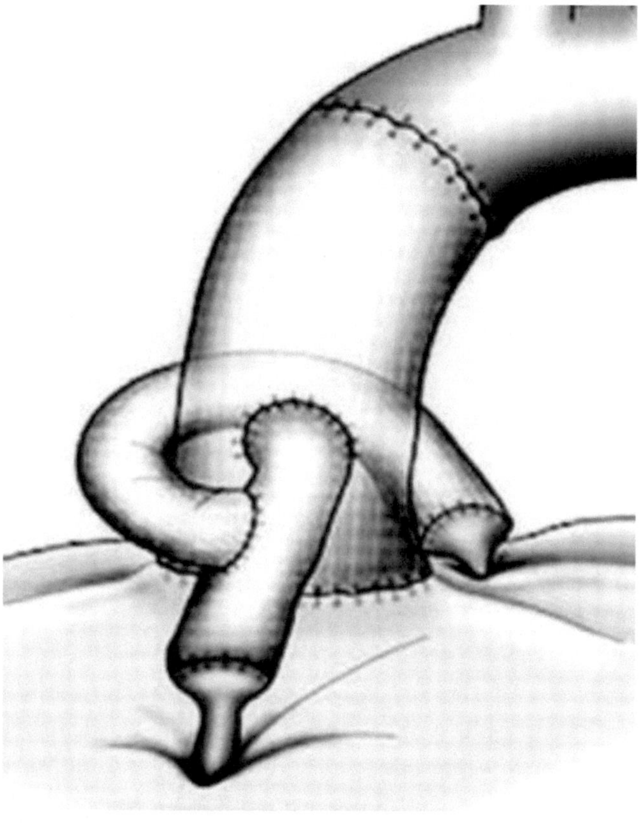

Figure 14. Aortic root replacement via the Cabrol technique. Coronary buttons are sutured side-to-side to a Dacron interposition graft during root replacement.[140]

There can be difficulty with mobilizing the coronary buttons and placing them in into the new root or they can be damaged. The Cabrol technique should then be deployed, (Figure 14) where a graft is sutured end to end to both the right and left coronary buttons then sutured side to side to the aorta.[140] Results have been mixed,[141,142] which may be due to difficulty orienting the graft. A second option is to place an interposition vein graft (Figure 15) between the coronary buttons and the graft.[143] This is our preferred method as we find the grafting to be easier. Lastly bypass-grafting can be done with ligation of the coronary arteries. This is typically is a last resort when bleeding and technical difficulties with the anastomosis are encountered.

Infected roots pose a major problem because of the amount of debridement and reconstruction that is required. The same surgical principles apply of removal of all infected and foreign tissue. Results have been promising using homograft replacements as demonstrated in peri-operative and with long-term follow-up studies.[128,129]

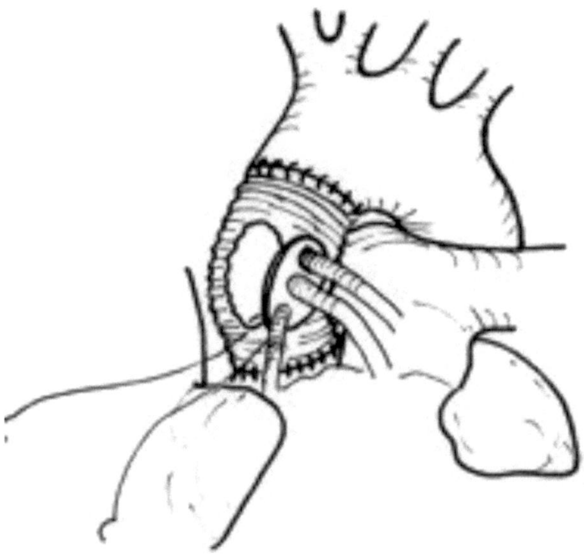

Figure 15. Vein graft interposition can be used as a conduit for coronary perfusion rather than using a Dacron interposition graft. This figure demonstrates venous conduits being sewn to the aortic root. 143

7. Conclusion

The anatomic complexity and serious pathology that affect the aortic root challenge the cardiac surgeon. Surgical procedures on the aortic root have drastically changed the lives of patients and extended their lifespan. Leaders in the field of cardiac surgery such as Bono, Bentall, Yacoub, and David have contributed greatly to our surgical armementaruium for treatment of aortic root pathology. These procedures will continue to evolve with improved graft material, improved valves, percutaneous approaches, and stem cell therapies.

Author details

B. Goslin
Grand Rapids Medical Education Partners, Michigan State University College of Human Medicine, USA

R. Hooker
Spectrum Health, Michigan State University, College of Human Medicine, West Michigan Cardiothoracic Surgeons, USA

8. References

[1] Ho, and Siew Yen. Structure and Anatomy of the Aortic Root. *Eur J Echocardiog* 2009;10(1):i3-i10.
[2] Sutton III JP, Ho SY, and Anderson RH. The Forgotten Interleaflet Triangles: A Review of the Surgical Anatomy of the Aortic Valve. *Ann Thorac Surg* 1995;59(2):419-427.
[3] Azadani AN, Chitsaz S, Matthews PB, et al. Comparison of Mechanical Properties of Human Ascending Aorta and Aortic Sinuses. *Ann Thorac Surg* 2012;93(1):87-94.
[4] Blanchard C, Lalande A, Sliwa T et al. Automatic Evaluation of the Valsalva Sinuses From Cine-MRI. *Mag Reson Mater Phy* 2011;24(6):359-370.
[5] Zhu D, and Zhao Q. Dynamic Normal Aortic Root Diameters: Implications for Aortic Root Reconstruction. *Ann Thorac Surg* 2011;91(2):485-489.
[6] D'Andrea A, Cocchia R, Riegler L, et al. Aortic Stiffness and Dispensability in Top-Level Athletes. *J Am Soc Echocardiog.* Epub Jan 2012.
[7] Rubinshtein R, Lerman A, Spoon DB, and Rihal CS. Anatomic Features of the Left Main Coronary Artery and Factors Associated with Its Bifurcation Angle: A 3-dimensional Quantitative Coronary Angiographic Study. *Catheter Cardio Inte* 2012:1-6.
[8] Pejkovic B, Krajnc I, and Anderhuber F. Anatomical Variations of Coronary Ostia, Aortocoronary Angles and Angles of Division of the Left Coronary Artery of the Human Heart. *J Int Med Res* 2008;36(5): 914-922.
[9] Evangelista A. Bicuspid Aortic Valve and Aortic Root Disease. *Cur Cardiol Rep* 2011;13(3): 234-241.
[10] Brandenburg RO, Tajik AJ, Edwards WD, et al. Accuracy of 2-dimensional echocardiographic diagnosis of congenitally bicuspid aortic valve: Echocardiographic-anatomic correlation in 115 patients. *Am J Cardiol* 1983;51:1469-1473.
[11] Alkadhi H, et al. Cardiac CT for the Differentiation of Bicuspid and Tricuspid Aortic Valves: Comparison With Echocardiography and Surgery. *Am J Rad* 2011;195(4):900-908.
[12] Davies MJ. Pathology of Cardiac Valves. London: Butterworths & Co; 1980. 51-61.
[13] Michelena HI, Khanna AD, Mahoney D, et al. Incidence of Aortic Complications in Patients with Bicuspid Aortic Valves. *J Am Med Assoc* 2011;306(10):1104-1112.
[14] Aldo C, Russo CF, and Vitali E. Bicuspid Aortic Valve: About Natural History of Ascending Aorta Aneurysms. *Ann Thorac Surg* 2008;85(1):362-363.

[15] Sood N, and Taub C. Unicuspid Aortic Valve: An Interesting Presentation. *Eur Heart J* 2008;29(10):1295.
[16] Mookadam F, Thota V, et al. Unicuspid aortic valve in children. *J Heart Valve Dis* 2010;19(6):678-683.
[17] Di Pino A, Gitto P, Silvia A, and Bianca I. Congenital Quadricuspid Aortic Valve in Children. *Cardiology in the Young* 2008;18(3):324-327.
[18] Rajamannan NM, Evans FJ, Aikawa E, et al. Calcific Aortic Valve Disease: Not Simply a Degenerative Process. *Circulation* 2011;124(16):1783-1791.
[19] LaPar DJ, Ailawadi G, Bhamidipati CM, et al. Small Prosthesis Size in Aortic Valve Replacement Does Not Affect Mortality. *Ann Thorac Surg* 2011;92(3):880-888.
[20] Davies RR, Kaple RK, Mandapati D, et al. Natural History of Ascending Aortic Aneurysms in the Setting of An Unreplaced Bicuspid Aortic Valve. *Ann Thorac Surg* 2007;83(4):1338-1344.
[21] Kallenbach K, Leyh RG, Salcher R, et al. Acute Aortic Dissection Versus Aortic Root Aneurysm: Comparison of Indications for Valve Sparing Aortic Root Reconstruction. *Eur J Cardio-thorac Surg* 2004;25(5):663-670.
[22] Davies, RR, Goldstein LJ, Coady MA, et al. Yearly Rupture or Dissection Rates for Thoracic Aortic Aneurysms: Simple Prediction Based on Size. *Ann Thorac Surg* 2002;73(1):17-28.
[23] Cannata, Aldo, Russo CF, and Vitali E. Bicuspid Aortic Valve: About Natural History of Ascending Aorta Aneurysms. *Ann Thorac Surg* 2008;85(1):362-363.
[24] David TE, Maganti M, and Armstrong S. Aortic Root Aneurysm: Principles of Repair and Long-term Follow-up. *J Thorac Cardiovasc Surg* 2010;140(6):S14-S19.
[25] Augoustides, JGT, Plappert T, and Bavaria JE. Aortic Decision-making in the Loeys–Dietz Syndrome: Aortic Root Aneurysm and a Normal-caliber Ascending Aorta and Aortic Arch. *J Thorac Cardiovasc Surg* 2009;138(2):502-503.
[26] Yuan SM, Jing H. Marfan's Syndrome- an overview. *Soa Paulo Med J* 2010:128(6):360-366.
[27] Keane MG, Pyeritz RE. Medical management of Marfan syndrome. *Circulation.* 2008;117:2802-2813.
[28] Song HK, Kindem M, Bavaria JE, et al. Long-term Implications of Emergency Versus Elective Proximal Aortic Surgery in Patients with Marfan Syndrome in the Genetically Triggered Thoracic Aortic Aneurysms and Cardiovascular Conditions Consortium Registry. *J Thorac Cardiovasc Surg* 2012;143(2):282-286.
[29] Loeys BL, Chen J, Neptune ER, et al. A syndrome of altered cardio-vascular, craniofacial, neurocognitive and skeletal development caused by mutations in TGFBR1 or TGFBR2. *Nat Genet* 2005;37(3):275-281.
[30] Atzinger CL, Meyer RA, Khoury PR, et al. Cross-Sectional and Longitudinal Assessment of Aortic Root Dilation and Valvular Anomalies in Hypermobile and Classic Ehlers-Danlos Syndrome. *J Ped* 2011;158(5):826-830.
[31] Siu SC, and Silversides CK. Bicuspid Aortic Valve Disease. *J Am Coll Cardiol* 2010;55(25): 2789-2800.

[32] Beroukhim RS, Kruzick TL, Taylor AL, Gao D, Yetman AT. Progression of aortic dilation in children with a functionally normal bicuspid aortic valve. *Am J Cardiol* 2006;98:828 -830.

[33] Liu G, Shupak R, and Chiu BY. Aortic Dissection in Giant-cell Arteritis. *Seminars in Arthritis and Rheumatism* 1995;25(3):160-171.

[34] Ostberg G: On arteritis: with special reference to polymyalgia arteritica. *Acta Pathol Microbiol Immunol Scand* 1973;237:1-59, 1973.

[35] Kerr GS, Hallahan CW, Giordano J, et al. Takayasu arteritis. *Ann Intern Med* 1994;120:919 -929.

[36] Robinson WP, Detterbeck FC, Hendren RL, and Keagy BA. Fulminant Development of Mega-aorta Due to Takayasu's Arteritis: Case Report and Review of the Literature. *Vascular* 2005;13(3):178-183.

[37] Song M, Nakayama T, Hattori K, et al. Aortic Root Aneurysm in Takayasu Arteritis Syndrome: Exploration in Active Phase and Repair in Inactive Phase. *J Thorac Cardiovasc Surg* 2008;136(4):1084-1085.

[38] O'Connor MB, Murphy E, O'Donovan E, et al. Takayasu's Arteritis Presenting As a Dissecting Aortic Aneurysm History: A Case Report. *Cases journal* 2008;1(1):52.

[39] Paulus HE, Pearson CM, and Pitts W. Aortic Insufficiency in Five Patients with Reiter's Syndrome: A Detailed Clinical and Pathologic Study. *The American Journal of Medicine* 1972;53(4):464-472.

[40] Roldan CA, Chavez J, Wiest PW, et al. Aortic Root Disease and Valve Disease Associated with Ankylosing Spondylitis. *J Am Coll Cardiol* 1998;32(5):1397-1404.

[41] Bruckner BA, DiBardino DJ, Cumbie TC, et al. Critical Evaluation of Chest Computed Tomography Scans for Blunt Descending Thoracic Aortic Injury. *Ann Thorac Surg* 2006;81(4):1339-1346.

[42] Dávila-Román VG, Murphy SF, Nickerson NJ, et al. Atherosclerosis of the Ascending Aorta Is An Independent Predictor of Long-term Neurologic Events and Mortality. *J Am Coll Cardiol* 1999;33(5):1308-1316.

[43] Lee S, and Cho SH. Huge Ascending Aortic Pseudoaneurysm Caused by a Penetrating Atherosclerotic Ulcer. *Circulation. Cardiovasc Imag* 2008;1(3):e19-e20.

[44] White CS, and Plotnick GD. Case 33: Sinus of Valsalva Aneurysm. *Radiology* 2001;219:82-85.

[45] Takach TJ, Reul GJ, Duncan JM, et al: Sinus of Valsalva aneurysm or fistula: Management and outcome. *Ann Thorac Surg* 1999;68:1573-1577.

[46] Chu SH, Hung CR, How SS, et al. Ruptured aneurysms of the sinus of Valsalva in Oriental patients. *J Thorac Cardiovasc Surg* 1999;99:288-298.

[47] Shah, AJ, Pocock JM, Belham M, et al. Aneurysm of the Sinus of Valsalva. *Cardiology Journal* 2009;16(6):312-313.

[48] Ott, David A. Aneurysm of the Sinus of Valsalva. *Seminars in Thoracic and Cardiovascular Surgery: Pediatric Cardiac Surgery Annual* 2006;9(1):165-176.

[49] Pearson R, Philips N, Hancock R, et al. Regional Wall Mechanics and Blunt Traumatic Aortic Rupture at the Isthmus. *European journal of cardio-thoracic surgery* 2008;34(3):616-622.

[50] Matthew JW, Tsai PI, Gilani R, and Mattox KL. Challenges in the Diagnosis and Management of Unusual Presentations of Blunt Injury to the Ascending Aorta and Aortic Sinuses. *J Surgi Res* 2010;163(2):176-178.

[51] Bruckner BA, DiBardino DJ, Cumbie TC, et al. Critical Evaluation of Chest Computed Tomography Scans for Blunt Descending Thoracic Aortic Injury. *Ann Thorac Surg* 2006;81(4):1339-1346.

[52] Smith MD, Cassidy JM, Souther S, et al. Transesophageal echocardiography in the diagnosis of traumatic rupture of the aorta. *N Engl J Med.* 1995;332:356-362.

[53] Saletta S, Lederman E, Fein S, and Fortune JB. Transesophageal echocardiography for the initial evaluation of the widened mediastinum in trauma patients. *J Trauma.* 1995;39:137-142.

[54] Brooks SW, Young JC, Cmolik B, et al. The use of transesophageal echocar-diography in the evaluation of chest trauma. *J Trauma.* 1992;32:761-768.

[55] Brasel KJ, and Weigelt JA. Blunt Thoracic Aortic Trauma. A Cost-utility Approach for Injury Detection. *Arch Surg.* 1960;131(6): 619-625.

[56] Symbas PJ, Horsley WS, and Symbas PN. Rupture of the Ascending Aorta Caused by Blunt Trauma. *Ann Thorac Surg* 1998;66(1):113-117.

[57] Lewis JV, Dunn JA, Compton RP. Injuries of the ascending aorta. *S Tenn Med Assoc* 1993;86:399-400.

[58] Mastroroberto P, Mizio GD, Colosimo F, and Ricci P. Occlusion of Left and Right Coronary Arteries and Coronary Sinus Following Blunt Chest Trauma. *J Forens Sci* 2011;56(5):1349-1351.

[59] Sandrelli L, Cavalotti C, Casati V, et al. Aortic valve repair for traumatic aortic insufficiency. *Ital Heart J* 2000;1(11):767-768.

[60] Schoen FJ. Surgical pathology of removed natural and prosthetic valves. *Hum Pathol* 1987;18:558.

[61] Robbins & Cotran, The Heart Chapter 12, p. 590.

[62] Bostrom K, Watson KE, Stanford WP, and Demer LL. Atherosclerotic calcification: relation to developmental osteogenesis. *Am J Cardiol* 1995;75:88B–91B.

[63] Carabello BA. Aortic Stenosis N Engl J Med 2002;346:677.

[64] Lakier JB, Copans H, Rosman HS, et al. Idiopathic Degeneration of the Aortic Valve: A Common Cause of Isolated Aortic Regurgitation. *J Am Coll Cardiol* 1985;5(2):347-351.

[65] Bermudez EA, Gaasch WH: Regurgitant lesions of the aortic and mitral valves: Considerations in determining the ideal timing of surgical intervention. *Heart Fail Clin* 2006; 2:473.

[66] Tornos P, Bonow RO: *Aortic regurgitation.* In: Otto CM, Bonow RO, ed. *Valvular Heart Disease: A Companion to Braunwald's Heart Disease,* Philadelphia: Saunders/Elsevier; 2009:155-168.

[67] Enriquez-Sarano M, Tajik AJ: Clinical practice. Aortic regurgitation. *N Engl J Med* 2004; 351:1539.

[68] Williams DM, Lee DY, Hamilton BH, et al. The dissected aorta. III. Anatomy and radiologic diagnosis of branch-vessel compromise. *Radiol* 1997;203(1):37–44.

[69] Hiratzka LF, Bakris GL, Beckman JA, et al. ACCF/AHA/AATS/ACR/ASA/SCA/SCAI/SIR/STS/SVM guidelines for the diagnosis and management of patients with Thoracic Aortic Disease: A report of the American College of Cardiology Foundation/American Heart Association Task Force on Practice Guidelines, American Association for Thoracic Surgery, American College of Radiology, American Stroke Association, Society of Cardiovascular Anesthesiologists, Society for Cardiovascular Angiography and Interventions, Society of Interventional Radiology, Society of Thoracic Surgeons, and Society for Vascular Medicine. *Circulation* 2010; 121:e266-e369.

[70] Williams DM, LePage MA, Lee DY The dissected aorta. I. Early anatomic changes in an in vitro model. *Radiol* 1997;203(1):23–31.

[71] Gilon D, Mehta RH, Oh JK, et al: Characteristics and in-hospital outcomes of patients with cardiac tamponade complicating type A acute aortic dissection. *Am J Cardiol* 2009; 103:1029.

[72] Bonderman D, Gharehbaghi-Schnell E, Wollenek G et al. Mechanisms underlying aortic dilatation in congenital aortic valve malformation. *Circulation* 1999;99:2138–2143.

[73] Nistri S, Grande-Allen J, Noale M et al. Aortic elasticity and size in bicuspid aortic valve syndrome. *Eur Heart J* 2008;29:472–479.

[74] Aydin A, Mortensen K, Rybczynski M, et al. Central pulse pressure and augmentation index in asymptomatic bicuspid aortic valve disease. *Int J Cardiol* 2011;147:466–468.

[75] Aydin A, Desai N, Bernhardt A, et al. Ascending aortic aneurysm and aortic valve dysfunction in bicuspid aortic valve disease. *Int J Cardiol* Epub, July 2011.

[76] Penco M, Paparoni S, Dagianti A, et al. Usefulness of Transesophageal Echocardiography in the Assessment of Aortic Dissection. *Am J Cardiology* 2000;86(4):53-56.

[77] Nienaber CA, Spielmann RP, Von Kodolisch Y, et al. Diagnosis of thoracic aortic dissection: magnetic resonance imaging versus transesophageal echocardiogra-phy. *Circulation* 1992;85:434-447.

[78] Simon P, Owen AN, Havel M, et al. Transesophageal echocardiography in the emergency surgical management of patients with aortic dissection. *J Thorac Cardiovasc Surg* 1992;103:1113-1118.

[79] Shiga T, Wajima Z, Apfel CC, Inoue T, and Ohe Y. Diagnostic Accuracy of Transesophageal Echocardiography, Helical Computed Tomography, and Magnetic Resonance Imaging for Suspected Thoracic Aortic Dissection: Systematic Review and Meta-analysis. *Arch Intern Med* 2006;166(13):1350-1356.

[80] Takahashi K, and Stanford W. Multidetector CT of the Thoracic Aorta. *Int JCardiovasc Imag* 2005;21(1):141-153.

[81] LePage MA, Quint LE, Sonnad SS, et al. Aortic dissection: CT features that distinguish true lumen from false lumen. *Am J Roentgenol* 2001; 177: 207-211.
[82] Pouleur A, le Polain J, Pasquet A, et al. Aortic Valve Area Assessment: Multidetector CT Compared with Cine MR Imaging and Transthoracic and Transesophageal Echocardiography. *Radiol* 2007;244(3):745-754.
[83] Cornily J, Gilard M, Bezon E, et al. Cardiac Multislice Spiral Computed Tomography As An Alternative to Coronary Angiography in the Preoperative Assessment of Coronary Artery Disease Before Aortic Valve Surgery: A Management Outcome Study. *Arch Cardiovasc Dis* 2010;103(3):170-175
[84] Gilard M, Cornily J, Pennec P, et al. Accuracy of Multislice Computed Tomography in the Preoperative Assessment of Coronary Disease in Patients with Aortic Valve Stenosis." *J Am Coll Cardiol* 2006;47(10):2020-2024.
[85] Krishnam MS, Tomasian A, Malik S, et al. Image Quality and Diagnostic Accuracy of Unenhanced SSFP MR Angiography Compared with Conventional Contrast-enhanced MR Angiography for the Assessment of Thoracic Aortic Diseases. *Eur Radiol* 2010;20(6):1311-1320.
[86] Gebker R, Gomaa O, Schnackenburg B, et al. Comparison of Different MRI Techniques for the Assessment of Thoracic Aortic Pathology: 3D Contrast Enhanced MR Angiography, Turbo Spin Echo and Balanced Steady State Free Precession. *Int J Cardiovasc Imag* 2007;23(6):747-756.
[87] Hamon M, Baron J, Viader F, and Hamon M. Periprocedural Stroke and Cardiac Catheterization. *Circulation* 2008;118(6):678-683.
[88] Bentall H, Bono A. A technique for complete replacement of the ascending aorta. *Thorax* 1968;23:338-339.
[89] http://www.destinationheart.com/ross_procedure.php
[90] Cartier PC, Dumesnil JG, Métras J, et al. Clinical and hemodynamic performance of the freestyle aortic root bioprosthesis. *Ann Thoracic Surg* 1999;67:345-349.
[91] El-Hamamsy I, Clark L, Stevens LM, et al. Late Outcomes Following Freestyle Versus Homograft Aortic Root Replacement. *J Am Coll Cardiol* 2010;55(4):368-376.
[92] Zehr, KJ, Orszulak TA, Mullany CJ, et al. Surgery for Aneurysms of the Aortic Root. *Circulation* 2004;110(11):1364-1371
[93] Tourmousoglou C, and Rokkas C. Is Aortic Valve-sparing Operation or Replacement with a Composite Graft the Best Option for Aortic Root and Ascending Aortic Aneurysm? *Interactive Cardiovascular and Thoracic Surgery* 2009;8(1):134-147.
[94] David TE, Feindel CM, Webb GD, et al. Jack M Colman, Susan Armstrong, and Manjula Maganti. Long-term Results of Aortic Valve-sparing Operations for Aortic Root Aneurysm. *J Thorac Cardiovasc Surg* 2006;132(2):347-354.
[95] Dias RR, Mejia OV, Carvalho EV, et al. Aortic Root Reconstruction Through Valve-sparing Operation: Critical Analysis of 11 Years of Follow-up. *Revista brasileira de cirurgia cardiovascular : órgão oficial da Sociedade Brasileira de Cirurgia Cardiovascular* 2005;25(1): 66-72.

[96] Elefteriades JA. Indications for Aortic Replacement. *The Journal of Thoracic and Cardiovascular Surgery* 2010;140(6):s5-s9.
[97] Guntheroth WG. A Critical Review of the American College of Cardiology/American Heart Association Practice Guidelines on Bicuspid Aortic Valve with Dilated Ascending Aorta. *Am J Cardio* 2008;102(1):107-110.
[98] Vahanian A, Baumgartner H, Bax J, et al. Guidelines on the management of valvular heart disease: The Task Force on the Management of Valvular Heart Disease of the European Society of Cardiology. *Eur Heart J* 2007;28(2):230-268.
[99] Warnes CA, Williams RG, Bashore TM, et al. ACC/AHA 2008 Guidelines for the Management of Adults with Congenital Heart Disease. *Circulation* 2008;118(23):e714-e833.
[100] Etz CD, Homann TM, Silovitz D, et al. Long-Term Survival After the Bentall Procedure in 206 Patients with Bicuspid Aortic Valve. *Ann Thorac Surg* 2007;84(4):1186-1194.
[101] Fazel SS, Mallidi HR, Lee RS, et al. The aortopathy of bicuspid aortic valve disease has distinctive patterns and usually involves the transverse aortic arch. *J Thorac Cardiovasc Surg* 2008;135:901-907.
[102] McKellar SH, Michelena HI, Li Z, et al. Long-Term Risk of Aortic Events Following Aortic Valve Replacement in Patients with Bicuspid Aortic Valves. *The American Journal of Cardiology* 2010;106(11):1626-1633.
[103] El-Hamamsy I, Ibrahim M, Stevens L, et al. Early and Long-term Results of Reoperative Total Aortic Root Replacement with Reimplantation of the Coronary Arteries. *The Journal of Thoracic and Cardiovascular Surgery* 2011;142(6):1473-1477.
[104] Gaudino M, Anselmi A, Glieca F, et al. Contemporary Results for Isolated Aortic Valve Surgery. *Thorac Cardiovasc Surg* 2011; 59(4): 229-232.
[105] Zehr KJ, Matloobi A, Connolly HM, et al. Surgical management of the aortic root in patients with Marfan syndrome. *J Heart Valve Dis* 2005;14(1):121-128.
[106] Borger MA, Prasongsukarn K, Armstrong S, et al. Stentless Aortic Valve Reoperations: A Surgical Challenge. *Ann Thorac Surg* 2007;84(3):737-743.
[107] Malvindi PG, van Putte BP, Leone A, et al. Aortic Reoperation After Freestanding Homograft and Pulmonary Autograft Root Replacement. *Ann Thorac Surg* 2011;91(4):1135-1140.
[108] Luciani GB, Mazzucco A. Aortic root disease after the Ross procedure. *Curr Opin Cardiol* 2006;21(6):555-560.
[109] Aicher D, Langer F, Kissinger A, Lausberg H, Fries R, Schafers HS. Valve-sparing aortic root replacement in bicuspid aortic valves: a reasonable option? *J Thorac Cardiovasc Surg* 2004;128:662-668.
[110] Achneck HE, Rizzo JA, Tranquilli M, and Elefteriades JA. Safety of Thoracic Aortic Surgery in the Present Era. *Ann Thorac Surg* 2007;84(4):1180-1185.

[111] van Putte BP, Ozturk S, Siddiqi S, et al. Early and Late Outcome After Aortic Root Replacement with a Mechanical Valve Prosthesis in a Series of 528 Patients. *Ann Thorac Surg* 2012;93(2):503-509.

[112] LeMarie SA, Green SY, Sharma K, et al. Aortic Root Replacement with Stentless Porcine Xenografts: Early and Late Outcomes in 132 Patients. *Ann Thorac Surg* 2009;87(2):503-513.

[113] Tanaka K, Makuuchi H, Naruse Y, et al. False Aneurysm Due to Suture Loosening After Aortic Arch Replacement. *Asian Cardiovasc Thorac Ann* 2002;10:346-348.

[114] Chen X, Huang F, Xu M, et al. The stented elephant trunk procedure combined total arch replacement for Debakey I aortic dissection: operative result and follow-up. *Interact CardioVasc Thorac Surg* 2010;11(5): 594-598.

[115] Shiono M, Hata M, Sezai A, et al. Validity of a Limited Ascending and Hemiarch Replacement for Acute Type A Aortic Dissection. *The Annals of Thoracic Surgery 2006;*82(5):1665-1669.

[116] Di Bartolomeo R, Pacini D, Savini C, et al. Complex Thoracic Aortic Disease: Single-stage Procedure with the Frozen Elephant Trunk Technique. *The Journal of Thoracic and Cardiovascular Surgery* 2010;140(6):S81-S91.

[117] Yacoub MH, Fagan A, Stassano P, et al. Results of valve conserving operations for aortic regurgitation. *Circulation* 1983;68:311–312.

[118] David T, Feindel C. An aortic valve-sparing operation for patients with aortic incompetence and aneurysm of the ascending aorta. *J Thorac Cardiovasc Surg* 1992;103(4):617–621

[119] Lansac E, Di Centa I, Varnous S, et al. External Aortic Annuloplasty Ring for Valve-Sparing Procedures. *Ann Thorac Surg* 2005;79(1):356-358.

[120] Matalanis G. Valve Sparing Aortic Root Repairs—An Anatomical Approach. *Heart Lung Circ* 2004;13(3):S13-S18.

[121] Kvitting JP, Ebbers T, Wigstrom L, et al. Flow patterns in the aortic root and the aorta studied with time-resolved, 3-dimensional, phase-contrast magnetic resonance imaging: implications for aortic valve-sparing surgery. *J Thorac Cardiovasc Surg* 2004; 127: 1602-1607.

[122] Baird CW , Myers PO, Nido PJ. Aortic Valve Reconstruction in the Young Infants and Children. *Seminars in Thoracic and Cardiovascular Surgery: Pediatric Cardiac Surgery Annual* 2012;15(1):9-19.

[123] Settepani F, Szeto WY, Bergonzini M, et al. Reimplantation Valve-sparing Aortic Root Replacement for Aortic Root Aneurysm in the Elderly: Are We Pushing the Limits? *J Cardiac Surg* 2010;25(1):56-61.

[124] Volguina, IV, Miller DC, LeMaire SA, et al. Valve-sparing and Valve-replacing Techniques for Aortic Root Replacement in Patients with Marfan Syndrome: Analysis of Early Outcome. *J Thorac Cardiovasc Surg* 2009;137(3):641-649.

[125] David TE, Armstrong S, Maganti M, et al. Long-term Results of Aortic Valve–sparing Operations in Patients with Marfan Syndrome. *J Thorac Cardiovasc Surg* 2009;138(4):859-864.

[126] Trimarchi S, Nienaber CA, Rampoldi V, et al. Contemporary Results of Surgery in Acute Type A Aortic Dissection: The International Registry of Acute Aortic Dissection Experience. *J Thorac Cardiovasc Surg* 2005;129(1);112-122.

[127] Lai DT, Miller DC, Mitchell RS, et al. Acute Type a Aortic Dissection Complicated by Aortic Regurgitation: Composite Valve Graft Versus Separate Valve Graft Versus Conservative Valve Repair. *J Thorac Cardiovasc Surg* 2003;126(6):1978-1985.

[128] Jassar, A, Bavaria JE, Szeto WY, et al. Graft Selection for Aortic Root Replacement in Complex Active Endocarditis: Does It Matter? *Ann Thorac Surg* 2012;93(2):480-487.

[129] Musci M, Weng Y, Hübler M, et al. Homograft Aortic Root Replacement in Native or Prosthetic Active Infective Endocarditis: Twenty-year Single-center Experience. *J Thorac Cardiovasc Surg* 139(3):665-673.

[130] Oswalt JD, Dewan SJ, Mueller MC, et al. Nelson S. Highlights of a ten-year experience with the Ross procedure. *Ann Thorac Surg*. 2001;71:S332-S335.

[131] Dávila-Román VG, Murphy SF, Nickerson NJ, et al. Atherosclerosis of the Ascending Aorta Is An Independent Predictor of Long-term Neurologic Events and Mortality. *J Am Coll Cardio* 1999;33(5):1308-1316.

[132] Takach TJ, Reul GJ, and Duncan JM. Sinus of valsalva aneurysm or fistula: management and outcome. *Ann Thorac Surg* 1999;68(5):1573-1577.

[133] Wang Z, Zou C, Li D, et al. Surgical Repair of Sinus of Valsalva Aneurysm in Asian Patients. *Ann Thorac Surg* 2007;84(1):156-160.

[134] Menon S, Kottayil B, Panicker V, et al. Ruptured Sinus of Valsalva Aneurysm: 10-year Indian Surgical Experience. *Asian Cardiovascular & Thoracic Annals* 2011;19(5):320.

[135] Murashita T, Kubota T, Kamikubo Y, Shiiya N, Yasuda K. Long-term results of aortic valve regurgitation after repair of ruptured sinus of Valsalva aneurysms. *Ann Thorac Surg* 2002;73:1466 -71.

[136] Stelzer, Paul. The Ross Procedure: State of the Art 2011. *Seminars in Thoracic and Cardiovascular Surgery* 2011;23(2):115-123.

[137] Charitos EI, Stierle U, Hanke T, et al. Long-Term Results of 203 Young and Middle-Aged Patients with More Than 10 Years of Follow-Up After the Original Subcoronary Ross Operation. *Ann Thorac Surg* 2012;93(2):495-502.

[138] Takkenberg, JJM, Zondervan PE, and van Herwerden LA. Progressive Pulmonary Autograft Root Dilatation and Failure After Ross Procedure. *Ann Thorac Surg* 1999;67(2):551-553.

[139] El-Hamamsy I, Clark L, Stevens LM, et al. Late Outcomes Following Freestyle Versus Homograft Aortic Root Replacement: Results From a Prospective Randomized Trial. *Journal of the American College of Cardiology* 2010;55(4):368-376.

[140] Kourliouros A, Grapsa J, Nihoyannopoulos P, and Athanasiou T. Modification of the Cabrol as a bailout procedure in complicated bicuspid valve aortopathy. *Interact Cardiovasc-Thorac Surg* 2011;12(2):199-201.

[141] Gelsomino S, Frassani R, Da Col P, et al. A long-term experience with the Cabrol root replacement technique for the management of ascending aortic aneurysms and dissections. *Ann Thorac Surg*. 2003;75(1):126-131.

[142] Garlicki M, Roguski K, Puchniewicz M, Ehrlich MP. Composite aortic root replacement using the classic or modified Cabrol coronary artery implantation technique. *Scand Cardiovasc J*. 2006;40(4):230-3.

[143] Yaku H, Fermanis GG, Macauley RJ, and Horton DA. Dissection of the Ascending Aorta: A Late Complication of Coronary Artery Bypass Grafting. *Ann Thorac Surg*. 1996;62:1834-1835.

Chapter 9

Robotic Resection of Left Atrial Myxoma

José Francisco Valderrama Marcos,
María Teresa González López and Julio Gutiérrez de Loma

Additional information is available at the end of the chapter

http://dx.doi.org/10.5772/50868

1. Introduction

1.1. General considerations

Cardiac myxoma is a benign primitive tumor of endocardial origin that occurs with an incidence of 40-50% of all detected primary cardiac neoplasms. The vast majority of them are manifest as cavitary gelatinous masses and they may have a smooth or rough surface or thrombus adherent. The tumor is constituted by primitive connective tissue cells form rings, cords and nests that are often associated with capillaries and they exist in a myxoid stroma that is composed of variable amounts of proteoglycans, elastin and collagen.

Approximately 90% are solitary and pedunculated and the most common site of attachment is at the border of the fossa ovalis in the left atrium (75-85%), although myxomas can also originate from the atrial appendage, 25% of cases are found in the right atrium and up to 7% arise in the ventricular cavities [1].

The etiology remains to be determined and most cases are sporadic. About 75% of sporadic myxomas occur in females and the mean age for these cases is 55 years. Myxomas are familial in only 5-7% of the cases, and they have atypical features such as multicentricity, atypical localization, recurrence after excision and association with Carney complex [2]. Although atrial myxomas are typically benign, local recurrence due to malignant change has also been reported [3].

The growth rate of these tumors has been cited as reaching 0.15 cm per month and the clinical presentation varies according to the size, tumor's location and mobility (depending on the extent of attachment to the interatrial septum) [4-5]. Left atrial myxomas may produce symptoms by mechanical interference of blood flow across the mitral valve or pulmonary venous drainage, symptoms associated with embolization, constitutional symptoms and arrhythmias. Embolism is a major feature of cardiac myxomas, with systemic embolism occurring in 30% to 40% of patients with a left atrial tumor, although in general terms, the site is dependent upon the location (left or right atrium). Signs of heart failure with pulmonary congestion or pulmonary embolism are presented in 22% and 20% of patients respectively, indicating a high-risk situation [6]. Sudden death may occur in 15% patients with atrial myxomas and it is typically caused by coronary embolization or obstruction of heart valves.

In about 20% of cases, myxoma may be asymptomatic and discovered as an incidental finding by imaging techniques, such as transthoracic or transesophageal echocardiography (TEE), cardiac magnetic resonance imaging or computed tomography (CT). Cardiac imaging along with a high index of suspicion plays an important role in the diagnosis and subsequent management of patients with cardiac myxomas who can potentially benefit from surgical treatment.

Although these tumors are histologically benign, they may be lethal because of their strategic position and, after the diagnosis has been established, surgery should be performed promptly because of the possibility of embolic complications or sudden death previously described. In the past, cardiac myxoma has been generally considered a surgical emergency. However, currently it tends to be observed in a more elderly and higher risk population, often at an early stage because of the development of cardiac imaging techniques and, because of this reason, emergency surgery is not appropriate in stable forms [6]. With the exception of real emergency situations, there is no reason why surgery for cardiac myxoma should not comply with the usual recommendations for preoperative routine assessment before any form of cardiac surgery.

Long-term follow-up is recommended and annual echocardiograms are useful for early detection of recurrent tumors after surgery.

1.2. Surgical considerations

Operative resection of atrial myxoma is the treatment of choice and it is a safe procedure, with an early postoperative mortality of 2% and an excellent long-term prognosis [7].

Surgery is usually curative and includes a complete resection with adequate margin. In most cases, cardiac myxomas can be removed easily because they are pedunculated. Simple resection is justified in the most of patients, avoiding a large resection of the atrial septum below the tumor implantation, although extensive resection appears to be mainly justified in high-risk cases of recurrence, such as familial myxomas [8]. Right atrial tumors are resected through the right atrium and left atrial tumors can be removed using a trans-septal or trans-atrial approach.

Optimal operative technique emphasizes minimal manipulation of the tumor before institution of cardiopulmonary bypass (CPB) to prevent fragmentation and embolization and the tumor must be removed intact. Recurrence is possible after surgery and it can be attributed to incomplete excision of the tumor, intracardiac implantation from the primary tumor or growth of a second focus.

Traditionally, surgery for cardiac myxomas has been performed by median sternotomy, which provides a generous exposure. However, a challenge is occurring and minimally invasive cardiac surgery has grown in last decade because of the observed benefits of minimal access surgery, such as reduced surgical trauma and decreased pain. Moreover, the advancements in three-dimensional (3D) video and robotic instrumentation have progressed to a point where a large number of cardiac procedures (including myxomas excision) are feasible by specially trained cardiac surgeons.

Currently, resection of atrial myxomas can be performed through small port sites with enhanced technological assistance rather than a traditional median sternotomy. The application of robotic telemanipulation systems enables the surgeon to provide the most effective and least invasive treatment option available for this condition, offering all the potential benefits of a minimally invasive procedure, including smaller incisions with minimal scarring, less trauma (including less pain and less bleeding), a decreased risk of infection, shorter hospital stay and recovery, and a quicker return to daily activities [9].

Removal of left atrial myxomas under robotic assistance has demonstrated to be safe and efficient with no limitations to resection of the tumor, allowing the surgeon generous access to the heart and surrounding structures. It can be done with reasonable cross clamp and perfusion times, conversions to open surgery are uncommon and excellent mid-term results can be achieved by well-trained surgical teams.

With this relatively new technology being more widespread, it is important to know about standard surgical procedure for resection of left atrial myxomas under robotic assistance, as well as acknowledge any related complications for this procedure.

2. Historical background

Prior to advances in robotic technology, a variety of smaller incisions were developed for endoscopic heart operations in the mid-1990s, such as coronary artery bypass grafting or valve surgery [10-11]. In 1998, Carpentier [12] and Mohr et al [13] performed endoscopic mitral procedures and coronary artery bypass grafting using peripheral perfusion and endoaortic cross-clamp techniques.

Minimally invasive approaches have also been applied for cardiac myxomas resection, such as right parasternal or partial sternotomy with standard cardioplegic techniques [14], right submammary port-access method with antegrade cardioplegia and ascending aortic balloon occlusion [15] or right submammary incision with femoro-femoral bypass and nonclamped ventricular fibrillation [16]. In general terms, video-assisted resection by using these approaches has been successfully described, providing satisfactory exposure for atrial and ventricular myxomas [17-19].

Nevertheless, endoscopic instrumentation (with four degrees of freedom) reduces the dexterity needed for delicate cardiac surgical procedures, along with the loss of depth perception by using two-dimensional viewing systems. Robotic technology provides a solution to these problems and it has been born to facilitate cardiac procedures, initially by providing enhanced endoscopic camera control and in the recent decade, by allowing the manipulation of surgical instruments through thoracoscopic port incisions.

In 2001, Torracca et al [20] first reported a series of atrial septal defect closure using robotic device in Europe and, in the last decade, surgical telemanipulation systems have expanded to coronary revascularization, left ventricular lead implantation, congenital heart surgery, valvular surgery, arrhythmia procedures (Cox-Maze III) and cardiac tumors. The American Heart Association identified robotic surgery as one of the top 10 research advancements of 2002 [21].

The first group of robots consisted of assisting tools that were used for holding and positioning the endoscope during surgery, such as the robot AESOP (Automatic Endoscopic System for Optimal Positioning; Computer Motion Inc, Goleta, CA) [22], although cardiac procedures have not obtained any relevant benefit from this system.

The second group comprises surgical telemanipulation systems, which are under the control of a surgeon who works at the console. The development of telemanipulation systems was performed in the late 1980s: the da Vinci Surgical System (Intuitive Surgical Inc, Sunnyvale, CA) and the ZEUS robotic system (Computer Motion Inc, Goleta, CA) [23]. In 2003, Intuitive Surgical and Computer Motion agreed to merge and the ZEUS system was phased out in favor of the da Vinci system.

The advantages of the da Vinci system include 3D-viewing system, the robotic wrist and it can provide up four robotic arms. These characteristics seems to be more advantageous in mammary artery harvesting for coronary artery bypass grafting, but are also interesting features for a number of cardiac procedures, such as atrial myxomas excision.

The initial experience with robot-assisted excision of left atrial myxomas has been reported using the da Vinci Surgical System and it is the most widely used for cardiac procedures. It comprises three components: a surgeon's console, an instrument cart (including two robotic operating arms with a diameter of 11 mm, their articulating instruments, the camera arm and an optional fourth arm) and a 3D-visioning platform for enabling natural depth perception with high-power magnification. The surgeon is seated in front of the computer console and operates the robotic arms while viewing the surgical field in 3D-image. The finger and wrist movements are registered digitally and the dual master controls translate them to the operation being performed on the patient with the surgical robotic arms, allowing various types of movements including rotating, sliding and squeezing. "Wrist-like" instrument articulation emulates the surgeon's actions at the tissue level, and dexterity becomes enhanced through combined tremor suppression and motion scaling. It minimizes opportunities for human error when compared with traditional approaches.

3. Application area

As mentioned above, robotic-assisted cardiac surgery using the da Vinci Surgical System has allowed performing selected coronary artery bypass surgery, mitral valve repair or replacement, atrial and ventricular septal defect repairs [24-25] and most recent totally endoscopic removal of atrial myxomas. Isolated cases of removal of uncommon cardiac tumors using robotic techniques have also been reported, such as aortic valve papillary fibroelastoma, with excellent results [26].

The first successful application of robotic technology for totally resection of left atrial myxoma with da Vinci Surgical System was reported in 2005 by Murphy and associates [27], through transeptal and left atrial approaches. In 2008, at Beijing (China), Changqing Gao et al reported a new successful resection of left atrial myxoma by using this technology [28]. To date, approximately 30 cases of cardiac myxomas excision under robotic assistance have been described [28-29] and this author have reported the largest single institution series of robotic resection of left atrial myxomas, with 19 consecutive patients undergoing this procedure with no operative deaths or strokes [30] and follow-up echocardiograms up to 18 months noted no recurrence or atrial septal defect.

To minimize patient risk in this setting, cardiac surgeons should have previous experimental training in robotic techniques (in vivo animal laboratory work and human cadavers can be used) and they must demonstrate clinical proficiency to operate the robotic equipment per FDA (Food and Drug Association) approved company testing.

4. Surgical procedure

4.1. Anesthetic considerations

Some anesthetic considerations must be done. Cardiac anesthesiologists must be trained in order to recognize potential complications and challenges posed by the use of robotic systems, such as long surgical times or problems with single-lung ventilation. Management of TEE and minimally invasive percutaneous CPB management are also desirable for the anesthesiology team.

Patient monitoring consisted of standard electrocardiography, oxygen saturation, end-tidal CO_2, bispectral index, urine output and nasopharyngeal and bladder temperatures. Arterial blood gas analysis for acid-base status, oxygen and CO_2 arterial pressures, hematocrit, haemoglobin, potassium and ionized calcium is performed during the procedure as needed.

TEE is a valuable adjunct in robotic cardiac surgery. During establishment of peripheral CPB, TEE is used to guide placement of the cannulas in the inferior and superior venae cavae and ascending aorta. When the midesophageal bicaval view (80-110º) is obtained, the venous cannula must be identified as two parallel lines surrounding the fluid-filled lumen. As example, the midesophageal aortic valve long-axis view (120-160º) can be obtained to assess the placement of the endoclamp for aortic occlusion when it is used.

After weaning from CPB, TEE is also used to evaluate the completeness of air removal. TEE identifies patients at risk for significant complications before they leave the operating room [31].

Other special anesthetic considerations required for robotic cardiac surgery, in order to maintain stable hemodynamic and oxygenation, are single-lung ventilation and carbon dioxide insufflation [32]. It may reduce cardiac output and result in hypercapnia and hypoxia. These characteristics are especially relevant for patients with chronic obstructive pulmonary disease because of the creation of a transpulmonary shunt through the collapsed lung, worsening arterial oxygenation.

An active communication between anesthesiologist and surgeon is key to ensure the success, timely execution and safety of cardiac robotic surgery.

4.2. Surgical approach

Robotic resection of left atrial myxomas is considered a good right-sided atrial approach with excellent visibility, which includes an adequate exposure of the attachment point of the tumor, excision of tissue margins and debridement, meticulous removal without fragmentation and a careful examination of intracardiac chambers. To date, robotic enhancement has been used to perform portions of intracardiac procedures via thoracotomy incisions as well as the application of this technology for totally endoscopic open heart surgery. For removal of left atrial myxomas, both approaches have been reported.

In first place, robotic arm placement and specialized equipment must be reviewed with the operating room staff.

Then, the patient is anesthetized and intubated with a dual-lumen endotracheal tube, allowing single left-lung ventilation; the lung needs to be deflated on the side of the chest that the robot is entering so visualization of the heart is not obstructed. Arterial pressure monitoring line and central venous catheter are inserted and transesophageal echocardiographic (TEE) study is performed. If an endoclamp for aortic occlusion is used, bilateral radial arterial catheters are required to monitor correctly balloon placement.

As there is limited access to the heart for direct defibrillation, external defibrillator pads are required.

The patient is positioned with the right chest elevated 30°–45° and the right arm positioned along the right side. This position permits direct access to the thoracic cavity and decreases the risk for brachial plexophaty. Patient positioning is of fundamental importance in decreasing patient-robot conflict during surgery, defined as a limitation in the free movement of the robot's telemanipulated arms by interference with the patient's body.

Percutaneous cannula (15-17 F) is inserted through the right internal jugular vein for drainage from superior cava vein under TEE assistance *(Figure 1)*.

After sterile preparation and draping the patient, a transverse right groin incision is made and femoral artery and vein are dissected and prepared for cannulation *(Figure 2)*.

When totally robotic resection of left atrial myxoma is performed [28], the da Vinci endoscope is inserted through a 12-15 mm port in the fourth intercostal space (ICS), approximately 2-cm lateral to the midclavicular line. The camera is then introduced through the endoscope port into the pleural space and a small working port (2 cm) is created in the same ICS upward from the camera port.

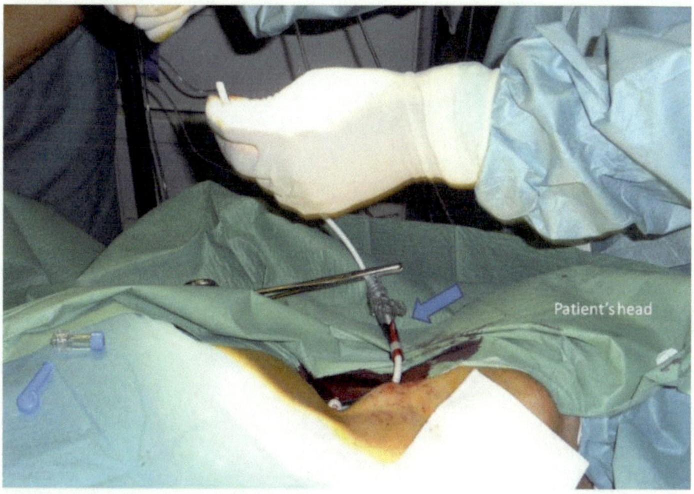

Figure 1. Percutaneous cannula through the right internal jugular vein. This venous cannula is advanced into the right atrium.

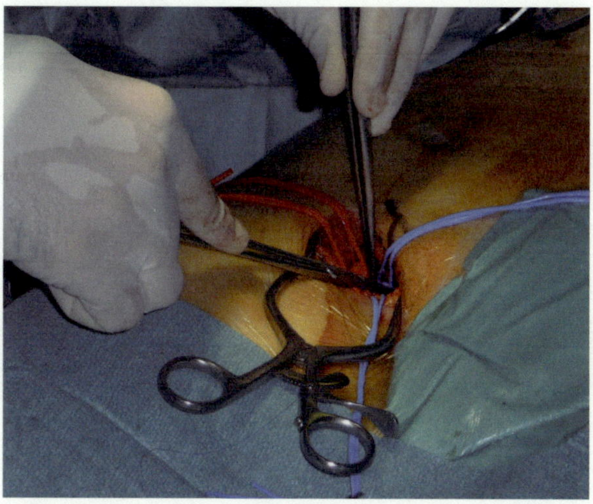

Figure 2. The common femoral artery and femoral vein are dissected free from the surrounding structures. Both are dissected circumferentially and vessel-loops are placed for bleeding control.

Then, the da Vinci instrument arms are inserted in their respective ports through three 1-cm trocar incisions in the right side (anterior axillary line): the right instrument arm is positioned 5 cm lateral to the working port in the 6th ICS; the left arm, medial and cephalad to the right arm in the 2nd or 3rd ICS; and the fourth arm trocar is placed in the midclavicular line in the 5th ICS (to achieve an optimal interatrial exposure). For this approach, no rib-spreading retractor is necessary.

In selected cases, this approach can be modified and removal of giant left atrial myxomas is performed via thoracotomy incision under robotic assistance *(Figure 3)*.

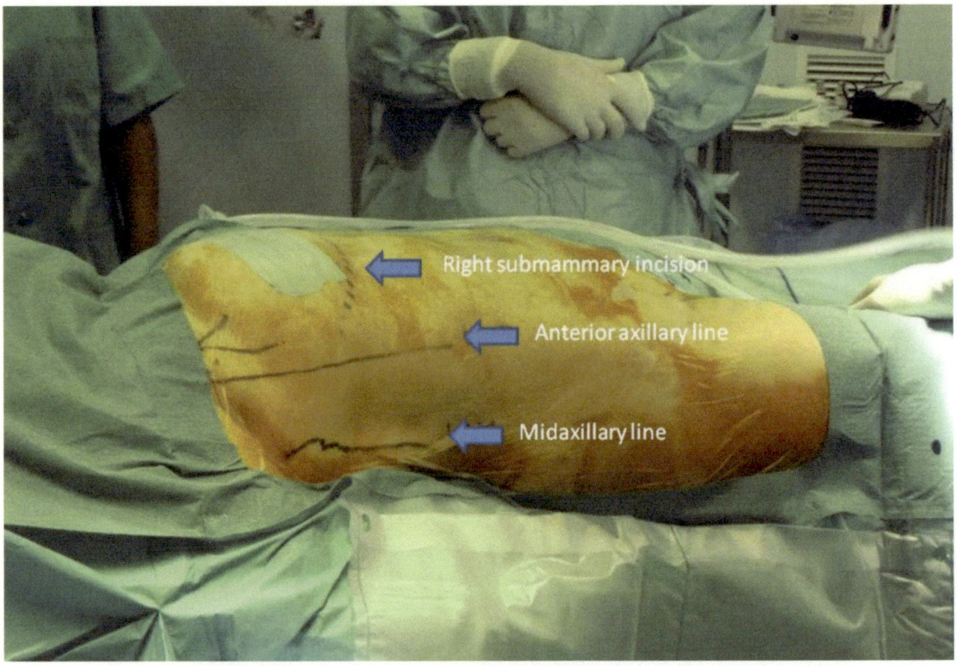

Figure 3. Positioning of the patient when anterolateral thoracotomy under robotic assistance is the selected approach.

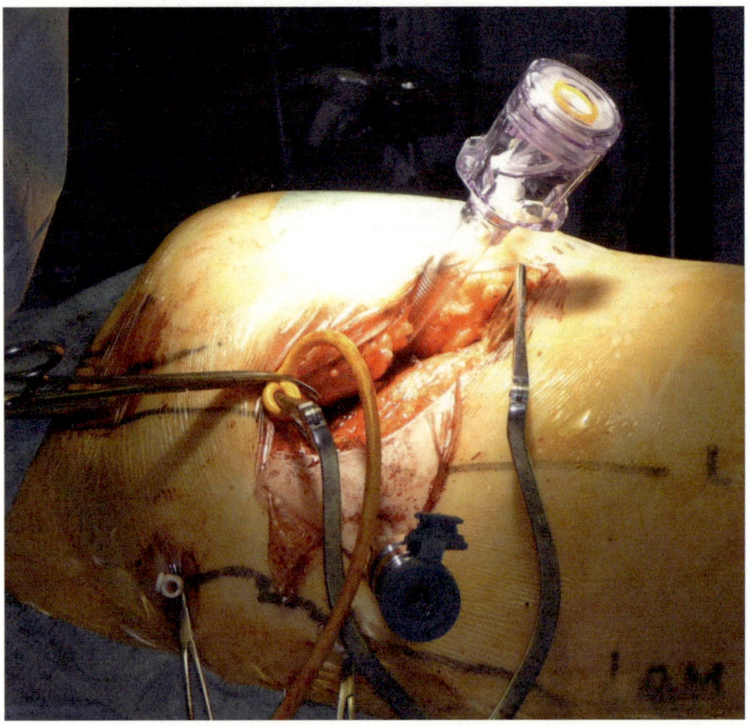

Figure 4. Anterolateral thoracotomy. The da Vinci endoscope is introduced through the incision.

For these cases, a right submammary skin incision (about 9-10 cm) is made with the aim of reaching the chest wall, retractor is used and the camera is then introduced *(Figure 4)*. This camera port and the working port can be fused together to be a new work-port for the intracardiac procedure.

For both approaches, after port insertion, the entire operation (including pericardiotomy, atriotomy and myxoma excision) are performed with robotic assistance.

After the selected approach has been initiated, the patient is heparinized and peripheral cannulation is performed as previously described for minimally invasive cardiac surgery [33] (bicaval venous drainage through the jugular and femoral cannulas along with arterial perfusion through femoral cannula placed into the ascending aorta). The sizes of the cannulas are determined by the patient's body surface area and circulatory requirements. Cannulas are inserted over the Seldinger guidewire, are confirmed to be in the correct placement by TEE and the guidewire is then removed.

After the da Vinci endoscope and instrument arms have been inserted *(Figure 5)*, pleural adhesions are rule out, the right pleural space is insufflated with carbon dioxide to create working space (intrapleural pressure of 5 to 10 mm Hg) and, via 4 port incisions and a working port, this procedure can be completed with a 30° angled endoscope facing upward with the da Vinci Surgical System.

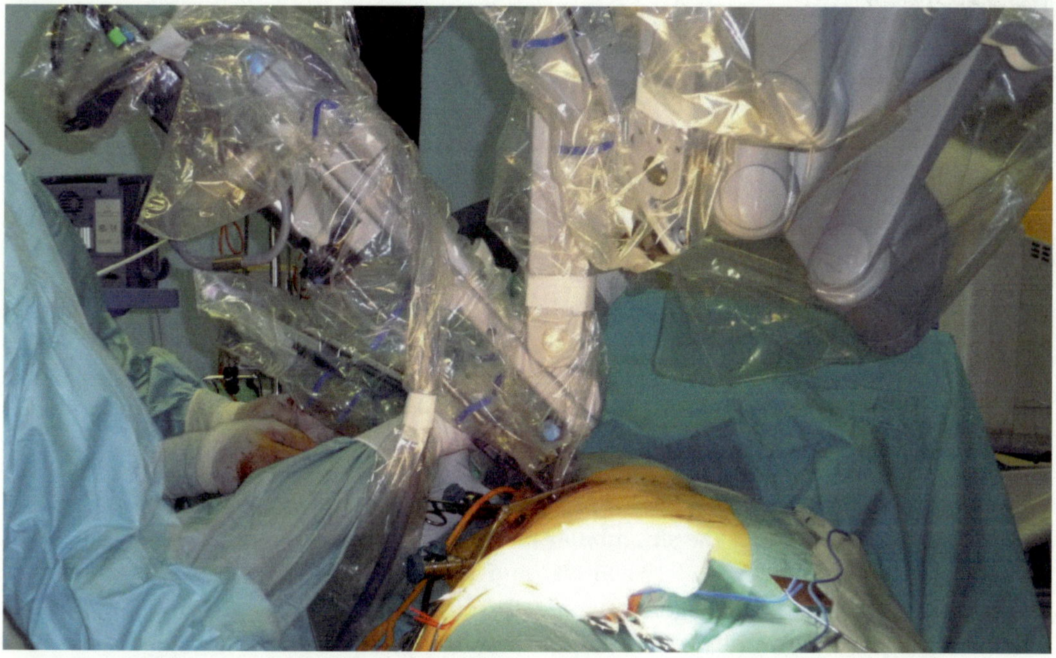

Figure 5. View of the da Vinci robotic system's arms positioned in the patient's chest, for robotic assistance when a thoracotomy incision has been made.

The operating surgeon is positioned at the operative console and begins the intrathoracic portion of the operation by controlling the robotic camera and surgical instrument arms. The patient-side assistant changes instruments, supplies and retrieves operative materials.

The pericardium is opened with direct visualization of the phrenic nerve (3-4 cm anterior to the nerve) and it is excised (for a possible atrial septal reconstruction). Traction sutures are placed low on the pericardium on the right side (usually three sutures are necessary for better visualization of the septal rim of the left atriotomy). This maneuver enables an optimal exposure of the left atrium.

The venae cavae are encircled with linen tapes and caval snares are placed using a long-tip forceps and passed out of the working port. Total CPB is started. Usually, CPB is established at 26 °C through peripheral vessels, using femoral arterial inflow and kinetic venous drainage through a femoral (21–23 Fr) and right internal jugular vein (15-17 Fr) cannula.

The management of extracorporeal circulation for robotically assisted cardiac surgery has suffered modifications from the standard procedures. As mentioned above, for most of the patients, extracorporeal circulation is established through a femoral arterial cannula, femoral venous cannula and right internal jugular venous cannula, with vacuum-assisted venous drainage and continuous blood gas monitoring. The femoral artery needs to be able to fit this cannula and provide adequate flow. A learning curve of perfusion technique is necessary for the establishment of this type of extracorporeal circulation system and adequate communication between the surgical team is essential.

There are different venous cannulas for peripheral cannulation in robotic surgery, such as 25 F Quickdraw (Edwards LifeSciences, CA, USA) or 21-23 F cannula (Medtronic, Inc, Minneapolis, Minnesota, USA). For arterial cannulation, different cannulas can be used. For endoaortic clamp, a 21-23 F EndoReturn cannula (Edwards LifeSciences, Irvine, CA, USA) is available. Any standard femoral access cannula may be used if cross-clamping is going to be achived. Finally, a remote access perfusion cannula has been developed to avoid both retrograde perfusion and cross-clamping (RAP Cannula, Estech Inc., Danville, CA, USA).

Aortic occlusion can be performed with a transthoracic cross-clamp, such as Chitwood (Scanlan International, Minneapolis, Minnesota, USA) developed by Chitwood, Elbeery and Moran [34], which enables central aortic occlusion without the use of an intra-aortic balloon. It is inserted through the 3rd or 4th ICS in the midaxillary line and is applied across the aorta. It is usually used for patients in whom use of endoaortic occlusion balloon is not indicated due to extensive calcification or tortuosity of aorto-iliac axis or aneurysmal disease.

When endoaortic clamping is going to be achieved, the aortic balloon is positioned in the ascending aorta (1 cm above the sinotubular junction) by TEE assistance. The aortic balloon is then inflated to a pressure of 250 to 300 mm Hg. The myocardium is protected with antegrade cold blood cardioplegia delivered through the distal lumen of the balloon, or directly through the second ICS working port with a 14 F angiocatheter if cross-clamping is used. Then, the heart is arrested. Repeat doses can be given when necessary during the procedure. Currently, the cardioplegia cannulas used in this setting are the dual-lumen antegrade cardioplegia cannula (Medtronic DLP, Minneapolis, MN), allowing for the simultaneous delivery of cardioplegia and aspiration of the aorta and left heart; or the RAP cannula (Estech, Inc, Danville, CA) mentioned above.

De-airing is ensured through the same angiocatheter for cardioplegia or with a left vent across the mitral valve.

When left atrial myxomas are attached to the interatrial septum, exploration can be achieved through an oblique right atriotomy for an optimal exposure of the atrial septum [27] and, when the point of attachment has been identified, the incision can be made in the septum (medial to the fossa ovalis) and it is extended 360º around the myxoma attachment following the entering to the left atrium. For this approach, margins of normal septal tissue must be maintained.

A left atriotomy through Sondergaard's groove (anterior to the pulmonary veins) has been also described for patients with tumor attachment to the posterior left atrial wall. Traction sutures can be placed at the left atriotomy and pulled upward, or and atrial retractor (Estech, Inc., Danville, CA, USA) can be used for achieving an optimal operative field.

For selected cases, an atrial EndoWrist retractor (Intuitive Surgical, Inc, CA) is placed through the fourth robotic arm for an adequate exploration of the atrial myxoma. This dynamic robotic atrial retractor makes the right side of the heart to rotate up and the left side to rotate down and, along with the magnification provided by the robotic optical system, enhances the exposure and visualization in the left atrium.

Then, excision can be achieved by dissecting a plane at the point of attachment and atrial septum is maintained. Calcified areas and adherences must be identified. When atrial myxomas are located in the right atrium, they can be completely resected from the beating heart with the superior and inferior venae cavae snared.

Resection of full-thickness wall or only an endocardial attachment is controversial, although a partial thickness resection of the area of tumor attachment when anatomically is necessary has been reported, without an increase in recurrence rate [35]. The base of the myxomas can also be cauterized to prevent recurrence when, despite to be anatomically necessary, it has not been completely resected.

Because myxomas are generally very friable, their removal through a small working port is an important step during the robotic procedure. Endoscopic specimen baskets have been developed and are routinely used for laparoscopic procedures with good results and its use to catch and remove atrial myxomas has demonstrated to be safe and without risk for the patient when a video-assisted myxoma excision is performed [17]. For robotic procedures, the tumor is removed and grasped by the tissue margins and is extracted using an Endopouch bag (Ethicon Endo-Surgery, Cincinnati, Ohio) through the service port without fragmentation in the pleural space.

A vacuum-extractor device has also been reported for this procedure [36], allowing the extraction of giant left atrial myxomas. The components for this device are the top of a plastic bottle of fluid serum (of 3-5 cm in diameter) connected to a flexible tube with a suction device. It is introduced and placed without aspiration through a thoracotomy incision, facilitated with the robotic magnification, and once the tumor is reached, it is removed with vacuum-traction under active aspiration *(Figure 6)*. This device allows the manipulation and a complete removal of the tumor, even if it is friable.

The interatrial septum can be removed with the tumor, but it seems to be indicated only in high-risk patients. When an atrial wall defect is created after excision (usually at the septum), it is repaired using the principles learned from endoscopic atrial septal defect repair. It can be repaired primarily by a running suture in the most of cases or by patch closure using autologous or bovine pericardium. After resection, empty left atrial and left ventricular chambers inspection is accomplished with the da Vinci endoscope.

The entire procedure can be performed with the da Vinci Surgical System, including left atrial closure with running suture, although the left atrium can be closed under direct vision to decrease operative times for selected patients.

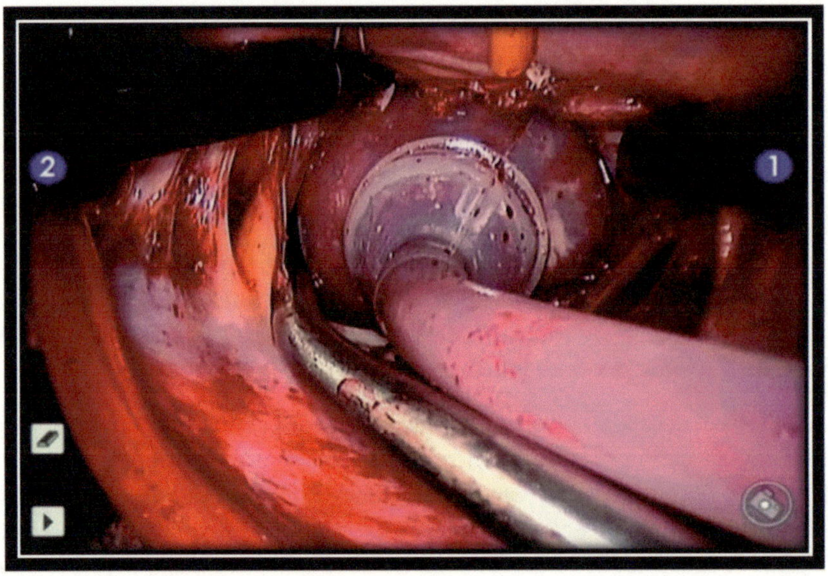

Figure 6. Resection of a giant atrial myxoma through a left atrial approach using the da Vinci Surgical System. Vacuum-extractor into the left atrium (viewing from the console's surgeon).

After de-airing, aortic cross-clamp is deflated and removed. TEE is used for proving the absence of tumor in cardiac chambers, adequate removal of air as well as residual atrial septal defect or mitral regurgitation *(Figure 7)*. Then, the patient is rewarmed and weaned from CPB.

Protamine is given and the femoral vessels are repaired once off CPB and the groin incision is closed. When cardioplegia has been infused through the second ICS, the site can be closed with extracorporeal knot tying through the working port and surgical close of the chest wall may be performed in the standard fashion.

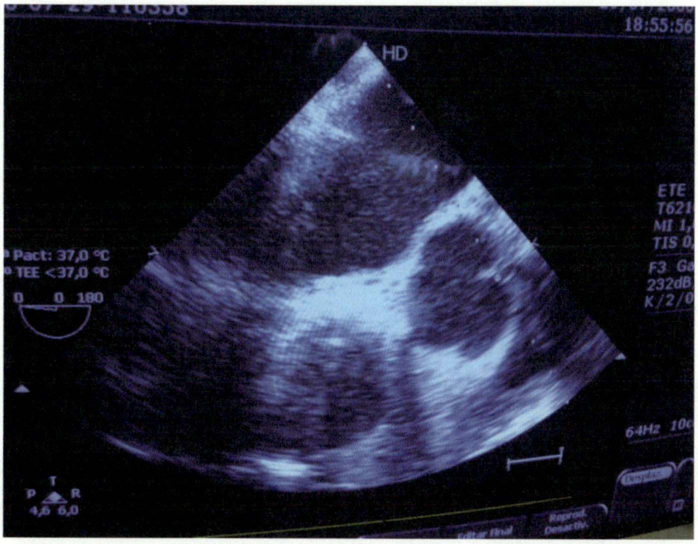

Figure 7. TEE allows for an exhaustive inspection the cardiac chambers after removal of the atrial myxoma.

In most of patients, temporary cardiac pacing wires are not routinely required. When this step is required, it must be performed previously to removal of aortic clamp. The chest tube (or Blake drain, depending on institution) is placed in an existing intercostals porthole and they are usually left in the pericardium and in the right pleural space. The double-lumen endobronchial tube can be changed to a single-lumen tube. In selected cases, the patient can be extubated in the operating room or shortly upon arrival to the intensive care unit.

5. Results

5.1. Current results

In general terms, although experience is limited, surgical results at a relatively large number of centres worldwide are optimal and this technology is of reproducible value with excellent cosmetic results. Despite successful cases reported of robotic-assisted excision of left atrial myxomas, most surgeons continue to use a median sternotomy approach.

An endoscopic approach to left atrial myxomas is appropriate only when the exposure of the attachment point of the tumor is optimal, excision of adequate tissue margins, removal with no fragmentation, reconstruction of atrial wall defects and an exhaustive inspection the cardiac chambers after removal of the atrial myxoma. These surgical tenets are achieved with the robotic technology.

Cross-clamp and perfusion times are longer under robotic assistance compared with conventional surgery [37-38], although a longer CPB time has not demonstrated any negative impact on operative and postoperative outcomes.

Increased total operative and cross-clamp times have been demonstrated for the endoaortic balloon versus the transthoracic clamp for valve surgery [39], but there are no studies for left atrial myxoma excision.

Learning curve can be long and minimally invasive surgery experience is desirable. The learning curve has demonstrated a progressive decline in cross-clamp, CPB, and overall operative times [40].

The perioperative results are similar to those obtained using traditional approaches and no serious complications during the robotic procedure have been reported in this setting. Necessity of conversion to sternotomy due to robotic system malfunction has not been described and to date, no operative mortality or neurologic complications have been observed [30].

The long incision in the midline of the chest, the risk of bleeding and infection and the relatively long recovery time after surgery seem to be avoided with robotic cardiac surgery. Usually, these patients benefit from low blood transfusion rate.

Intensive care unit stay duration is reduced in several studies [41-42]. Moreover, the patients are usually ready to be discharged on the third or fourth postoperative day and patient education regarding to sternotomy precautions is not needed for totally endoscopic cardiac surgery. Most patients can return to work in two or three weeks. Excellent quality of life has been demonstrated and, after discharge, these patients must be scheduled for a follow-up echocardiogram to rule out any recurrence of the myxoma.

Mid-term follow-up comparative studies between conventional and robotic surgery for removal of atrial myxomas are not yet available and data that include mid- and long-term follow-up are required.

5.2. Pitfalls and complications

It is important to keep in mind the potential complications for robotic extraction of left atrial myxomas. The working ports are only 2-2.5 cm in length and, during tumor resection through these small incisions, care must be taken to excise the mass entirely, given the friability of myxomas. Any fragment dropped during removal creates a high risk of systemic embolization and stroke [43]. When a left atrial approach is used, a "non-touch" technique (not possible with a conventional biatrial approach) is achieved, decreasing the risk for fragmentation of the tumor.

Vascular injuries from peripheral cannulation include arterial occlusion or aortic dissection (although extremely rare, but devastating).

In general terms, cardiac surgeons must be prepared to convert to a lateral thoracotomy or full sternotomy in case of unsuccessful result or emergency during the robotic procedure. For this reason, they must plan the alternative surgical procedure and choose the optimal access in advance.

5.3. Limitations

The early clinical experience with computer-enhanced telemanipulation systems has defined many of the limitations of this approach despite rapid procedural success. Limitations can include an incomplete and delayed motion tracking, although this limitation might negatively affect the quality of an anastomosis in beating-heart surgery, such as coronary artery bypass grafting [44], and it does not seem relevant for intra-cardiac tumor resection. Lack of tactile feedback has demonstrated to be also a limitation: the visual force feedback primarily benefits inexperienced robot-assisted surgeons, with diminishing benefits among experienced surgeons [45].

The operation is demanding, expensive and it is only suitable for a selected patient population, but elevated costs of instruments and maintenance may be justified by a speed of recovery and reduction in hospital stay [46]. It is necessary to determine the cost of these systems by virtue of their measured benefits.

Longer operative times and learning curve, above mentioned, are due to the complexity of the system and because of this reason, this technology must be concentrated in a few reference centres with a high volume and expertise cardiac surgeons.

6. Further research

To date, literature about feasibility of robotic resection of left atrial myxomas is focused on small series or isolated case reports, and the world experience is mostly retrospective and noncontrolled.

There are no randomized studies comparing robotic to either video-assisted or sternotomy or thoracotomy left atrial myxoma excision and, although it is generally believed that patient morbidity is significantly reduced with this minimally invasive approach, further studies are needed to support this hypothesis. Despite early procedural success, future refinements in these devices such as "haptic" technology, which provide tactile and resistance feedback to the surgeon, are needed to apply this new technology more widely in this era of cardiac surgery.

The results of robotic procedures should be at least equivalent to those of conventional methods and the time required should be comparable to conventional surgery. Long-term results are needed to determine whether robotic technology could become a new standard in cardiac tumors excision.

7. Conclusion

Computer-aided robotic surgical technology is a safe procedure and can be used to perform open-heart procedures such as atrial myxomas excision with a totally endoscopic approach.

Atrial myxoma resection using surgical telemanipulation systems such as the da Vinci Surgical System have achieved excellent results and provide an attractive cosmetic advantage over traditional approaches.

Adults with atrial myxomas are a small but constant and growing population of patients who can benefit of this minimally invasive approach.

Decreased postoperative pain and recovery times along with improved cosmetic results are the main benefits for this approach.

Further research is necessary to demonstrate the reproducible value for this technology in patients with cardiac tumors on a larger scale.

Author details

José Francisco Valderrama Marcos, María Teresa González López
and Julio Gutiérrez de Loma
Cardiovascular Surgery Department, Carlos Haya Regional Hospital, Málaga, Spain

8. References

[1] Larsson S, Lepore V, Kennergren C. Atrial myxomas: results of 25 years' experience and review of literature. Surgery 1989;105:695-8.
[2] Stajevic MS, Vukomanovic VA, Kuburovic VD, Djuricic SM. Early recurrent left atrial myxoma in a teenager with the novo mutation of Carney complex. Indian J Hum Genet 2011;17:108-10.
[3] Hou YC, Chang S, Lo HM, Hsiao CH, Lin FY. Recurent cardiac myxoma with multiple distant metastasis and malignant change. J Formos Med Assoc 2001;100:63-5.
[4] Rendón F, Agosti J, Llorente A, Rodrigo D, Montes K. Intramural cardiac myxoma in left ventricular wall: an unusual location. Asian Cardiovasc Thorac Ann 2002;10:170-2.
[5] Van Gelder HM, O'Brien DJ, Staples ED, Alexander JA. Familial cardiac myxoma. Ann Thorac Surg 1992;53:419–24.
[6] Selkane C, Amahzoune B, Chavanis N. Changing management of cardiac myxoma based on a series of 40 cases with long-term follow-up. Ann Thorac Surg 2003;76:1935-1938.
[7] Bjessmo S, Ivert T. Cardiac myxoma: 40 years' experience in 63 patients. Ann Thorac Surg 1997;63:697-700.
[8] Meyns B, Vancleemput J, Flameng W, Daenen W. Surgery for cardiac myxoma: a 20-year experience with long-term follow-up. Eur J Cardiothorac Surg 1993;7:437–40.
[9] Rodríguez E, Chitwood WR. Robotics in cardiac surgery. Scand J Surg 2009;98:120-4.
[10] Arom K, Emery R, Kshettry V, Janey P. Comparison between port-access and less invasive valve surgery. Ann Thorac Surg 1999;68:1525-1528.
[11] Navia J, Cosgrove D. Minimally invasive mitral valve operations. Ann Thorac Surg 1996;62:1542-1544.
[12] Carpentier A, Loulmet D. Open heart operation under videosurgery and minithoracotomy. First case (mitral valvuloplasty) operated with success. C R Acad Sci III 1996;319:219-223.

[13] Mohr FW, Falk V, Diegeler A. Minimally invasive port-access mitral valve surgery. J Thorac Cardiovasc Surg 1998;115:567-571.

[14] Ravikumar E, Pawar N, Gnanamuthu R, Sundar P, Cherian M, Thomas S. Minimal access approach for surgical management of cardiac tumors. Ann Thorac Surg 2000;70:1077-9.

[15] Gulbins h, Reichenspurner H, Wintersperger BJ. Minimally invasive extirpation of a left ventricular myxoma. J Thorac Cardiovasc Surg 1999;47:129-30.

[16] Ko PJ, Chang CH, Lin PJ, Chu JJ, Tsai FC, Hsueh C. Video-assisted minimal access in excision of left atrial myxoma. Ann Thorac Surg 1998;66:1301-5.

[17] Panos A, Myers PO. Video-assisted cardiac myxoma resection: basket technique for complete and safe removal from the heart. Ann Thorac Surg 2012;93:109-10.

[18] Greco E, Mestres CA, Castañá R. Video-assisted cardioscopy for removal of primary left ventricular myxoma. Eur J Cardiothorac Surg 1999;16:677-678.

[19] Li JY, Lin FY, Hsu RB, Chu SH. Video-assisted cardioscopic resection of recurrent left ventricular myxoma. J Thorac Cardiovasc Surg 1996;112:1673-74.

[20] Torracca L, Ismeno G, Alfieri O. Totally endoscopic computer-enhanced arterial septal defect closure in six patients. Ann Thorac Surg 2001;72:1354-1357.

[21] 2002 Heart and Stroke Statistical Update. Dallas, Tex: American Heart Association 2002.

[22] Jacobs LK, Shayani V, Sackier JM. Determination of the learning curve of the AESOP robot. Surg Endosc 1997;11:54-5.

[23] Pugin F, Bucher P, Morel P. History of robotic surgery: from AESOP and ZEUS to da Vinci. J Visc Surg 2011;148:3-8.

[24] Gao C, Yang M, Wang G, Xiao C, Wang J, Zhao Y. Totally endoscopic robotic ventricular septal defect repair in the adult. J Thorac Cardiovasc Surg 2012;[in press].

[25] Argenziano M, Oz MC, Kohmoto T, Morgan J, Dimitui J, Mongero L. Totally endoscopic atrial septal defect repair with robotic assistance. Circulation 2003;108:191-4.

[26] Woo YJ, Grand TJ, Weiss SJ. Robotic resection of an aortic valve papillary fibroelastoma. Ann Thorac Surg 2005;80:1100-1102.

[27] Murphy DA, Miller JS, Langford DA. Robot-assisted endoscopic excision of left atrial myxomas. J Thorac Cardiovasc Surg 2005;130:596-7.

[28] Gao C, Yang M, Wang G, Wang J. Totally robotic resection of myxoma and atrial septal defect repair. Interact Cardiovasc Thorac Surg 2008;7:947-950.

[29] Hassan M, Smith JM. Robotic assisted excision of a left ventricular myxoma. Interact Cardiovasc Thorac Surg 2012;14:113-114.

[30] Gao C, Yang M, Wang G et al. Excision of atrial myxoma using robotic technology. J Thorac Cardiovasc Surg 2010;139:1282-1285.

[31] Wang Yao, Gao C, Wang J, Yang M. The role of intraoperative transesophageal echocardiography in robotic mitral valve repair. Echocardiography 2011;28:85-91.

[32] Wang G, Gao C, Zhou Q, Chen T, Wang Y, Li J. Anesthesia management of totally endoscopic atrial septal defect repair with robotic surgical system. J Clin Anesth 2011;23:621-625.

[33] Grossi EA, Galloway AC, LaPietra A et al. Minimally invasive mitral valve surgery: a 6-year experience with 714 patients.

[34] Chitwood WR, Elbeery JR, Moran JM. Minimally invasive mitral valve repair; using a mini-thoracotomy and transthoracic aortic occlusion. Ann Thorac Surg 1997;62:1477-9.
[35] Actis Dato GM, De Benedictus M, Actis Dato A, Ricci A, Sommarival L, De Paulis R. Long-term follow-up of cardiac myxoma (7-31 years). J Cardiovasc Thorac Surg (Torino) 1993;34:41-3.
[36] Gutiérrez de Loma J, Valderrama Marcos J.F, Melero Tejedor J.M, González González S. Left atrial myxoma: extraction by robotic and vacuum assistance. Innovations 2009;4:351-353.
[37] Falk V, Diegeler A, Walther T. Developments in robotic cardiac surgery. Curr Opin Cardiol 2000;15:378-387.
[38] Autschbach R, Onnasch JF, Falk V. The Leipzig experience with robotic valve surgery. J Card Surg 2000;15:82-87.
[39] Reichenspurner H, Detter C, Deuse T. Video and robotic-assisted minimally invasive mitral valve surgery: a comparison of the port-access and transthoracic clamp techniques. Ann Thorac Surg 2005;79:485-490.
[40] Bonaros N, Schachner T, Oehlinger A, Ruetzler E, Kolbitsch C. Robotically assisted totally endoscopic atrial septal defect repair: insights from operative times, learning curves and clinical outcome. Ann Thorac Surg 2006;82:687-93.
[41] Chitwood WR. Video-assisted and robotic mitral valve surgery. Semin Thorac Cardiovasc Surg 1999;11:194-205.
[42] Reichenspurner H, Boehm D, Reichart B. Minimally invasive mitral valve surgery using three-dimensional video and robotic assistance. Semin Thorac Cardiovasc Surg 1999;11:235-243.
[43] Disesa VJ, Collins JJ, Cohn LH. Considerations in the surgical management of left atrial myxoma. J Card Surg 1988;3:15-22.
[44] Modi P, Rodríguez E, Chitwood R. Robot-assisted cardiac surgery. Interact Cardiovasc Thorac Surg 2009;9:500-505.
[45] Reiley CE, Akinbiyi T, Burschka D, Chang DC, Okamura AM, Yuh DD. Effects of visual force feedback on robot-assisted surgical task performance. J Thorac Cardiovasc Surg 2008;135:196-202.
[46] Morgan JA, Thornton BA, Peacock JC, Hollingsworth KW, Smith CR, Oz MC, Argenziano M. Does robotic technology make minimally invasive cardiac surgery too expensive? A hospital cost analysis of robotic and conventional techniques. J Cardiac Surg 2005;20:246-251.

Chapter 10

Thoracic Reconstruction

Christodoulos Kaoutzanis, Tiffany N.S. Ballard and Paul S. Cederna

Additional information is available at the end of the chapter

http://dx.doi.org/10.5772/54137

1. Introduction

The chest wall is a stable yet flexible structure that provides protection for the intrathoracic organs and plays an important role in respiratory function. The integrity of the chest wall can be affected by a variety of congenital conditions, pathologic processes, or traumatic injuries. The principal goals of reconstruction are to restore the functional and structural integrity of the chest wall to protect the underlying vital organs. It is also essential to consider the aesthetic outcome of the reconstruction, particularly in situations where there are no functional deformities. In every reconstruction, no matter what caused the underlying cause of the chest wall deformity, the bony thorax and the soft tissues must always be considered and addressed. Despite significant improvements in surgical techniques and perioperative care, the management of patients requiring chest wall reconstruction remains an ongoing challenge for any surgeon. Close collaboration between thoracic and reconstructive plastic surgeons is essential in obtaining optimal functional and aesthetic outcomes.

2. Anatomy of the chest wall

The skeleton of the thorax is an osseo-cartilaginous cage with a conical shape. It consists of the sternum, the clavicles, the scapulae, twelve pairs of ribs, and twelve thoracic vertebrae. The anterior surface is formed by the sternum and costal cartilages (Figure 1). Posteriorly, it is formed by the twelve thoracic vertebrae, the posterior portions of the ribs, and the paired scapulae. The ribs are separated by the intercostal spaces to form the lateral chest wall.

All twelve pairs of ribs are connected posteriorly with the vertebral column. The first seven rib pairs, which are also called "true" ribs, are secured to the sternum anteriorly through intervention of the costal cartilages. The remaining five rib pairs, which are also called "false" ribs, do not directly articulate with the sternum. Of these, the 8th, 9th and 10th ribs have confluent attachments of their cartilage with one another at the costal margin. The last two ribs are also known as "floating" ribs; they are only attached to the posterior vertebrae and remain free anteriorly. Each rib has a head, a neck and a shaft (Figure 2). The head has two facets. The superior facet is used for articulation with the upper vertebrae, whereas the inferior facet is used for articulation with its own vertebrae creating the costovertebral joint. The facet tubercle of the neck of the rib articulates with the transverse process of its own vertebra creating the costotransverse joint. The inferior aspect of the shaft encompasses the costal groove, where the intercostal vessels and nerve run.

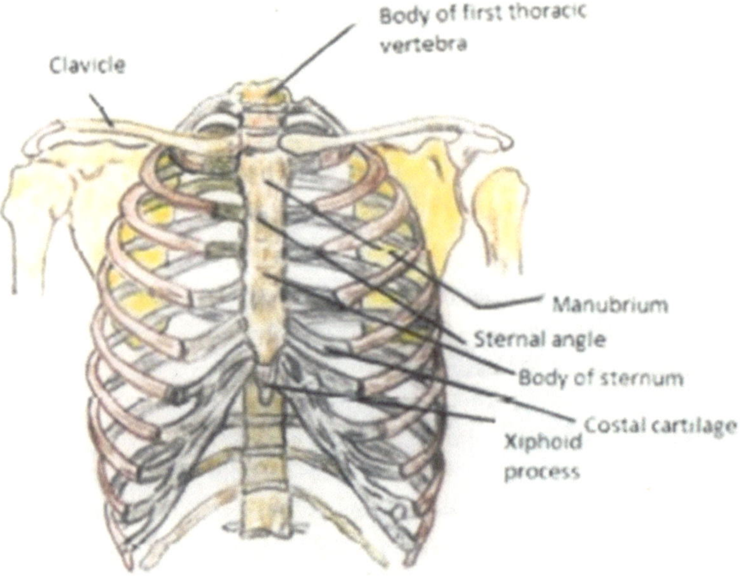

Figure 1. Anterior view of the skeleton of the thorax.

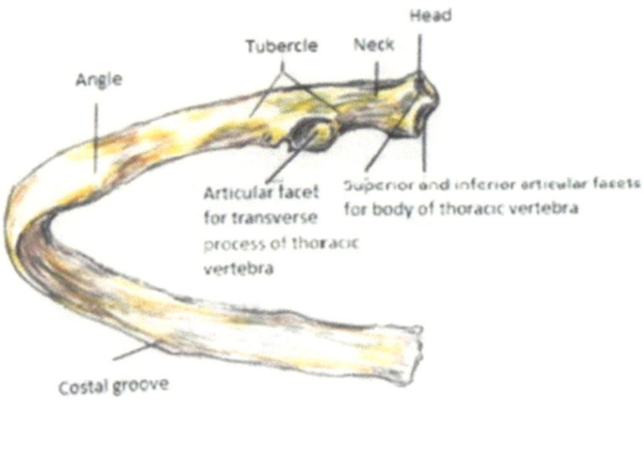

Figure 2. Posterior view of a typical rib.

The spaces between the ribs are filled by the intercostal musculature, which consists of three layers. The external intercostal muscles, with fibers oriented inferoanteriorly, extend from the tubercles of the ribs posteriorly to the costochondral articulation anteriorly. They terminate in thin membranes, the anterior intercostal membranes, which are connected medially with the sternum. The intermediate layer is formed by the internal intercostal muscles, which have fibers that are oriented superoanteriorly. The muscles extend from the sternum to the angle of the ribs posteriorly, where they are connected to the vertebral column by thin aponeuroses called the posterior intercostal membranes. The innermost intercostal muscle is the least developed layer and has fibers oriented vertically or almost parallel to those of the internal intercostal muscle. The internal intercostal muscle extends from the plane of the costochondral articulations anteriorly to the plane of the medial margin of the scapula posteriorly.

The intercostal neurovascular bundle lies beneath the internal intercostal muscles. It is comprised of intercostal arteries, veins and nerves. The anterior and posterior intercostal arteries originate from different vessels but anastomose with each other. The anterior intercostal arteries arise from the internal mammary arteries. The first two posterior intercostal arteries usually arise from the costocervical trunk, which is a branch of the subclavian artery. The remaining nine arteries are branches of the thoracic aorta. The intercostal veins are found superior to the arteries but follow the course of the arteries along the inferior aspect of each rib. They drain into the azygous, hemiazygous and accessory hemiazygous veins.

The dynamic elasticity of the bony and soft tissue components of the chest wall allow for changes in the intrathoracic cavity, hence maintaining the mechanics of ventilation. The muscles of the chest wall play a significant role in this process. The diaphragm and the intercostal muscles represent the primary muscles of respiration, whereas the serratus, pectoralis major and minor, scalenes, latissimus dorsi, trapezius, sternocleidomastoids, and deltoid muscles constitute the main secondary respiratory muscles.

During quiet respiration, inspiration occurs when the diaphragm and the external intercostal muscles contract. The diaphragm is responsible for approximately 75% of the work of breathing, and the intercostal muscles for the remaining 25%. Contraction of the diaphragm causes an increase in the vertical dimensions of the thoracic cavity, while contraction of the external intercostal muscles elevates the ribs and expands the transverse dimensions of the thorax. This reduces the intrathoracic pressure, resulting in flow of atmospheric air into the lungs. Expiration is a passive process that is facilitated by the elastic recoil of the lungs. This increases intrathoracic pressure, which in turn leads to an increase in intrapulmonary pressure above the atmospheric pressure. At that point outflow of air from the lungs occurs. The secondary muscles of respiration are used in addition to the primary respiratory muscles during periods of respiratory distress. Several chest wall muscles have been reported to facilitate inspiration including the serratus, pectoralis, scalenes, latissimus dorsi, deltoid, and trapezius. Active expiration is achieved with contraction of the internal and innermost intercostal muscles as well as the abdominal muscles.

3. Etiology of chest wall defects

Chest wall defects can be divided into acquired and congenital defects. They can involve bony structures, soft tissues, or a combination of both. Several pathological processes can contribute to the development of acquired defects such as neoplasm, infection, radiation injury, and trauma. Congenital defects, although less common and usually asymptomatic, do occasionally cause cardiopulmonary compromise and can be a reconstructive challenge.

3.1. Congenital chest wall deformities

Congenital chest wall anomalies include pectus excavatum (funnel chest), pectus carinatum (pigeon chest), Poland syndrome, asphyxiating thoracic dystrophy (Jeune syndrome), and assorted sternal anomalies such as sternal clefts and sternal hypoplasia. Pectus excavatum is the most common congenital chest wall anomaly (90 percent), followed by pectus carinatum (5 to 7 percent), cleft sternum, pentalogy of Cantrell, asphyxiating thoracic dystrophy, and spondylothoracic dysplasia [1].

Pectus excavatum is a congenital chest wall deformity of unknown etiology, which produces a concave appearance in the anterior chest wall (Figure 3). It is believed that the sternum is pushed in by abnormal growth at the articulation with the cartilage and the ribs. Two different forms of this chest wall deformity have been described. The most common form is seen as an acute posterior curve of the sternum with its deepest point just above the xiphoid process and sharp curvatures in the lower costal cartilages on each side of the sternum. The second type is characterized by a widespread superficial anomaly between the two nipples. The manubrium can be depressed, and there is usually depth asymmetry with one side being deeper than the opposite side. Other associated deformities can be observed during childhood development such as a broad thin chest lateral to the anterior pectus deformity, internally rotated and depressed shoulders, flaring of the costal margins, protuberant abdomen, kyphosis, and scoliosis.

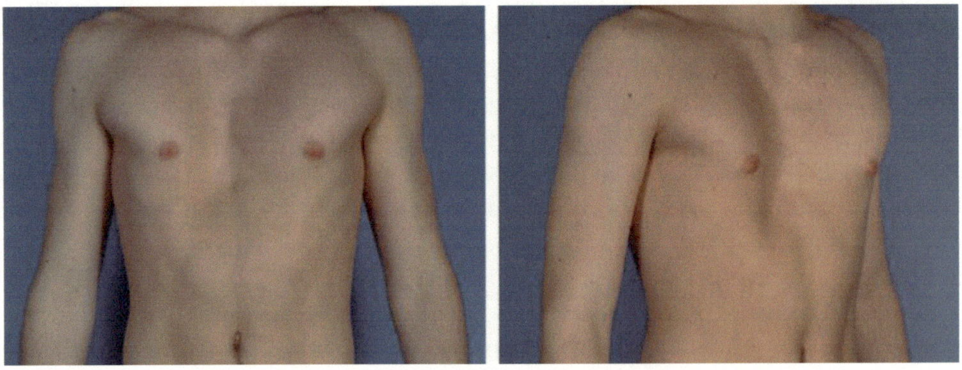

Figure 3. A 15-year-old male with a symmetric pectus excavatum deformity.

The condition is generally noticed at birth and the majority of cases are diagnosed in the first year of life. It is typically asymptomatic during early childhood unless the patient's sternal depression is unusually severe leading to cardiac or pulmonary compromise. It is not uncommon for patients to first present to the surgeon following the rapid skeletal growth of adolescence, which can worsen the pectus excavatum deformity and make the condition symptomatic. Some affected individuals develop chest and back pain, which is believed to be musculoskeletal in origin or posture related. With regard to the pulmonary function of affected individuals, there is scientific evidence to suggest that dyspnea upon exertion in patients with the deformity is predominantly due to the decrease in pulmonary reserve [2-4]. Although it has been advocated that the decrease in intrathoracic volume may be a contributing factor in the pulmonary impairment seen with the deformity, this association is difficult to prove given the wide variation of pulmonary function amongst healthy individuals, as well as the correlation of pulmonary function with body habitus and physical activity. In patients with severe pectus excavatum, the heart may be displaced into the left chest causing compression of the right ventricle and dramatic impedance of right ventricular outflow. Dr. Ravitch was one of the first to make these observations [5,6]. Several more recent studies have demonstrated improvement in the cardiac function following operative repair of the pectus deformity [7,8].

There are opposing beliefs regarding whether pectus excavatum is a predominantly cosmetic problem or a disorder that leads to significant physiologic impairment. Affected individuals frequently desire correction for aesthetic purposes. The distorted appearance of the chest, especially in young teenagers, can be very distressing resulting in problems with psychosocial well-being, emotional functioning, body image perception, and self-esteem. However, adolescent patients also often present with compression-like discomfort in the anterior chest, dyspnea on exertion, exercise-induced wheezing, palpitations, and tachycardia. The recognition of symptoms and the recommendation for surgical correction remain controversial.

Pectus carinatum represents a spectrum of anterior chest wall protrusion deformities. The classical deformity, also known as "chicken breast" or "pigeon breast" (chondrogladiolar), is characterized by anterior protrusion of the median and lower portions of the sternum associated with lower bilateral costal depression. A less common type, also known as "Pouter pigeon breast" (chondromanubrial), is seen with anterior protrusion of the manubriosternal joint with depression of the body of the sternum. There is accompanying protrusion of the second to the ninth costal cartilages, bilaterally. Lateral deformities have also been reported such as unilateral protrusion of the costal cartilages with sternal rotation about its long axis to the opposite side. Pectus carinatum is primarily a symmetrical deformity, but in about one-third of the cases, asymmetric or mixed deformities are identified.

Pectus carinatum occurs approximately one-tenth as often as pectus excavatum. Unlike pectus excavatum, it is rarely noticed at birth. It is typically identified in mid-childhood and accentuated during the rapid skeletal growth in early adolescence. Although the etiology remains unclear, a congenital component with abnormalities in connective tissue development has been postulated given the increased incidence of positive family history and associated anomalies such as Marfan's syndrome and congenital heart disease. A recent review of 260 cases with pectus carinatum revealed the presence of positive family history of chest wall deformities in at least 25% of patients [9]. Clinical manifestations of pectus carinatum are quite common and include dyspnea, exertional tachypnea, decreased endurance, and asthmatic-like symptoms [9,10]. Cardiac and hemodynamic changes have also been reported [11]. The psychosocial and aesthetic impairment associated with the deformity is one of the main reasons for patients to seek medical attention and should not be underestimated.

Poland syndrome is a severe form of chest wall and breast hypoplasia. It was first described in the 18th century but the label was not used until 1962 when Clarkson operated on a patient with similar anomalies to that described by Dr. Poland [12]. The initial description included absence of the pectoralis major and minor muscles associated with syndactyly of the ipsilateral hand [13]. Numerous other components of the syndrome have been described, and each of these components can occur with variable severity. The chest wall involvement may include hypoplasia or aplasia of the pectoralis major and minor muscles. Other components of the syndrome include absence of the anterior portions of the second to fifth ribs and associated costal cartilages, as well as hypoplasia or aplasia of the the latissimus dorsi, deltoid, infraspinatus and supraspinatus muscles. The overlying skin and subcutaneous tissue abnormalities include limited subcutaneous chest wall fat, absence of axillary hair, and hypoplasia or aplasia of the breast and nipple. The most common upper extremity abnormalities include syndactyly and brachydactyly, primarily involving the central three digits. The extent of the involvement however, can range from hypoplasia or absence of a single digit to complete agenesis of the arm. Poland syndrome may also be associated with several other anomalies such as Sprengel deformity (winging of the scapula), pectus excavatum, scoliosis, foot anomalies, dextrocardia, renal hyperplasia, and blood dyscrasias.

Most cases of Poland syndrome are sporadic, but familial patterns of inheritance have been reported [14,15]. The etiology of Poland Syndrome is unknown. The syndrome is present from birth, but because the functional disability is usually mild, patients usually present late for evaluation and treatment of the chest deformity and breast asymmetry [16]. Three main factors impact the timing and options for reconstruction: breast development, existence of a latissimus dorsi muscle, and degree of chest wall deformity.

Asphyxiating thoracic dystrophy (Jeune's syndrome) is a rare autosomal recessive disorder characterized by skeletal dysplasias, with respiratory, renal and hepatic manifestations [17-19]. It causes dwarfism with short ribs, short limbs, and characteristic radiologic changes in the ribs and pelvis. There is variability in the severity of clinical and radiologic features. The narrow, bell-shaped thorax and protuberant abdomen together with the short, horizontally placed ribs significantly restrict chest expansion and promote alveolar hypoventilation. The extent of pulmonary impairment varies from negligible to rapidly fatal. Other features include abundant and irregular costal cartilages, high transversely placed clavicles, a small hypoplastic pelvis, variable micromelia, and short digits.

Sternal cleft is an entity within the spectrum of sternal defects related to failure of ventral fusion of the sternum. It is rare and the least severe of the four main congenital chest wall anomalies. The other three groups of sternal defects include thoracic ectopia cordis, thoracoabdominal ectopia cordis, and cervical ectopia cordis.

Sternal cleft results from failure of fusion of the sternal bars that typically occurs by the eighth week of gestation. The anomaly is characterized by partial or complete separation of the sternum with a normally positioned intrathoracic heart [20]. Despite the sternal separation, skin coverage is intact with normal pericardium and diaphragm. In most infants, the deformity is asymptomatic. Occasionally, functional problems can arise such as respiratory impairment from the paradoxical movement of the sternal defect. Most affected individuals have an upper sternal cleft with a V- or U-shape appearance. Rarely, this can extend down to the xiphoid or be complete. Lower sternal defects are much less common and are primarily associated with thoracic and thoracoabdominal ectopia cordis [20].

Several differences exist between the sternal cleft and the other three conditions. Most importantly, the heart is in the normal position in individuals with sternal cleft, but displaced in the other three conditions. In addition, intrinsic congenital heart disease is rarely seen in sternal clefts as opposed to individuals with the other sternal defects.

3.2. Chest wall tumors

Chest wall tumors include a wide spectrum of bony, soft tissue and cartilaginous neoplasms that can present a diagnostic and therapeutic challenge. They can be classified as primary, locally invasive or metastatic. Primary tumors of the bony skeleton or soft tissues can be further classified as benign or malignant. Chest wall tumors may also result from cancers of contiguous structures, such as the pleura, mediastinum, muscle, lung, breast, and skin. These malignancies can invade adjacent tissues either locally or regionally. The sternum, ribs, clavicles and chest wall soft tissues are common areas of metastasis from primary malignant processes of distant primary sites, such as the breast, lungs, kidneys, and thyroid gland. Benign nonneoplastic conditions, such as cysts and inflammation, can also present as chest wall tumors. All primary tumors of the chest wall, including skeletal and soft tissue neoplasms, account for only 2% of all body tumors. However, more than 50% of these tumors are malignant, thus making their prompt recognition essential in the management and treatment process [21]. Some of the common types of primary benign and malignant tumors will be discussed below.

In general, chest wall tumors start as asymptomatic slowly enlarging nodules that usually progress to painful and sometimes ulcerating lesions. Malignant tumors are much more likely to cause pain as opposed to benign disease. Appropriate diagnostic evaluation includes a thorough patient history and physical examination, as well as evaluation of laboratory parameters and radiological studies. Plain chest radiographs, computed tomography (CT) and bone scans as well as magnetic resonance imaging (MRI) are the most common imaging modalities used. Tissue diagnosis by histologic examination is also usually warranted. The diagnostic yield of the available techniques is inversely related to the invasiveness of the procedure. Fine needle aspiration has a poor diagnostic yield, core needle biopsy has a good diagnostic yield, incisional biopsy has an excellent diagnostic yield, and excisional biopsy allows for a definitive diagnosis. Selection of the biopsy technique must be individualized and several factors, such as the tumor type and size, should be considered.

The surgical treatment of the majority of chest wall tumors requires careful planning and execution. When surgery is curative, the objective is a wide excision to extirpate the tumor with adequate margins. The extent of the resection should not be restricted by the size of the resulting defect as multiple reconstrucive options are generally available. The en bloc resection includes the skin and soft tissue overlying the tumor, the involved sternum, primarily involved and/or adjacent ribs, as well as any attached structures such as the lung, pleura and pericardium. Similar basic principles apply for chest wall resection of any infectious or inflammatory process. Resection should be wide enough to obtain healthy viable tissue at the edges of the wound for proper healing. In certain occasions, if the lesion is deep and the overlying skin is intact, it may be appropriate to spare the skin to facilitate closure.

3.2.1. Benign bone tumors

Fibrous dysplasia is a slowly-enlarging painless lesion. It accounts for approximately 30% of benign chest wall tumors. It originates from the rib shaft and is characterized by fibrous replacement of the medullary cavity of the rib. Radiographically, it has a characteristic ground-glass appearance on plain films. In the presence of multiple lesions associated with skin pigmentation and precocious puberty, Albright's syndrome should be suspected. Conservative management is the treatment of choice. However, if the lesion becomes large enough to cause pressure symptoms and/or pathologic fractures, surgical excision should be considered.

Chondroma is a slowly growing asymptomatic mass arising from the costochondral junction anteriorly. It tends to occur during the second or third decade of life and constitutes about 15% of all benign bony neoplasms of the chest wall. Radiographically, chondroma appears as a lytic lesion with sclerotic margins, thus making a distinction from its malignant counterpart, chondrosarcoma, quite difficult. Often, chondromas cannot be distinguished from chondrosarcomas even on incisional biopsy. Therefore, these lesions should be managed as if they were malignant and complete surgical excision should be performed.

Osteochondroma is the most common benign bone tumor accounting for about 50% of benign chest wall tumors. It originates from the metaphyseal component of the rib and presents as a pedunculated mass capped by viable cartilage. Stippled calcification is often present within the tumor and gives a characteristic radiological appearance. Familial osteochondromatosis is a recognized variant that manifests with multiple rib lesions. Multiple lesions can also be encountered throughout the body in the triad of Albright's syndrome. Surgical resection of an osteochondroma is indicated when the lesion increases in size or becomes symptomatic. The onset of pain in a previously asymptomatic lesion should alert the treating physician to the possibility of malignant degeneration of the tumor.

3.2.2. *Malignant bone tumors*

Chondrosarcoma is one of the most common primary malignant bone neoplasms, accounting for approximately 30% of such tumors. It tends to occur after the third or fourth decade of life and typically presents with a slowly enlarging painful anterior chest wall mass involving the anterior costochondral junctions of the sternum. The etiology is unknown, however, an association with local trauma to the chest has been made. It has also been suggested that it could arise secondary to malignant degeneration of benign cartilaginous tumors such as chondromas and osteochondromas. Radiographically, a chondrosarcoma has a characteristic appearance as a lobulated mass with poorly defined margins, destroying cortical bone. The radiographic appearance tends to be very similar to that of a benign chondroma. Definitive diagnosis can only be made pathologically, but at times, histological findings can resemble that of chondromas, making the diagnosis challenging. Resection with a 4cm margin is recommended to provide the best chance of local control. Five-year survival after complete resection has been reported to be 70% [22].

Osteogenic sarcomas (osteosarcomas) usually occur in the long bones of the extremities, but can originate from the ribs and account for about 10% of all primary malignant bone neoplasms. They commonly affect teenagers and young adults. They are typically associated with pain. Unlike chondrosarcomas, they are rapidly enlarging and metastases are often present at initial evaluation. They have a characteristic "sunburst" pattern on chest radiographs. Metastatic work up is often indicated prior to the initiation of treatment. The treatment of osteogenic sarcomas includes wide resection of the tumor including the involved bone and adjacent soft tissues. Prognosis is poor and the five-year survival rate after complete excision can be as low as 20% [22]. Adjuvant chemotherapy has been reported to increase the survival rate up to 60% [23].

Ewing's sarcoma can involve the ribs and accounts for approximately 10% of all primary malignant tumors of the chest wall. Patients usually present with a painful enlarging mass. Fever, malaise, anemia and leukocytosis may also be present. Radiographically, an "onion peel" appearance from periosteal elevation and bone remodeling is typically seen, which is characteristic but not pathognomonic. A large proportion of patients with apparently localized disease at diagnosis have occult metastatic disease. Metastases display a preference for the lung and central nervous system. Treatment incorporates chemotherapy with surgery and/or radiation therapy. Local disease control is critical to long-term cure and definitive surgical margins are desirable. Radiation therapy is considered for local control in poor surgical candidates.

3.2.3. *Soft tissue tumors*

A variety of benign soft tissue tumors of the chest wall have been reported including fibromas, lipomas, giant cell tumors, connective tissue tumors, neurogenic tumors, and vascular tumors such as hemangiomas. Local excision is typically the treatment of choice.

Desmoid tumors can arise in any skeletal muscle but more than one-third develop in the shoulder and chest wall. They present as poorly circumscribed lesions and can encase nerves or vascular structures. Whatever the cause, there is a high risk of tumor recurrence if inadequately resected [24]. Therefore, aggressive wide surgical excision with negative margins is the most successful primary treatment modality for these tumors.

Sarcomas are the most common malignant soft tissue chest wall tumors. Pleomorphic undifferentiated sarcoma, previously known as malignant fibrous histiocytoma, and rhabdomyosarcoma are the most frequent types. Unlike pleomorphic undifferentiated sarcoma, which typically presents in late adult life with a painless slowly growing mass, rhabdomyosarcoma occurs most frequently in children and young adults as a painless rapidly enlarging mass. Other tumors of the soft tissue chest wall include liposarcomas, neurofibrosarcomas and leiomyosarcomas. Surgical resection with wide margins is typically the standard treatment for all the above-mentioned tumors for local disease control.

3.3. Infection

Chest wall infections can be classified as primary and secondary. Primary infections occur spontaneously, whereas secondary infections can be caused by the progression of a preexisting disease process or as a complication of a previous procedure. Management of these infections must not be overlooked and intervention in a timely fashion is necessary to prevent or minimize potentially devastating consequences. Some of these infections are particularly challenging to treat due to their proximity to major vascular structures and the lack of substantial overlying soft tissues. Treatment options vary from antibiotic administration to complex resections with reconstruction.

The chest wall covers approximately 20% of the total body surface area and can be affected by all the common nonspecific soft tissue infections such as boils and furuncles. Soft tissue abscesses of the chest wall present with the same symptoms and signs of an abscess located anywhere else in the body. Abscesses involving the subpectoral or subscapular spaces can lead to a serious infection. In the majority of cases antibiotic therapy with incision and drainage of the abscess is sufficient treatment. Necrotizing soft tissue infections rarely occur but are rapidly spreading and highly lethal. They may occur postoperatively or as a complication of an empyema or trauma. A high index of suspicion, early diagnosis, and aggressive treatment with appropriate antibiotics and radical debridements are essential to their successful management. Delayed wound closure with skin grafting or muscle transfer has been used [25].

Sternal osteomyelitis, once a rare disorder, has become more common in the last few decades due to the increased frequency of coronary artery bypass grafting and prevalence of intravenous drug abuse. Primary infection is typically seen in intravenous drug abusers, whereas secondary infection is associated with coronary artery bypass grafting. Overall, the most common pathogen is *Staphylococcus aureus*, but *Pseudomonas aeruginosa* is the most common cause in intravenous drug abusers [26]. Several factors have been implicated in the development of poststernotomy osteomyelitis including diabetes, prolonged perfusion time, a depressed cardiac output, excessive postoperative bleeding, re-exploration for the control of hemorrhage, length of postoperative intubation, and use of bilateral internal mammary arteries for cardiac revascularization [27,28]. Patients with poststernotomy osteomyelitis usually present with pain and drainage at the site. Occasionally, there is a palpable mass overlying the incision. Sternal instability may also be evident. The infection can extend deeply into the mediastinum. CT scan of the chest is the diagnostic study of choice. Treatment with antibiotics and aggressive surgical debridement of the infected area followed by muscle flap reconstruction yields the best clinical outcome [29].

The complexity of *median sternotomy wound infections* has challenged cardiothoracic and plastic surgeons over the last few decades. Prompt identification and treatment are crucial to prevent potentially lethal consequences such as extension to cardiac and aortic suture lines and intracardiac prostheses. It is well known that the surface appearance of the wound may look deceivingly insignificant in a patient with a sternal infection. For instance, severe mediastinitis with sternal disruption may be hidden under a small draining sinus tract. Although sternotomy wound infections manifest as a continuum of clinical entities, Jones et al. divided them into three types [30]. Type 1a represents the patient with a suture abscess or infected wound hematoma superficial to the deep fascia, whereas type 1b is associated with exposure of the deep fascial suture layer. Treatment consists of wound drainage and wound packing to allow closure by secondary intention. Sometimes they may be secondarily closed when clean. Type 2a typifies a deeper process with an exposed stable sternotomy, while type 2b is associated with an unstable sternotomy. If the sternum is stable and there is no evidence of bacterial contamination of the parasternal fluid, debridement and closure of the wound may be appropriate. If the sternum is unstable but sterile with intact bilateral sternal blood supply, rewiring can be considered. However, if there is any doubt about the ability of the sternal bone stock to withstand rewiring, sternectomy with muscle flap closure is the safest option. Type 3a is characterized by complete sternal disruption and suppurative mediastinitis with exposure of the heart. Type 3b is associated with any of the types 2a, 2b or 3a and septicemia. All these wounds must be widely debrided and may require delayed closure, particularly when septicemia is present, or when the patient is hemodynamically unstable. Closure of the wound is accomplished with muscle flaps.

Osteomyelitis of the rib is a rare cause of chest wall infection. Diagnosis is usually delayed but the condition commonly presents with fever, pain, and a palpable mass overlying the infected rib segment. A draining sinus tract can also be present. It predominantly occurs from contiguous spread, but the hematogenous route has also been reported [31]. Treatment consists of excision of the diseased bone with care taken to avoid penetration and contamination of the adjacent pleural cavity during resection. Reconstruction with soft tissue coverage is often used for the remaining defect.

Sternoclavicular osteomyelitis usually presents with fever, joint pain, and an associated palpable mass. Several gram-positive and gram-negative organisms have been identified. Sternoclavicular osteomyelitis has been frequently associated with intravenous drug abuse, indwelling central venous catheters, and trauma [32-34]. The majority of patients also have a long-term immunosuppresion related to diabetes mellitus, steroid use, human immunodeficiency virus or an overwhelming acute illness from a distant site [35]. These infections are managed with intravenous antibiotics, aggressive surgical resection and often, soft tissue reconstruction. The joint's proximity to major neurovascular structures and the lack of substantial overlying soft tissues makes surgical management more challenging. A successful approach involves resection of the sternoclavicular joint with partial resection of the manubrium, medial clavicle, anterior first rib and in some cases, an involved portion of the anterior second rib [35]. Reconstruction is typically accomplished with an ipsilateral pectoralis major muscle flap [35,36].

3.4. Radiation

Radiation therapy has saved many lives and plays an important role in the treatment of malignant neoplasms that involve the chest wall. Examples of neoplasms in which radiation therapy is well-established include breast and lung cancer as well as some types of sarcomas and lymphomas. Radiation therapy works by damaging the targeted cells through complicated intracellular processes. The tissues that are included in the field of radiation can potentially suffer both early and late adverse effects. Early adverse effects typically occur within the first few weeks following treatment and may present as erythema, skin hyperpigmentation or desquamation. These changes are generally self-limiting and resolve with moisturizers and local wound care. On the other hand, chronic adverse effects can be progressive, permanent, debilitating and even life-threatening. Some of these late injuries include delayed wound healing, ulceration, infection, tissue fibrosis, malignant transformation, osteoradionecrosis, and constrictive microangiopathic changes to small and medium sized vessels. Management of several of these late injuries such as infected wounds, radiation ulcers and new or recurrent neoplasms, often requires the attention of a reconstructive surgeon. It has been reported that a significant number of patients undergoing chest wall reconstruction will receive radiation therapy in the course of their treatment [37].

The first step in evaluating a patient with a wound related to a late radiation injury is to rule out the presence of a new or recurrent tumor. This is usually accomplished by obtaining imaging studies such as a chest radiograph, computed tomography or magnetic resonance imaging, and possibly bronchoscopy. The two latter imaging studies will also allow better understanding of the extent of radiation injury in adjacent tissues. Once the extent of the disease is determined, an appropriate treatment approach can be proposed.

If there is a mass or an open wound, further work up and evaluation by the extirpative surgeon may be required. Subsequently, the tumor must be completely excised with negative pathologic margins before considering reconstruction of the remaining defect. If tumor is not present, the radiation-induced ulcer or infected wound should be completely resected and debrided. All fibrotic tissue and foreign bodies must be carefully removed, because sternal wires, retained sutures or persistently infected non-viable cartilage and bone may be sources of a chronic sinus tract or open wound. Inadequate debridement with retention of any of the aforementioned non-viable materials or tissues is usually the source of recurrent infections and wound healing problems. Also, the extent of radiation injury is often underestimated and difficult to appreciate, and therefore, several debridements may be required to establish a clean wound with a well-vascularized bed and edges before proceeding with reconstruction.

The chest wall is a fairly thin structure and most chest wall defects are full thickness following thorough debridement. Therefore, chest wall reconstruction is often required to obtain an airtight seal and preserve respiratory function. Soft tissue coverage is then achieved generally with a musculocutaneous flap or a muscle flap with a skin graft. The most commonly used flaps include the pectoralis major, rectus abdominis, latissimus dorsi, and greater omentum flaps.

4. General principles of reconstruction of composite chest wall defects

Reconstruction of the chest wall has evolved over the last century to be an integral component of therapy for patients with chest wall defects. Developments in therapy include the introduction of tracheal intubation and positive-pressure ventilation, the description of the latissimus dorsi musculocutaneous flap for coverage of an anterior chest wall defect and the discussion of the use of fascia lata grafts for stabilizing the skeletal structures and greater omentum transposition for reconstruction of chest wall defects [38-41]. Since 1970, several authors have made remarkable contributions to the reconstructive field by describing the use of several muscle and musculocutaneous flaps such as the pectoralis major, latissimus dorsi, rectus abdominis, serratus anterior, and external oblique. More recently, free microvascular transfers of muscle or musculocutaneous units have been described, when local flaps were not available.

Chest wall reconstruction can be complex and continues to pose a formidable challenge. Close collaboration between the reconstructive surgeon and the thoracic surgeon can ensure appropriate management of this patient population in order to safely accomplish a desirable and durable outcome. The primary goals of reconstruction are maintenance of structural stability and preservation of physiologic function, as well as an acceptable cosmetic result without compromising the cancer or other primary operation. Two components may be involved; the bony thorax and the soft tissues. Reconstruction of these two components will be discussed in great detail later in the chapter.

Preoperative evaluation is essential in patients undergoing chest wall resection and reconstruction given the extensive nature of these procedures and the potential for life-threatening complications. A simple history and physical examination, as well as laboratory and radiological studies can help identify patients at high risk for developing postoperative complications. Understanding the patient's preoperative pulmonary status is critical and must be comprehensively evaluated preoperatively to determine the presence of respiratory symptoms, history of tobacco use, and exposure to pulmonary irritants. Typically, pulmonary function tests are an essential component of most preoperative workups.

The goals of the reconstruction and the expectations should be discussed with the patient. A teenager with pectus excavatum may have different expectations than an elderly person with a malignant chest wall tumor. Multiple factors dictate the type of reconstruction of a chest wall defect. These include the patient's history and co-morbid conditions, physical stability and hemodymamic status, as well as the ultimate prognosis. A comprehensive understanding of both the anatomy of the defect and the availability of regional tissue for reconstruction of the defect is essential. The location, extent and etiology of the defect will determine the technique that should be used for reconstruction. Subsequently, the reconstructive surgeon can apply the concepts of the reconstructive ladder and select amongst several techniques including tissue expansion, standard flap transposition, and microsurgical composite tissue transplantation.

4.1. Location of the defect

Defining the location of the chest wall defect is important in the decision-making process regarding technique selection for reconstruction. The chest wall covers a large body surface area and can be divided into several different regions, each with a specific series of reconstructive needs and flap options.

The *anterior chest* area is located between the parasternal and the anterior axillary lines and extends from the clavicle to the inferior costal margin [42]. The breast is included in this area, but for the purpose of this discussion, breast reconstruction will not be analyzed. The skeletal structure of the anterior chest protects intra-thoracic organs, and its semi-rigidity maintains relative negative pressure for inspiration and positive pressure for expiration. Resection of 4 or more consecutive ribs or a defect that is larger than 5 cm in diameter may result in a flail segment and hence "paradoxical chest wall motion", leading to impairment of the respiratory mechanics. Skeletal reconstruction is typically recommended in these cases to restore chest wall stability. Absence of the pectoralis major muscle at the defect base may require a regional flap for wound coverage.

The *sternal* area is located between the two parasternal lines and extends from the jugular notch between the sternal heads of the sternocleidomastoid muscles to the xiphisternal junction [42]. Sternal defects may result in anterior mediastinal exposure, and chest wall instability may develop with possible functional impairment. In the past, it was believed that the extent of sternal components lost can affect the pulmonary status of the patient. However, several authors have examined the functional impact of sternal resections and concluded that sternal resection with or without soft tissue reconstruction is a well-tolerated procedure and in general shows no significant change in postoperative pulmonary function [43-45]. There is a signficant amount of controversy which exists regarding the need to reconstruct sternal defects. However, most surgeons would agree that if a patient is experiencing sternal pain from instability, rigid fixation in the midline may improve their symptoms. In addition, the anterior chest wall also provides a rigid base for upper extremity movement. Loss of skeletal chest wall support in patients with sternal wounds may reduce upper extremity and shoulder girdle function [46]. Indeed, the location and size of the sternal defect will have an impact on the stability and physiologic integrity of the chest wall. The physiologic deficit is minimal with loss of the upper sternal body and associated ribs, is moderate with loss of the entire sternal body and associated ribs, and may be more significant with loss of the manubrium, upper sternal body and associated ribs. However, this does not predict the need for structural reconstruction in these situations. More comprehensive physiologic assessments of outcomes in this patient population are required to answer this difficult question. For now, there is no conclusive evidence to support the necessity for reconstruction of sternal wounds following resection.

The *superior chest* area is located between the deltopectoral groove of the anterior chest and the spine of the scapula of the posterior chest and extends between the base of the neck to the acromioclavicular joints [42]. Chest wall stability should not be compromised with the absence of the clavicle or acromioclavicular joint. Skeletal reconstruction is generally not required for functional reasons because of the natural parietal suspension provided by the sternum, scapula, and attached wide muscles of the thorax. It should be noted that the subclavian artery and vein as well as the brachial plexus may be exposed with defects in the superior chest wall, and under these circumstances, soft tissue reconstruction will be required.

The *lateral chest* area is located between the anterior and posterior axillary lines [42]. The area extends between the apex of the axilla and the inferior costal margin. In general, lateral chest defects extend into either the anterior or posterior thorax or both. Reconstruction to restore skeletal wall stability is often required for extensive rib defects. Bone graft or vascularized bone has been utilized for this purpose. However, the associated donor-site morbidity has led to the more extensive use of alloplastic materials such as Prolene or Marlex mesh, GoreTex patches and methylmethacrylate sandwiches, which will be discussed below. Subsequent coverage of these materials with vascularized soft tissue is necessary. Isolated defects involving the lateral chest wall are uncommon, unless they extend into the axilla. Several neurovascular structures, including the axillary artery and vein and the median and ulnar nerves, could potentially be exposed with such defects. A variety of flaps can be used for closure of axillary defects such as serratus anterior, pectoralis major, and latissimus dorsi muscle flaps. The use of perforator flaps (e.g. thoracodorsal artery perforator flap) has also been proposed given their numerous advantages such as longer vascular pedicle, flexible arc of rotation, and preservation of the integrity of functional limb girdle muscles.

The *posterior chest* area is located between the two posterior axillary lines and extends between the level of the spine of the scapula to the posterior costal margin at the L1 level. Defects of the posterior thorax are typically characterized by a deep dead space. The wound base of the defect may be covered by muscle given the presence of several large muscle groups in this area such as the latissimus dorsi, trapezius and shoulder girdle muscles. Unless the defect extends to adjacent territories, chest wall instability secondary to the absence of ribs is rare due to good muscular support. Exposure of bone and hardware is occasionally seen with central posterior defects. The objectives for reconstruction are to fill the dead space, cover the exposed bone, as well as any exposed hardware or vascular prostheses that cannot be removed, and avoid formation of debilitating axillary and neck contractures. A tension-free reconstruction is desirable. Perforator flaps have been utilized for these purposes. Their advantages include leaving the underlying muscle intact, consequently preserving function. Also, their flexible long vascular pedicles enable transposition and coverage of defects that cannot be reached by conventional musculocutaneous flaps. In contrast, muscle and musculocutaneous flaps will more reliably cover large deep defects as well as exposed hardware and vascular prostheses. Although reconstruction of the posterior thorax is usually achieved with pedicled flaps, microvascular free-tissue transfer is sometimes necessary. Free flaps are mainly used for large defects that are difficult to reach with pedicled flaps or when regional flaps are unavailable due to extirpation of the muscle or damage of the vascular pedicles following surgical ablation, radiation therapy, or trauma.

4.2. Size of the defect

The size of the chest wall defect is an important determining factor when considering the necessity of soft tissue and/or skeletal reconstruction. Partial thickness defects of the chest wall are usually limited to the skin and subcutaneous tissues with viable muscle in the wound base. These defects can be simply closed with skin grafts or local skin flaps.

Full thickness defects are more challenging. Small full thickness defects of the chest wall can often be closed primarily. Large full thickness defects are readily covered with regional muscle and musculocutaneous flaps or omental pedicled flaps with the aim of obliterating the dead space, controlling infection, and covering any prosthetic materials used in skeletal reconstruction. Microvascular reconstruction with free flaps is occasionally used in cases where the pedicled flaps are either unable to reach the defect or compromised secondary to extirpation, radiation therapy, or trauma. Skin grafts may be used for coverage of muscle flaps to avoid inclusion of a large skin paddle, hence allowing primary closure of the flap donor site. In cases of very large defects, use of a single flap may not provide adequate coverage, and use of chimeric flaps is an option.

4.3. Timing of reconstruction

Contemporary approaches to the management of complex chest wall defects typically requires a multidisciplinary approach involing both the thoracic and reconstructive surgeons. Certainly, an important consideration in the decision-making process is the timing of the reconstruction. Although immediate chest wall reconstruction can be achieved successfully for the majority of the defects, a more careful approach should be adopted for specific conditions such as sternal wound infections, radiation wounds and chronically draining empyemas.

Sternal wound infections are classically seen following cardiac procedures. As mentioned earlier, the surface appearance of these wounds can be deceptive, and delayed recognition and treatment can lead to life-threatening complications. Single-stage repair with sternal debridement and flap closure has been shown to be appropriate in most cases without an increase in either morbidity or mortality [30]. Antibiotics tailored to the offending organisms should be used judiciously. As a general principle, adequate debridement of the necrotic tissue, evacuation of blood clots, removal of foreign bodies, and excision of devascularized bone and exposed cartilage should be performed prior to considering soft tissue coverage. In cases of inadequate debridement or suppurative mediastinitis, the wound must be left open with frequent dressing changes and the closure must be delayed for at least 48 hours or later if necessary, particularly when septicemia is present or when the patient is hemodynamically unstable [30]. Once the wound is clean, soft tissue reconstruction is usually achieved with regional flaps. The most commonly used flaps are the pectoralis major and rectus abdominis. Other less frequently used flaps include the omentum and latissimus dorsi. It should be noted that, the longer the period of time that elapses between debridement and soft tissue coverage, the greater the risk of damage to vital structures, such as coronary or aortic grafts.

Radiation wounds are another type of chest wall defect that deserve special attention with regard to timing of reconstruction. These wounds may represent soft tissue ulceration or osteoradionecrosis but can also be related to a recurrent tumor or a new primary malignancy. If tumor is present, it should be completely excised with negative pathologic margins before proceeding with reconstruction. If tumor is not present, the key to obtaining a well-healed chest wall reconstruction relies on wide excision and thorough debridement of all nonviable irradiated tissues as well as removal of foreign bodies. Numerous debridements are usually required to establish a clean wound with well-vascularized margins before reconstruction of the resulting defect is considered. This is important for various reasons as a poorly vascularized and fibrotic irradiated wound bed may lead to failure of an attempted primary closure or skin grafting as well as suboptimal healing of a transposed muscle flap. It should also be remembered that the degree of radiation injury often extends beyond the initially established edges of damaged tissue, making serial debridements necessary.

Empyema is the development of infection within the pleural space and can be due to many different etiologies. Postsurgical empyema accounts for 20% of all cases of empyema and most frequently follows pneumonectomy [47]. Although empyemas can occur several years after the initial surgery, they are most frequently encountered in the early postoperative period.

Post-surgical empyemas are generally treated with correction of the underlying cause, appropriate antibiotics, and drainage with chest tube thoracostomy. The response to this treatment for empyemas complicating pulmonary resections highly depends on the state of the remaining lung and its location. If the pleural space is not completely filled by expansion of the remaining lung, elevation of the diaphragm or shifting of the mediastinum, the empyema will likely persist. The previously mentioned treatment is almost never sufficient for the treatment of empyemas which occur after upper lobectomies and pneumonectomies, resulting in chronically draining empyemas. Bronchopleural fistulas may also be present in about 40% of the cases, making treatment more complex [47]. General management of empyemas associated with pulmonary resections includes initial drainage and sterilization of the infected pleural space. Subsequently, the bronchopleural fistula is closed if present, and the pleural space is obliterated with either a muscle flap or antibiotic solution. A variety of extrathoracic pedicled flaps have been used to obliterate the pleural space including latissimus dorsi muscle, serratus anterior muscle, pectoralis major or minor muscle, rectus abdominis muscle, and omentum.

An important issue in the management of pleural cavities with empyema is the timing of the reconstruction, whether with a muscle flap or antibiotic solution. In general, the initial treatment of an empyema with closed drainage of the pleural space is required for 1-2 weeks until the mediastinum becomes stabilized. It should be noted that open drainage of the pleural space may be considered at any point if the patient becomes medically unstable. If a bronchopleural fistula is identified during the initial period, open drainage is also performed with possible closure of the fistula. Once the patient is medically stable and has entered into the chronic phase after the initial 2-week period, obliteration of the pleural space may be undertaken. There is no established scientific evidence as to the best timing of the closure. Some authors advocate closure at approximately 3 months for benign disease and 6 months to 1 year for malignant disease, whereas others suggest obliteration of the pleural space anytime between 6 weeks and 3 months [47].

The timing of reconstruction is also important for certain *congenital anomalies* such as Poland syndrome. Although some believe that prepubertal patients with the syndrome are candidates for repair, others support the idea of delaying reconstruction until late adolescence [48,49]. Several reasons have been given to support the delayed approach, including the risk of growth inhibition with early intervention and the need for multiple revisions to maintain pace with breast and chest wall growth. Reconstruction of the female breast deformity in Poland syndrome remains controversial. Many females with the condition seek consultation early in development. Some advocate delaying reconstruction until the breasts are fully mature. However, this is a very sensitive age in young women, and if left untreated, the condition may lead to severe psyschological and behavioral problems. Therefore, it is often advisable to address the defect with insertion of a tissue expander on the affected side which is then filled to the volume to match the contralateral breast as the young woman matures. Periodic expansion of the breast tissue expander allows adjustment of breast size to match the unaffected contralateral breast until sexual maturity is reached. At that point, the expander can be replaced with a permanent implant.

The timing for repair and reconstruction of pectus deformities can also pose a challenge. A consideration in favor of skeletal reconstruction is the presence of cardiopulmonary compromise, or psychological and behavioral problems caused by the chest wall deformity. However, it should be remembered that severe disability may ensue due to limitaton of the growth of the thorax and associated severe chest wall constriction. Therefore, resectional repairs should be delayed, if possible, until after the age of 16 years. In addition, children and young adolescents who present before their growth spurts are not ideal candidates for implant correction. Breast reconstruction in female patients with pectus deformities is usually deferred until patients are well into their pubertal growth. As for all elective procedures, involving the patient in the decision-making process is critical to ensure a successful reconstruction and a satisfied patient.

5. Skeletal reconstruction

The bony thorax plays a vital role in the dynamic stability of the chest and respiratory mechanics. Skeletal reconstruction not only restores skeletal rigidity but also protects the vital organs and vascular structures contained within the thorax. Furthermore, it prevents herniation of thoracic organs, counteracts considerable shrinking of the operated side of the thorax, and maintains an acceptable chest shape while preserving the mechanical forces that enable respiration. The size and location of the skeletal defect generally determine whether skeletal reconstruction is required. The classic teaching is that the loss of two ribs can be compensated by adequate soft tissue reconstruction. However, structural wall support is required when defects involve the loss of more than four consecutive ribs or are greater than 5 cm in diameter to prevent the development of chest wall flail. Larger defects located posteriorly may be an exception, as the overlying scapula can provide support, but if the defect is near the tip of the scapula, reconstruction may be required to prevent entrapment with movement of the arm. In addition, in patients who have undergone radiation, as many as five ribs may be resected without requiring skeletal reconstruction as the resulting radiation fibrosis produces chest wall stiffness and affords inherent stability. Throughout the years, a variety of autogenous and prosthetic grafts have been used to restore the structural integrity of the chest wall.

5.1. Autogenous options

Traditionally, skeletal reconstruction was performed utilizing autogenous materials, such as fascial or split-rib grafts, with limited success. The tensor fascia lata muscle has a long fascial extension that can be easily harvested in the supine position. The fascia lata graft can be taken up to 28 cm in length, and 16 cm in width. It can provide a semirigid skeletal substitute, and has been used with bone chips or bone grafts. The use of fascia lata grafts is limited because they are prone to infections and have been shown to become flaccid over time, decreasing their ability to provide stable skeletal support [40,50]. Autogenous bone grafts are another option for reconstruction of the chest wall skeleton. For successful reconstruction, the bone graft must be opposed to a large surface area of trabecular bone adjacent to the chest wall defect in order to enhance graft survival and osteoconduction [50]. Several donor sites have been reported including the ribs, iliac crest, and fibula. Rib grafts are technically difficult to harvest and produce donor site morbidity, but are useful in preventing flail chests.

5.2. Prosthetic options

One of the most significant developments in chest wall surgery and reconstruction has been the increasing use of synthetic materials. Prior to the creation of these materials, cadaveric bone or the patient's own fascial or split-rib grafts were used for structural support, as described above. The ideal characteristics of a prosthetic material for skeletal reconstruction include rigidity, malleability, inertness, and radiolucency. Today, synthetic materials such as Prolene mesh, Marlex mesh, Gore-Tex, Vicryl mesh, and methylmethacrylate have all but eliminated the use of cadaveric or autogenous materials [51]. These prosthetic materials are widely available, reliable, and can be easily used to reconstruct the chest wall skeleton, conforming to any size or shape of defect. Their main disadvantage is the potential for infection.

The selection of which synthetic material to use is largely based on the surgeon's preferences as all available materials work reasonably well. Prolene and Marlex mesh are monofilament polypropylene, are porous, and are structurally sound. Prolene is double knitted and can withstand 150 pounds of pressure. A fibrous reaction occurs at the interface between the mesh and flap to provide permanent stability and incorporation into the surrounding tissue. Methylmethacrylate can be used alone or incorporated between two layers of Marlex mesh in a sandwich fashion in situations where rigidity is necessary. Methylmethacrylate is lightweight, versatile, and radiolucent, allowing for subsequent evaluation of the lungs. It undergoes an exothermic reaction during hardening, and therefore the Marlex sandwich is prepared on a side table and only sewn in place after the composite graft has cooled sufficiently [52]. Gore-Tex, which is reinforced polytetrafluoroethylene, has a smooth, nonporous surface, creating a more watertight closure to prevent movement of fluid and air across the reconstructed chest wall. The smooth surface also prevents adhesion formation and incorporation. Gore-Tex is considered easier to suture, stretch, and mold into the wound. Vicryl, or polyglactin 910, is an absorable mesh with limited strength and is often used for temporary coverage in cases where wound contamination or infection is present [42]. Acellularized dermal matrices (ADM) are newer biologic, nonimmunogenic materials which may be useful in situations where reconstructive material must be placed directly over viscera or into an irradiated or infected operative site. ADM becomes vascularized and undergoes remodeling into the autologous tissue following implantation. Initial studies show that it produces a strong, stable repair, resists infection, and causes minimal adhesions [53]. Following stabilization of the chest with prosthetic mesh, the alloplastic material must be covered with healthy, well-vascularized tissue, often in the form of a muscle or myocutaneous flap.

6. Soft tissue reconstruction

In general, the nature of full thickness chest wall defects requires the recruitment of healthy skin and soft tissue for reconstruction. This includes several options, from local and regional muscle or myocutaneous flaps to more advanced reconstructive techniques such as microsurgical free tissue transfer. The excellent vascularity of these flaps provides the most reliable means of reconstructing complex chest wall defects, enabling the maintenance of physiologic functions and decreasing the risk of infection. Of note, a detailed preoperative history should be obtained regarding which surgical procedures a patient has had in the past to determine which flaps are available for use.

6.1. Muscle and myocutaneous flaps

Pectoralis Major

The pectoralis major muscle flap is the most commonly used muscle flap for reconstruction of sternal, anterosuperior chest, intrathoracic, and neck wounds. It is an ideal flap based on its proximity, reliability, and versatility. It is a thick, fan-shaped muscle that originates from the anterior surface of the medial aspect of the clavicle, anterior surface of the sternum, and the superior six costal cartilages. The fibers converge laterally and insert as a tendon on the intertubercular groove of the humerus. The muscle creates the anterior axillary fold. It is innervated by the medial and lateral pectoral nerves, and functions to adduct and medially rotate the humerus. The sternocostal head also contributes to extension of the humerus, while the clavicular head flexes the humerus.

It is classified as having a Mathes-Nahai Type V vascular supply, with both a dominant and segmental blood supply, and may be reliably raised on either. The dominant blood supply is derived from the thoracoacromial artery, which arises from the axillary artery. The segmental blood supply comes from the first through sixth intercostal perforating branches of the internal mammary artery. The muscle has a highly consistent vascular anatomy, and the multiple pedicles affords it significant reliability and versatility. When the flap is based on the thoracoacromial pedicle, its reach can be increased by dividing its humeral and clavicular attachments. The flap may be harvested as muscle alone or as a myocutaneous flap, but rates of skin paddle necrosis may be as high as 30% [54-56]. Transposition of the flap results in loss of pectoralis motor function except in cases where the humeral insertion and motor nerves are left intact in reconstruction of the upper sternum. The pectoralis can also be used to fill intrathoracic defects by passing it between the superior ribs. When based on its segmental supply, it is raised as a turnover flap, which requires the division of the humeral and clavicular attachments and may necessitate ligation of the thoracromial vessels to increase its mobility. The turnover flap is particuarly useful for midline sternal defects and in cases in which the thoracoacromial vessels are absent or damaged. However, the left pectoralis muscle cannot be based on the segmental supply if the patient has previously had a bypass using the left internal mammary artery. The use of only the medial two-thirds of the muscle as a turnover flap enables the lateral third and anterior axillary fold to be spared, decreasing donor site morbidity.

Rectus Abdominis

The rectus abdominis is a paired muscle running vertically on each side of the anterior abdomen. The muscle originates from the pubis and inserts into the costal cartilages of the fifth through seventh ribs and the xyphoid process. It is innervated segmentally by the thoracoabdominal nerves of the seventh through twelfth thoracic vertebrae. It functions to flex the lumbar spine. It may be harvested as a muscle or myocutaneous flap, and these flaps are useful in the reconstruction of anterior and anterolateral chest wall defects and are also a mainstay in autologous breast reconstruction [57].

The rectus abdominis has a Mathes-Nahai Type III vascular supply, with two dominant pedicles consisting of the superior and deep inferior epigastric arteries. The superior epigastric artery is a branch of the internal mammary artery, while the deep inferior epigastric artery arises from the external iliac artery. The superior and inferior epigastric vessels anastomose through a choke zone periumbilically. In patients who have undergone bypass using the left internal mammary artery (LIMA), the left rectus abdominis can be based on the eighth intercostal vessel, but the risk for flap loss is increased due to the decreased vascularity. The flap may be pedicled on the superior epigastric vessels or transferred as a free flap based on the inferior epigastric vessels. The overlying skin is supplied by musculocutaneous perforators arising from the deep inferior epigastric system. The skin paddle may be oriented transversely (TRAM) or vertically (VRAM). The transverse orientation allows for harvest of a larger skin paddle, and the donor site can be closed primarily and the transverse scar is well-concealed in the lower abdomen. The skin paddle of the VRAM is oriented directly over the muscle and encompasses a maximal number of perforators, and therefore has a better blood supply than the TRAM (Figure 4). A disadvantage of using the rectus abdominis muscles in chest wall reconstruction is that harvest of the rectus abdominis muscle can lead to abdominal morbidity including abdominal wall weakness, abdominal bulges, and hernias. Perforator flaps, like the deep inferior epigastric perforator flap (DIEP), have been designed to minimize rectus abdominis muscle harvest and the corresponding donor site morbidity, and have become increasingly popular in breast reconstruction. However, these flaps have less utility in chest wall reconstruction due to their less reliable vascularity, and potentially devastating consequences if flap loss occurs.

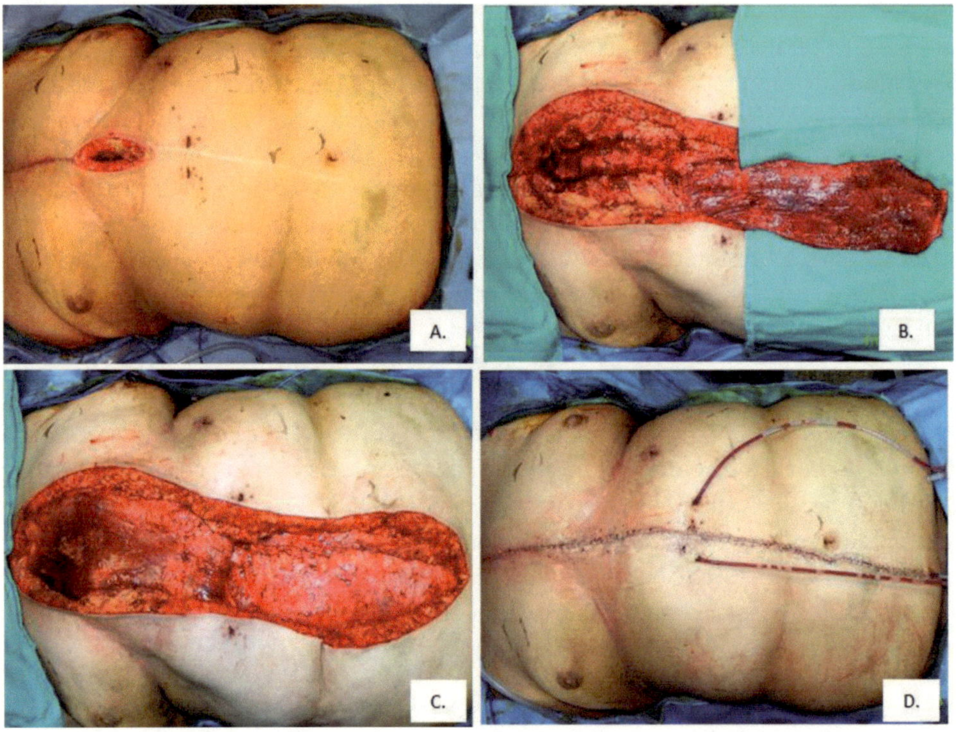

Figure 4. Vertical rectus abdominis muscle (VRAM) flap for closure of a sternal wound. (A) A 68-year-old female developed a median sternotomy wound infection following coronary artery bypass grafting. (B) A right vertical rectus abdominis muscle is elevated and divided from its attachments to the pubis. (C) The rectus abdominis muscle is transpositioned into the defect. (D) Final appearance of the anterior trunk following incision closure and placement of two abdominal drains.

Latissimus Dorsi

Tansini first described the use of a pedicled latissimus dorsi flap in 1906 to cover an anterior chest wall defect following mastectomy [39]. It remains a workhouse flap in chest wall reconstruction due to its reliability, size, and location and can be harvested as muscle alone or as a myocutaneous flap with a skin paddle to reconstruct full-thickness defects. The muscle is thin and broad and fans out from its origin on the thoracic, lumbar, and sacral vertebrae and posterior iliac crest to insert on the intertubercular groove of the humerus. Minor attachments to the inferior angle of the scapula and interdigitations with the external oblique at the anterolateral aspect are also present. It functions to extend, adduct, and medially rotate the upper extremity. In the absence of this muscle, these functions are generally well-compensated for by the other mucles of the shoulder girdle, including the pectoralis major, teres major, subscapularis, and deltoid muscles. The muscle is innervated by the thoracodorsal nerve, which arises from the posterior cord of the brachial plexus.

The muscle has a Mathes-Nahai Type V vascular supply, with one major vascular pedicle and secondary segmental vascular pedicles. The major blood supply is the thoracodorsal artery. The axillary atery gives off the subscapular artery, which then gives off two branches, first the circumflex scapular artery and then the thoracodorsal artery. The thoracodorsal vessels arise from the subscapular system in 94% of cases, 5% of the time they arise directly from the axillary vessels and the remaining 1% from the lateral thoracic vessels [58]. The thoracodorsal artery also gives off a branch to the serratus anterior. The pedicle enters on the deep aspect of the latissimus dorsi approximately 10 cm from the insertion of the muscle into the humerus and is accompanied by one or two venae comitantes and the thoracodorsal nerve. The significance of the serratus branch is that the latissimus can survive on this collateral if the thoracodorsal artery has been divided, which may occur, for example, during an axillary lymph node dissection. However, in patients with a history of radiation, there is an increased incidence of flap loss when it is based on retrograde flow through the serratus branch. The serratus branch can also be divided to lengthen the vascular pedicle from 7 cm to more than 10 cm [59]. The secondary segmental vascular pedicle is supplied by the ninth to eleventh posterior intercostal and lumbar arteries and associated veins. The latissimus can also survive on this secondary pedicle, and in this case the flap is raised as a turnover flap with the arc of rotation limited to the posterior central trunk. These dual arcs of rotation make the latissimus dorsi flap quite versatile based on the thoradorsal artery or segmental perforators.

As a result of its versatility, the latissimus flap can be utilized to reconstruct both anterior and posterior ipsilateral chest wall defects as well as neck and shoulder defects (Figure 5). In addition to dividing the serratus branch, the insertion on the humerus can be divided and the pedicle dissected from its investing fascia to increase the reach of the flap. The flap can be elevated as a myocutaneous flap with a skin island that can have any orientation. Primary closure of the donor site is usually possible if the width of the skin island is limited to 8 to 10 cm. If a larger skin island is required for reconstruction, the posterior donor site can be closed with a split thickness skin graft (Figure 5C). Due to its long pedicle and caliber of the thoracodorsal artery and vessels, the muscle is also an ideal choice for microsurgical free tissue transfer when indicated.

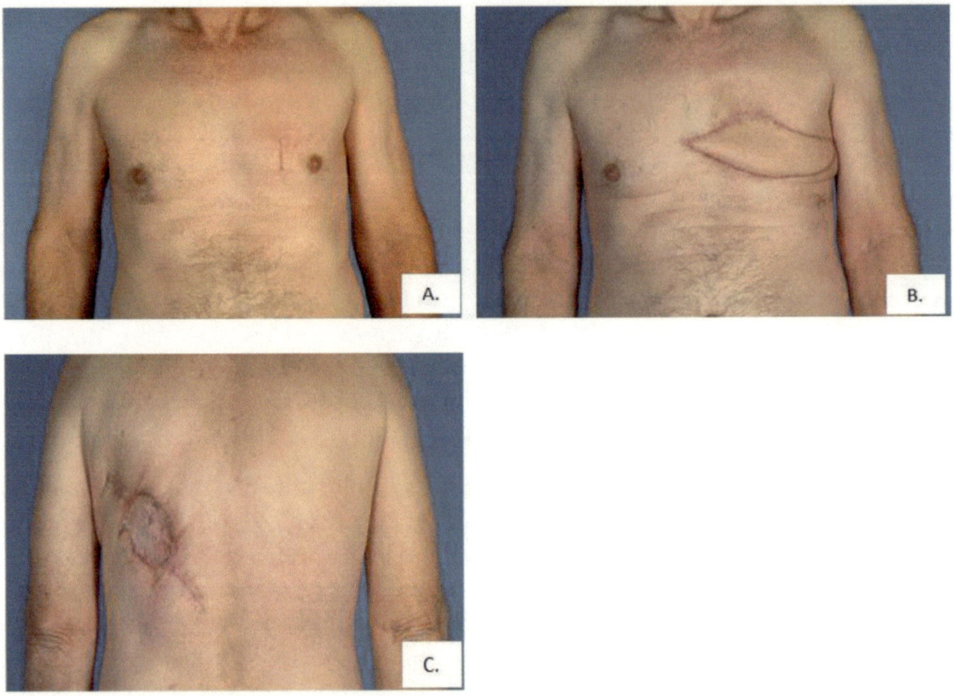

Figure 5. Latissimus dorsi musculocutaneous flap for anterior chest wall reconstruction. (A) A 59-year-old male with a desmoid tumor involving the left anterior chest wall. (B) Appearance of the left anterior chest wall three months following tumor resection and reconstruction with a left latissimus dorsi musculocutaneous flap. (C) Appearance following closure of the donor site with a split thickness skin graft.

The flap is harvested with the patient in the lateral thoracotomy position, with the arm prepped into the field to allow for manipulation during the procedure. A disadvantage of the latissimus is that the patient may need to be repositioned into this position intraoperatively for flap harvest. Donor site seroma rates are also very high, with one series reporting a 79% seroma rate, and donor site incision dehiscence rates are approximately 3% [60,61]. The harvest places a conspicous scar on the back, may leave a contour irregularity, and may require a skin graft for coverage of the donor site. The functional disability following flap harvest is generally minimal. Functional testing has revealed that the most significant deficit is weakness of the arm and that this is more significant in women than men. However, alternative flaps should be considered in patients who are crutch, walker, or wheelchair dependent and rely on the strength and function of the latissimus dorsi for mobility and for performance of activities of daily living.

External Oblique

The external oblique flap is an option to cover defects located in the lower anterior chest region up to the third intercostal space. It is a broad, thin muscle that originates from the fifth through twelfth ribs and inserts on the inguinal ligament and iliac crest. Its blood supply consists of the lateral cutaneous branches of the inferior eight posterior intercostal arteries, which provide a segmental blood supply to the muscle. The vessels enter the muscle posteriorly at the midaxillary line and send multiple perforating branches to the overlying skin. Traditionally, dissection included the anterior rectus sheath with the external oblique flap. However, this increases the risk of abdominal morbidity such as the development of abdominal hernias, especially if below the arcuate line, and may necessitate the use of prosthetic or bioprosthetic mesh to close the donor site. Studies have shown that the flap can be safely raised without the anterior rectus sheath by establishing the plane between the external and internal oblique muscles medially, then continuing the dissection laterally until the intercostal neurovascular bundles are encountered [62].

Trapezius

The trapezius flap can be utilized for reconstruction of defects of the upper mid-back, the base of the neck, and the shoulders. It is a broad, diamond-shaped superficial muscle located on the posterior thorax. It originates on the external occipital protuberance, the nuchal ligament, the medial superior nuchal line, and the spinous processes of C7-T12. It inserts on the lateral third of the clavicle, the acromion process, and the scapular spine. It is innervated by the eleventh cranial nerve, the spinal accessory nerve, and functions to move the scapula in a variety of directions. The dominant blood supply to the trapezius is the transverse cervical artery, which is a branch of the thyrocervical trunk arising from the subclavian artery. The overlying skin is supplied by musculocutaneous perforators, and the flap can be harvested as a muscular or myocutaneous flap. The cutaneous portion may extend up to 10 cm below the inferior edge of the muscle flap itself as long as one-third of the skin paddle overlies the trapezius muscle. Primary closure of the donor site is possible if the width of the skin paddle is less than 10 cm. To prevent dehiscence of the donor site closure, shoulder rotation and abduction should be minimized postoperatively for 4 to 6 weeks. Donor site morbidity is decreased if the surgeon preserves the superior 4 cm of the muscle, the spinal accessory nerve, and the insertion at the acromion [63].

Serratus Anterior

The serratus anterior is generally not used as an isolated muscle in chest wall reconstruction. It originates on the surface of the superior eight or nine ribs and inserts on the costal aspect of the medial margin of the scapula. The superior portion of the muscle is supplied by the lateral thoracic artery and the inferior by the thoracodorsal artery. It is innervated by the long thoracic nerve, and injury to this nerve results in the classic winged scapula. It is primarily used for intrathoracic defects and may also be elevated with the latissimus dorsi to carry additional skin and tissue to the anterior surface of the chest for reconstruction.

6.2. Microsurgical free tissue transfer

Local, pedicled flap options are the first choice for reconstruction of chest wall wounds in the majority of patients. However, factors such as trauma, recurrent disease, prior radiotherapy, or previous surgery may reduce or eliminate the possiblity of using local or regional flaps. Microsurgical free transfer is therefore a valuable technique in these patients to expand the choices for chest wall reconstruction. The most commonly used flaps include the latissimus dorsi, rectus abdominis, and omental flaps. Common lower extremity flaps, such as the anterolateral thigh flap or vastus lateralis, are also available. The recipient vessels available include the internal mammary vessels, thoracodorsal vessels, and branches of the thoracoacromial and thyrocervical trunks. Not all patients are suitable candidates for free flap reconstruction, either due to a poor prognosis or medical comorbidities, and therefore patient selection is critically important.

The *anterolateral thigh (ALT) flap* is a versatile fasciocutaneous flap based on the descending branch of the lateral femoral circumflex artery, which arises from the profunda femoris. It has a reliable vascularity and is relatively easy to harvest, making it an ideal choice for microsurgery. The donor site can be closed primarily when the skin paddle is less than 8 x 25 cm. Other advantages of this flap include a lengthy pedicle with good caliber vessels, and the possibility of being harvested as a sensate flap based on the lateral femoral cutaneous nerve of the thigh. Harvest does not require intraoperative repositioning of the patient, affording a two-team approach, and donor site morbidity is low.

6.3. Other methods of reconstruction

Omental Flap

The greater omentum consists of a large fold of peritoneum containing variable amounts of fat and lymphoid tissue. It is associated with the transverse colon and greater curvature of the stomach. It is highly vascularized, with an extensive vascular network supplied by the right and left gastroepiploic arteries, and the short gastric vessels. It may be as large as 36 x 46 cm^2 and can therefore cover large surface area defects and fill large cavities [64]. The large number of vessels supplying the omentum not only bring in a reliable blood supply, but can also afford a great deal of flexibility with regards to flap design. For coverage of low midline defects, all of the vascular anastomoses may be left intact. The pedicled flap can also be based on either the right or left gastroepiploic artery with its vascular arcade, and divided from the transverse colon and stomach to reach defects located anywhere on the anterior chest. The arc of rotation is 5-10 cm greater when the right gastroepiploic artery is utilized [65]. Once the omentum is transported to its new location, it is covered with a skin graft.

One disadvantage of the omental flap is that harvest requires a laparotomy, although laparoscopic flap harvest has been described. Associated intra-abdominal morbidity includes the potential for development of an abdominal hernia when the omentum is passed into the chest defect via a subcutaneous tunnel. The incidence of hernia development is as high as 21% when this approach is utilized. Therefore, a transdiaphragmatic route is preferred [66]. Flap inset is challenging due to the friable nature of omental tissue. It is also difficult to predict the size of the omentum preoperatively, as the volume of the greater omentum has no direct correlation with a patient's body habitus.

Chimeric Flaps

Chimeric flaps refer to two or more individual flaps that derive their blood supply from separate branches of the same vessel. They are utilized in chest wall reconstruction when coverage of a large surface area is required. One of the most useful examples is a combination of tissues based on the subscapular trunk, and may include the latissimus dorsi, serratus anterior, and a cutaneous portion based on the circumflex scapular vessels. It is also possible to include a bony component from the scapula. Since all of the branches converge on a single vascular trunk, the subscapular in this case, pedicled transposition on this vessel is possible. Further, free tissue transfer requires only one set of anastomoses. Preoperative angiography is useful for surgical planning to evaluate an individual patient's vascular anatomy.

Skin Grafts

Skin grafts have a limited role in chest wall reconstruction, but are a simple and straightforward means of reconstruction in select cases. They may be utilized for partial thickness defects that involve only the skin and subcutaneous tissues of the chest. They may also be used as an adjunct for coverage of muscle flaps when a skin island is not included in the flap or is not large enough to close the entire defect. When used alone, however, they will not provide the bulk, durability, or vascularity of a muscle flap. In addition, skin grafts will contract during healing, resulting in a poorer aesthetic outcome and potential scar contractures. Lastly, skin grafts may not take when utilized in a radiated field, or may break down in a wound if postoperative radiation therapy is required.

Tissue Expansion

Tissue expansion is a well-established means of stretching skin adjacent to a defect, enabling the use of chest wall tissue for reconstruction of chest wall wounds, thus avoiding distant donor site scars. Its indications in chest wall reconstruction are restricted to partial thickness chest wall defects in which optimal form and contour are required. The skin adjacent to a defect must be suitable to use as advancement flaps following expansion. It is contraindicated for defects associated with chronic infection or radiation-induced injury. The process involves placement of tissue expanders in a subcutaneous pocket beneath healthy skin and gradually inflating the expanders with saline over several months.

Negative Pressure Wound Therapy

Negative pressure wound therapy (NPWT), or vaccum-assisted closure, has become a popular modality for the treatment of a variety of wounds, including sternal wounds. The system involves a pump that applies either continuous or intermittent negative pressure that is connected to an open cell foam covered with a semi-occlusive drape. The exact mechanism of action is unknown, but is possibly due to the induction of cell division, proliferation, and angiogenesis secondary to the mechanical forces transmitted through the foam to the wound surface. The negative pressure also leads to the removal of interstitial edema, promoting blood flow to the wound by decreasing capillary compression. NPWT may be used in the initial management of a wound as a temporary dressing when definitive closure or flap coverage has to be delayed. It can also be utilized as a bolster over skin grafts post-operatively to increase the surface contact, stabilize the graft, and promote take. One advantage of NPWT is that the dressing can be changed approximately every 48-72 hours, decreasing the number of dressing changes for patients. Absolute contraindications of NPWT include using the dressing over exposed blood vessels or organs, and relative contraindications include the use of the device in wounds containing malignant tumors, untreated osteomyelitis, necrotic tissue, and non-enteric or unexplored fistulas.

Author details

Christodoulos Kaoutzanis
Department of Surgery, Saint Joseph Mercy Health System, Ann Arbor, MI, USA

Tiffany N.S. Ballard
Section of Plastic Surgery, Department of Surgery, University of Michigan Health System, Ann Arbor, MI, USA

Paul S. Cederna
Section of Plastic Surgery, Department of Biomedical Engineering, Department of Surgery, University of Michigan Health System, Ann Arbor, MI, USA

Acknowledgement

We would like to thank Doros Polydorou, M.D. for producing the schematic illustrations for Figures 1 and 2.

7. References

[1] Van Aalst JA, Phillips JD, Sadove AM (2009) Pediatric chest wall and breast deformities. Plast Reconstr Surg. 124: 38e-49e.
[2] Cahill JL, Lees GM, Robertson HT (1984) A summary of preoperative and postoperative cardiorespiratory performance in patients undergoing pectus excavatum and carinatum repair. J Pediatr Surg. 19: 430-433.
[3] Weg JG, Krumholz RA, Harkleroad LE (1967) Pulmonary dysfunction in pectus excavatum. Am Rev Respir Dis. 96: 936-945.
[4] Quigley PM, Haller JA, Jelus KL, Loughlin GM, Marcus CL (1996) Cardiorespiratory function before and after corrective surgery in pectus excavatum. J Pediatr. 128: 638-643.
[5] Ravitch MM (1951) Pectus excavatum and heart failure. Surgery. 30: 178–194.
[6] Ravitch MM (1961) Operative treatment of congenital deformities of the chest. Am J Surg. 19: 588–597.
[7] Fonkalsrud EW, DeUgarte D, Choi E (2002) Repair of pectus excavatum and carinatum deformities in 116 adults. Ann Surg. 236: 304-312; discussion 312-314.
[8] Peterson RJ, Young WG, Godwin JD, Sabiston DC Jr, Jones RH (1985) Noninvasive assessment of exercise cardiac function before and after pectus excavatum repair. J Thorac Cardiovasc Surg. 90: 251-260.
[9] Fonkalsrud EW (2008) Surgical correction of pectus carinatum: lessons learned from 260 patients. J Pediatr Surg. 43: 1235-1243.

[10] Fonkalsrud EW, Beanes S (2001) Surgical management of pectus carinatum: 30 years' experience. World J Surg. 25: 898–903.
[11] Iakovlev VM, Nechaeva GI, Viktorova IA (1990) Clinical function of the myocardium and cardio- and hemodynamics in patients with pectus carinatum deformity. Ter Arkh. 62: 69-72.
[12] Clarkson P (1962) Poland's syndactyly. Guys Hosp Rep. 111: 335-346.
[13] Poland A (1841) Deficiency of the pectoral muscles. Guys Hosp Rep. 6: 191-193.
[14] Shalev SA, Hall JG (2003) Poland anomaly: Report of an unusual family. Am J Med Genet. 118A: 180–183.
[15] Darian VB, Argenta LC, Pasyk KA (1989) Familial Poland's syndrome. Ann Plast Surg. 23: 531-537.
[16] Moir CR, Johnson CH (2008) Poland's syndrome. Semin Pediatr Surg. 17: 161-166.
[17] O'Connor MB, Gallagher DP, Mulloy E (2008) Jeune syndrome. Postgrad Med J. 84: 559.
[18] de Vries J, Yntema JL, van Die CE, Crama N, Cornelissen EA, Hamel BC (2010) Jeune syndrome: description of 13 cases and a proposal for follow-up protocol. Eur J Pediatr. 169: 77-88.
[19] Yang SS, Langer LO Jr, Cacciarelli A, Dahms BB, Unger ER, Roskamp J, Dinno ND, Chen H (1987) Three conditions in neonatal asphyxiating thoracic dysplasia (Jeune) and short rib-polydactyly syndrome spectrum: a clinicopathologic study. Am J Med Genet Suppl. 3: 191-207.
[20] Shamberger RC (2000) Chest Wall Deformities. In: Shields TW, LoCicero J III, Ponn RB, editors. General Thoracic Surgery. Vol 1, 5th ed. Philadelphia: Lippincott Williams and Wilkins. pp. 535-561.
[21] Pairolero PC (2000) Chest Wall Tumors. In: Shields TW, LoCicero J III, Ponn RB, editors. General Thoracic Surgery. Vol 1, 5th ed. Philadelphia: Lippincott Williams and Wilkins. pp. 589-598.
[22] Burt M, Fulton M, Wessner-Dunlap S, Karpeh M, Huvos AG, Bains MS, Martini N, McCormack PM, Rusch VW, Ginsberg RJ (1992) Primary bony and cartilaginous sarcomas of the chest wall: results of therapy. Ann Thorac Surg. 54: 226-232.
[23] Douglas YL, Meuzelaar KJ, Van Der Lei B, Pras B, Hoekstra HJ (1997) Osteosarcoma of the sternum. Eur J Surg Oncol. 23: 90-91.
[24] Buitendijk S, van de Ven CP, Dumans TG, den Hollander JC, Nowak PJ, Tissing WJ, Pieters R, van den Heuvel-Eibrink MM (2005) Pediatric aggressive fibromatosis: a retrospective analysis of 13 patients and review of literature. Cancer. 104: 1090-1099.
[25] Losanoff JE, Richman BW, Jones JW (2002) Necrotizing soft tissue infection of the chest wall. J Cardiovasc Surg (Torino). 43: 549-552.
[26] Gill EA Jr, Stevens DL (1989) Primary sternal osteomyelitis. West J Med. 151: 199-203.
[27] Culliford AT, Cunningham JN Jr, Zeff RH, Isom OW, Teiko P, Spencer FC (1976) Sternal and costochondral infections following open-heart surgery-A review of 2,594 cases. J Thorac Cardiovasc Surg. 72: 714-726.
[28] Ridderstolpe L, Gill H, Granfeldt H, Ahlfeldt H, Rutberg H (2001) Superficial and deep sternal wound complications: incidence, risk factors and mortality. Eur J Cardiothorac Surg. 20: 1168-1175.

[29] Johnson P, Frederiksen JW, Sanders JH, Lewis V, Michaelis LL (1985) Management of chronic sternal osteomyelitis. Ann Thorac Surg. 40: 69-72.

[30] Jones G, Jurkiewicz MJ, Bostwick J, Wood R, Bried JT, Culbertson J, Howell R, Eaves F, Carlson G, Nahai F (1997) Management of the infected median sternotomy wound with muscle flaps. The Emory 20-year experience. Ann Surg. 225: 766-776; discussion 776-778.

[31] Bishara J, Gartman-Israel D, Weinberger M, Maimon S, Tamir G, Pitlik S (2000) Osteomyelitis of the ribs in the antibiotic era. Scand J Infect Dis. 32: 223-227.

[32] Carlos GN, Kesler KA, Coleman JJ, Broderick L, Terrentine MW, Brown JW (1997) Aggressive surgical management of sternoclavicular joint infections. J Thorac Cardiovasc Surg. 113: 242-247.

[33] Bayer AS, Chow AW, Louie JS, Guze LB (1977) Sternoarticular pyoarthrosis due to gram-negative bacilli. Report of eight cases. Arch Intern Med. 137:1036-1040.

[34] Ross JJ, Shamsuddin H (2004) Sternoclavicular septic arthritis: review of 180 cases. Medicine (Baltimore). 83: 139-148.

[35] Song HK, Guy TS, Kaiser LR, Shrager JB (2002) Current presentation and optimal surgical management of sternoclavicular joint infections. *Ann Thorac Surg.* 73: 427-431.

[36] Zehr KJ, Heitmiller RF, Yang SC (1999) Split pectoralis major muscle flap reconstruction after clavicular-manubrial resection. Ann Thorac Surg. 67: 1507-1508.

[37] Chang RR, Mehrara BJ, Hu QY, Disa JJ, Cordeiro PG (2004) Reconstruction of complex oncologic chest wall defects: a 10-year experience. Ann Plast Surg. 52: 471-479; discussion 479.

[38] O'Dwyer J (1887) Fifty cases of croup in private practice treated by intubation of the larynx, with a description of the method and of the dangers incident thereto. *Med Rec.* 32: 557-561.

[39] Tansini I (1906) Sopra il mio nuovo processo di amputazione della mammella. *Gazz Med ltal Torino.* 57: 141.

[40] Watson WL, James AG (1947) Fascia lata grafts for the chest wall defects. *J Thorac Surg.* 16: 399-406.

[41] Kiricuta I (1963) The use of the great omentum in the surgery of breast cancer. Presse Med. 71: 15-17.

[42] Mathes SJ (1995) Chest wall reconstruction. Clin Plast Surg. 22: 187-198.

[43] Larson DL, McMurtrey MJ (1984) Musculocutaneous flap reconstruction of chest-wall defects: An experience with 50 patients. Plast Reconstr Surg. 73: 734-740.

[44] Kohman LJ, Auchincloss JH, Gilbert R, Beshara M (1991) Functional results of muscle flap closure for sternal infection. Ann Thorac Surg. 52: 102-106.

[45] Meadows JA 3rd, Staats BA, Pairolero PC, Rodarte JR, Arnold PG (1985) Effect of resection of the sternum and manubrium in conjunction with muscle transposition on pulmonary function. Mayo Clin Proc. 60: 604-609.

[46] Netscher DT, Eladoumikdachi F, McHugh PM, Thornby J, Soltero E (2003) Sternal wound debridement and muscle flap reconstruction: Functional implications. Ann Plast Surg. 51: 115-122; discussion 123-125.

[47] Miller JI Jr (2000) Postsurgical Empyema. In: Shields TW, LoCicero J III, Ponn RB, editors. General Thoracic Surgery. Vol 1, 5th ed. Philadelphia: Lippincott Williams and Wilkins. pp. 709-715.
[48] Fonkalsrud EW, Beanes S, Hebra A, Adamson W, Tagge E (2002) Comparison of minimally invasive and modified Ravitch pectus excavatum repair. J Pediatr Surg. 37: 413-417.
[49] Schaarschmidt K, Kolberg-Schwerdt A, Dimitrov G, Straubeta J (2002) Submuscular bar, multiple pericostal bar fixation, bilateral thoracoscopy: a modified Nuss repair in adolescents. J Pediatr Surg. 37: 1276-1280.
[50] McCormack PM (1989) Use of prosthetic materials in chest wall reconstruction. Assets and liabilities. Surg Clin N Am. 69: 965-976.
[51] Losken A, Thourani V, Carlson G, Jones G, Culbertson J, Miller J, Mansour K (2004) A reconstructive algorithm for plastic surgery following extensive chest wall resection. Br J Plast Surg. 57: 295-302.
[52] Anderson B, Burt M (1994) Chest wall neoplasms and their management. Ann Thorac Surg. 58: 1774-1781.
[53] Netscher D, Baumholtz M (2009) Chest reconstruction I: Anterior and anterolateral chest wall and wounds affecting respiratory function. Plast Reconstr Surg. 124: 240-252.
[54] Mehta S, Sarkar S, Kavarana N, Bhathena H, Mehta A (1996) Complications of the pectoralis major myocutaneous flap in the oral cavity: A prospective evaluation of 220 cases. Plast Reconstr Surg. 98: 31-37.
[55] Kroll S, Reece G, Miller M, Schusterman M (1992) Comparison of the rectus abdominis free flap with the pectoralis major myocutaneous flap for reconstruction in the head and neck. Am J Surg. 164: 615-618.
[56] Castelli M, Pecorari G, Succo G, Bena A, Andreis M, Sartoris A (2001) Pectoralis major myocutaneous flaps: Analysis of complications in difficult patients. Eur Arch Otorhinolaryngol. 258: 542-545.
[57] Hartrampf C, Scheflan M, Black P (1982) Breast reconstruction with a transverse abdominal island flap. Plast Reconstr Surg. 69: 216-225.
[58] Rowsell A, Eisenberg N, Davies D, Taylor G (1986) The anatomy of the thoracodorsal artery within the latissimus dorsi muscle. Br J Plast Surg. 39: 206-209.
[59] Moelleken B, Mathes S, Chang N (1989) Latissimus dorsi muscle-musculocutaneous flap in chest wall reconstruction. Surg Clin North Am. 69: 977-990.
[60] Delay E, Gounot N, Bouillot A, Zlatoff P, Rivoire M (1998) Autologous lastissimus dorsi breast reconstruction: A 3-year clinical experience with 100 patients. Plast Reconst Surg. 102: 1461-1478.
[61] Menke H, Erkens M, Olbrisch R. (2001) Evolving concepts in breast reconstruction with latissimus dorsi flaps: Results and follow up of 121 consecutive patients. Ann Plast Surg. 47: 107-114.
[62] Moschella F, Cordova A (1999) A new extended external oblique musculocutaneous flap for reconstruction of large chest wall defects. 103: 1278-1385.
[63] Villa M, Chang D (2010) Muscle and omental flaps for chest wall reconstruction. Thorac Surg Clin 20: 543-550.

[64] Mathisen D, Grillo H, Vlahakes G, Daggett W (1988) The omentum in the management of complicated cardiothoracic problems. J Thorac Cardiovasc Surg. 95: 677-684.

[65] Das S (1976) The size of the human omentum and methods of lengthening it for transplantation. Br J Plast Surg. 29: 144-170.

[66] Weinzweig N, Yetman R (1995) Transposition of the greater omentum for recalcitrant median sternotomy wound infections. Ann Plast Surg. 34: 471-477.

Chapter 11

Thoracic Trauma

Slobodan Milisavljević, Marko Spasić and Miloš Arsenijević

Additional information is available at the end of the chapter

http://dx.doi.org/10.5772/54139

1. Introduction

Thoracic trauma is a significant cause of morbidity and mortality in both adults and children. It is a leading cause of death in approximately 25% of multiple trauma patients and, when associated with other injuries, it causes death in additional 50% of multiple trauma patients, usually as a result of hypoxia and hypovolemia. When cardiac trauma is not involved, mortality from isolated penetrating chest injury is low (<1%), but if cardiac trauma is present, mortality rises to about 20%. The most important issue with thoracic trauma is to prevent lethal outcomes, because many of these wounds are fatal shortly after the injury or a few hours afterwards. Thoracic injury may occur in isolation (isolated thoracic trauma), or in the presence of polytrauma. According to etiology, thoracic injuries are divided into: blunt traumas and penetrating chest wounds. Specific injuries are: pulmonary barotraumas, burns of the tracheobronchial tree resulted from aspiration, blast lung injury, parenchymal lung damage from aspiration, and iatrogenic injury. Fractures associated with the chest wall may be caused by a direct force, and the tissues and organs of the chest may be damaged including contusions, lacerations or rupture. In addition, traumatic forces can act indirectly; in such cases the effect of a traumatic force is manifested after the disintegration of the tissue (air embolism resulting from the entrance of air into the pulmonary veins after lung laceration).[1]

The most common mechanisms of blunt trauma are road traffic accidents (70%), while drivers and front seat passengers in motor vehicles are most exposed to risk, and motorcycle drivers are much less frequently injured (10%), but with the highest percentage of death at the site of accidents (30%).[2,3] There are five types of motor vehicle-related injuries: head-on collision, side impact crashes, rear impact crashes, rotational impact and rollover, and injuries resulted from deceleration (deceleration injury) and crushing (crush injuries). At deceleration, a rapidly moving body is brought to a sudden halt, and injuries occur at the time of the abrupt impact of the body, damaging the chest wall, while internal organ injuries result from reflex glottic closure and therefore rapidly increasing intra-thoracic pressure. The transverse thoracic diameter increased rapidly, and when the traumatic force overcomes the elastic limit of the lungs the tracheobronchial tree injuries occur along with the injuries of the lung parenchyma, diaphragm, and mediastinal structures. The mechanism of deceleration injury is identical to the falls. [3]

Penetrating thoracic wounds occur as a consequence of side arms or firearms and are classified into three groups:

1. " Sleeper " wounds (no exit wound)
2. Perforating wounds (entrance wound and exit wound)
3. Wounds in which the projectile penetrates through the whole intra-thoracic cavity and remains in the subcutaneous tissue.

A common feature of all penetrating wounds is in direct communication between the external environment and the pleural space. If a defect in the chest wall is large, an open pneumothorax occurs. In small defects, wounds close spontaneously due to the contraction of muscle or blood clotting. However, it should be always borne in mind that establishing communication between the external environment and the pleural space leads to suction of air and devitalised tissue in the pleural space, favouring the infection development and further complicating the clinical management of the injuries.[4-6]

2. Pathophyslogy of thoracic trauma

Traumatic force with thoracic trauma impairs lung function by causing:

1. Disorder in the mechanics of breathing
2. Disruption in ventilation-perfusion relationship
3. Gas exchange abnormalities of alveolocapillary membrane

3. Disorder in the mechanics of breathing

Disorders in the mechanics of breathing with thoracic trauma are caused by blunt trauma related to rib fractures and flail chest and are accompanied with hypoventilation, atelectasis, difficult expectoration of sputum from the tracheobronchial tree, the development of bronchopneumonic complications, acute respiratory failure and even death, especially with elderly patients with penetrating injuries with direct communication between the external environment and the pleural space, leading to the occurrence of pneumothorax, haemothorax, traumatic diaphragmatic rupture and ruptured large airway. The presence of air or blood in the pleural space leads to the collapse of the lungs, the development of arteriovenous shunt and hypoxia. Disorder of breathing mechanics may threaten the life of the injured because it leads to respiratory disturbance, hypoxia and cyanosis, as in the case of tension pneumothorax.[1-6]

4. Disruption in ventilation - perfusion relationship

Normal blood oxygenation and elimination of CO_2 depends on the ventilation-perfusion relationship in the lungs. In thoracic trauma the disorder in ventilation-perfusion relationship appears with the lung collapse or mechanical obstruction of the large airway. Lobar collapse or the whole lung collapse is accompanied by perfusion through collapsed parenchyma, but since oxygenation is not maintained, it leads to systemic hypoxia. Impaired lung perfusion may appear following vascular thrombosis in damaged lung parenchyma and/or massive fat microembolism, disseminated intravascular coagulation (DIC) and acute respiratory distress syndrome (ARDS).[1-6]

5. Gas exchange abnormalities of alveolocapillary membrane

The alveolocapillary membrane is composed of the surfactant layer, the surface of macrophages, alveolar epithelium, the interstitial space and the capillary endothelium. In thoracic trauma direct damage to the alveolocapillary membrane may occur, as in the case of lung contusion, smoke inhalation, aspiration of gastric contents, heart failure and pulmonary interstitial oedema due to the excessive use of infusion solutions and blood transfusion. The most important factors that later damage the alveolar membrane are: ARDS, the development of hyaline membrane and alveolar oedema, terminal airway collapse and occlusion of blood capillaries, acid-base disturbance due to hypoxemia and hypercapnia, pulmonary hypertension, increased interstitial fluid pressure which increases the capillary resistance and disseminated intravascular coagulation.[2-6]

6. General surgical assessment of thoracic trauma

6.1. Introduction

A comprehensive and thorough examination of the injured and the assessing the injury severity must be done shortly, sometimes during the immediate treatment of potentially lethal injuries. Upon the arrival to the surgery, initial examination and assessment are important. It is of decisive importance for the injured, regardless of difficulties that may arise from the very beginning. The main task of a surgeon is to assess the state of the injured in order to detect or prevent life-threatening conditions. Conditions in case of thoracic trauma require medical emergency care, often immediately upon the patient's admission to hospital. These are:[7]

- airway obstruction
- massive haemothorax
- tension pneumothorax
- open pneumothorax
- flail chest
- cardiac tamponade

These states should be distinguished from other possible severe lesions that need to be treated by surgery. The surgeon must perform a physical examination and must ensure quick resolution, when the situation is complex and laboratory tests and a chest X-ray are time-consuming. Physical examination and clinical judgment are needed to decide upon the necessity for tracheostomy, chest drainage, emergency pericardiocentesis or thoracotomy. In certain cases, the information gained from arterial blood gas analysis directs towards the diagnosis of acidosis, hypoxemia, or alkalosis. Physical examination is important regarding the patient health history. Such information may result in the proper assessing the injury-related condition, and also may be a guideline for additional therapeutic procedures which are not directly due to trauma. Data on hypertension, cardiac arrhythmias, cardiomegaly, diabetes, renal failure, peripheral arterial occlusive disease, phlebothrombosis, hepatomegaly and splenomegaly, pulmonary emphysema and chronic obstructive pulmonary disease, possible alcoholism or alcoholism findings, and taking drugs or sedatives may be very significant.

6.2. Attitudes in thoracic trauma surgery

The first priority in the evaluation and treatment of thoracic injury is restoring of the airway passages, safety of lung ventilation and cardiovascular stability. Blood gas analysis can provide useful information when the circulatory system is preserved. The decision regarding the widening of airway passages can be made only on the basis of clinical observation. Tachypnoea (respiratory rate >30 breaths per minute) or clinical signs of increased respiratory muscle fatigue are common symptoms of respiratory insufficiency which requires urgent consideration. Endotracheal intubation and mechanical ventilation are indicated in patients with clinical signs of respiratory fatigue and tachypnea of over 35 breaths per minute, in patients in a state of shock, and in patients with associated craniocerebral injuries. Circulatory status is evaluated and adjusted simultaneously with the widening of the airway passages. In patients with hypotension it is necessary to evaluate the state of intra-thoracic organs in order to identify the cause of shock [8-10] induced by:

- tension pneumothorax
- haemothorax
- cardiac tamponade
- cardiac dysfunction after myocardial contusion
- air embolism
- large intra-thoracic vessel injuries
- massive contusion of lung parenchyma
- rupture of the diaphragm

Data on the mechanism of injury may be valuable for surgeons while assessing the types and characteristics of thoracic injuries. For example, patients who were run over in road traffic accidents or those crushed in motor vehicle accidents are expected to have severe intra-thoracic injuries. Deceleration injuries indicate potential injuries to large blood vessels (aortic arch and thoracic aorta) or large airway (trachea and main bronchi). In patients admitted with symptoms of hypotension diagnostic procedure begins with the examination of the neck veins. Distended (swollen) neck veins may point to possible cardiac compression shock, caused by tension pneumothorax or cardiac tamponade, while hypovolaemic shock is mainly associated with the neck vein collapse. Examining the chest wall during spontaneous respiration may indicate paradoxical breathing due to flail chest. Palpation may reveal the unstable chest wall integrity due to fractures or subcutaneous emphysema crepitation, which may be associated with the development of pneumothorax. Pain and tenderness may occur over the rib, sternum and clavicle fractures. Isolated chest trauma resulting from blunt trauma is very rare. Blunt thoracic trauma in polytraumatized patients is mainly associated with extra-thoracic injuries. The most common injuries among the associated extra-thoracic injuries and chest injuries are:

- Cranial injuries
- Abdominal injuries
- Extremity fractures
- Pelvic fractures
- Vertebral fractures

Associated extra-thoracic injuries occur in approximately two thirds of multiple trauma patients (Shor et al, 1987; Besson and Saegesser 1983; Glinz 1991) [3,11,12]. Main cause of haemodynamic instability in half of the injured patients with systolic pressure less than 100 mm Hg on admission to hospital is in severe intra-abdominal injury. Localization of penetrating thoracic injuries is important; entrance and/or exit wounds should be observed, but such wounds should not be probed. If the entrance penetrating injury is below the fifth rib, it is necessary to investigate the possibility of diaphragmatic rupture and intra-abdominal organ injury. The integrity of the diaphragm may be checked by using different techniques: video-assisted thoracoscopy, thoracoscopy, laparoscopy, laparotomy, and thoracotomy. Exploration of the abdomen in haemodynamically unstable patients with multiple chest and abdominal injuries is recommended first. Then abdominal bleeding is controlled, providing the intra-thoracic organs are stable. Finding the cause of intra-abdominal bleeding, the chest organ injuries may be explored and treated. Chest radiography is necessary if there is no need for emergency thoracotomy or if developing tension pneumothorax is excluded. Besides the investigation of the usual effects of thoracic trauma, particular attention is paid to possible injury-related complications or injuries that may be easily overlooked in the initial evaluation. The most common injuries that may be overlooked on the initial chest radiography in multiple trauma patients are:

- soft tissue injury
- bone injury
- ruptured diaphragm
- mediastinal expansion
- foreign body
- pneumomediastinum

Up to 35% of the patients with thoracic trauma along with a ruptured diaphragm appear to have normal or nearly normal results on initial radiographic findings. In patients with penetrating injuries it is useful to mark the entrance wound with an X-ray sensitive marker. It is useful to mark the initial localization of the foreign body inside the chest because it may move later, or cause embolism. Low-speed projectile wounds cause minimal injury to the chest wall, except when associated with intercostal vascular injury or internal mammary artery. Penetrating chest wall injuries are treated conservatively for possible massive bleeding. In the case of bleeding vessels, the therapy should include thoracotomy and ligation of the injured vessels. High-speed projectiles and firearms at close range have high penetrating power causing the considerable destruction in the projectile trajectory and surrounding tissue. Surgical treatment and debridement of the devitalised tissue is indicated in most cases. Chest wall trauma often indicates possible associated intra-abdominal injuries. According to some authors, diaphragmatic rupture and abdominal organ injuries are possible in such cases.[13] In such haemodynamically stable patients the integrity of the diaphragm may be assessed using laparoscopy. Similarly, in cases where diaphragmatic rupture is initially recognized, laparotomy is performed to inspect the abdomen and treat the diaphragmatic rupture. Laparotomy is also indicated in haemodynamically unstable patients with penetrating trauma to the chest wall and in patients with blunt trauma in the same area, since in such cases intra-abdominal injury may be expected. Chest wall injuries and intra-thoracic injuries are common in road accidents. In such cases common extra-thoracic injuries significantly complicate the patient's condition. It is not rare that other injuries are even more severe than the thoracic injury itself.[14] Complex polytrauma requires multiple specialist input, but output is often uncertain, especially in patients with severe intra-thoracic and craniocerebral injuries. After the initial treatment of life-threatening conditions, thoracic trauma is further managed with pain control and chest physiotherapy. Poor thoracic pain management and insufficient chest physiotherapy, i.e. poor respiratory hygiene, necessarily lead to various pulmonary complications.

Thoracotomy or thoracoscopy are indicated in the cases of: [15-18]

- open pneumothorax
- penetrating injuries due to foreign bodies or suspected foreign bodies
- bleeding complications of chest drain
- massive haemoptysis
- continuous air leak from the chest drain and permanent collapse of the lung
- tracheobronchial injury
- cardiac tamponade
- damage to large blood vessels and heart injuries
- diaphragm injuries and oesophagus injuries
- Thoracoabdominal injuries associated with intra-thoracic organ injuries
- complication of the injury - evacuation of coagulum or decortication (empyema)

7. Diagnostic procedures with thoracic trauma

7.1. Chest radiography and other techniques in the diagnosis of chest trauma

Chest radiography is the first-line diagnostic tool providing additional information in the diagnosis and evaluation of thoracic injuries.[19] The initial radiograph includes assessment of the injury and disorders directly or potentially threatening to a patient's life. Notwithstanding the objective limitations of the methods on the basis of clinical and radiographic findings, in many cases the surgeon may decide about the appropriate surgical treatment. In unconscious patients with multiple traumas chest radiography is useful immediately after the admission, after the establishment of airway passages (usually endotracheal intubation) and the insertion of nasogastric or orogastric tubes (used to determine the position of the mediastinum). In patients with penetrating injuries entrance and exit wounds should be marked with radiosensitive markers. Radiographs are normally taken in the AP or PA views. It is desirable to take a radiograph in inspiring, but if taken during expirium it may be useful in detecting small pneumothorax. Native radiographs may be used for evaluation of chest wall integrity, primarily to detect rib fractures and to examine the spine and mediastinum. Lateral decubitus radiographs are useful for the detection of air and liquid collection. Patient's position during exposure may be important in evaluation findings. A surgeon carefully and systematically interprets chest radiographs in order not to overlook some possible injuries. Then, the surgeon must check: [20]

1. **The correct placement of the endotracheal tube**: A surgeon must be sure that the tube is not positioned too high in the trachea, just below the vocal cords, as there is a risk of pulling it out while dealing with the patient; or the tube may be placed too deep – commonly in the right main bronchus to prevent the ventilation of the left lung.
2. **Pneumothorax**: The finding can easily be overlooked in the rush or when the radiograph is not carefully analyzed. Special attention must be paid to the lateral side of the chest and the possible costophrenic angles with increased lucency.
3. **Tension pneumothorax**: a typical radiograph shows increased lucency in the ipsylateral hemithorax, along with the diaphragm depression and shift of the trachea and mediastinum to the opposite side (easily noticeable if nasogastric tube is placed).
4. **Haemothorax**: Shaded area of hemithorax can be seen in X-ray findings. An X-ray reveals a shadow in the hemithorax due to persistent bleeding. However, in minor bleeding there is no characteristic radiographic finding and the interpretation is more difficult. In such cases, it is useful to compare the findings of both hemithoraces and spot X-ray shadowed areas, particularly in the costophrenic angles. When the radiograph is taken in the supine position, the blood may spread in the posterior part of hemithorax, which appears as the slight shadow of hemithorax on the X-ray through which the normal lung pattern is shown.
5. **Mediastinal emphysema**: There is no air in the mediastinum under usual conditions. When the X-ray shows the presence of air in the mediastinum and neck, especially when it is associated with pneumothorax (chest drain does not encourage lung re-expansion), tracheobronchial rupture should be considered.
6. **Lung contusion**: It cannot be seen on initial radiographs, but it is indicated by lung parenchyma diffuse shadows.
7. **The protrusion of intra-abdominal organs into the thorax**: Diaphragm injury is followed by herniation of intra-abdominal organs into the chest. On the left side the finding of hydroaeric collection may be mistaken for hydropneumothorax. Therefore, it is useful to place a nasogastric tube indicating the character of the injury. Radiographic diagnosis of diaphragmatic rupture on the right side is sometimes very difficult. The liver is most commonly herniated organ, and then the only possible finding is the elevation of the right hemi-diaphragm.

8. **Fractures**: Rib fractures are sometimes difficult to recognize in the native radiographs. Therefore, a detailed physical examination is necessary. However, multiple fractures such as flail chest are easily detectable. Attention should be paid to possible fractures or vertebral dislocation, fractures of clavicle and humeral condylar fractures.
9. **Projectiles in the thorax**: Any penetrating wound of the chest should be examined radiographically, especially in order to understand the direction of projectile penetration, the scope of organ damage and the position of the projectile in the chest. When a projectile enters from one side of the body to the other, or when it passes through the mediastinum, additional examination of the oesophagus, aorta and trachea should be performed for potential harm. Laparotomy is indicated when the projectile is located under the diaphragm and the entrance wound is above it.
10. **Mediastinal expansion**: Extended mediastinal shadow is a major finding indicating aortic rupture. When the initial radiograph shows extended mediastinal shadow, especially in the supine position, it is necessary and useful to take a posterolateral radiograph in the standing position. Mediastinal shadow wider than 8 cm most likely indicates the transection of the aorta and aortography should follow. Other radiographic findings indicating the aortic rupture are shadowing in the aortopulmonary window, depression of the left main bronchus, nasogastric tube deviation to the right, fractured ribs on the left side and left haemothorax.

In some cases, when the patient's condition is relatively stable, it is recommended to use thoracic computed tomography (chest CT) in additional diagnostic procedure. Using CT scan with contrast pleural space, lung parenchyma and mediastinum can be evaluated more precisely.

Another useful method is ultrasound scan of the abdomen and chest, especially for evaluation of the subdiaphragmatic space findings and when small collections of fluid in the pleural space are detected, and also for cardiac evaluation, especially when blood is present in the pericardial space. Ultrasound scan is simple, fast, non-invasive and reliable technique applicable to different body parts, such as the abdomen and thorax (evaluation of the subdiaphragmatic space including the liver, spleen, pancreas, retroperitoneal space, kidney, diaphragm; detection of the subphrenic collection; detection of small collections of fluid in the pleural space that cannot be seen in standard chest radiographs). Echocardiography, transesophageal echocardiography (used to assess the functional state of the heart and collection of blood in the pericardial space), and Color Doppler (used for the evaluation and detection of injuries to the brachiocephalic vessels) are also in current use. Ultrasound of the abdomen and thorax is becoming a routine diagnostic method that is used along with chest radiography. Fast and careful radiographic evaluation is indicated in patients with thoracic trauma. Native thoracic radiography is still the primary diagnostic tool. However, in modern and well equipped facilities chest CT and MSCT and ultrasound scan of the abdomen and chest have an important role in the diagnosis of thoracic trauma. Quick and qualitative diagnostics and therapeutics are possible only in direct cooperation between surgeons and radiologists, not only in taking and interpretation of radiographic or ultrasonographic findings, but also in monitoring the effects of the therapy applied or dealing with possible complications. VATS (Video-Assisted Thoracoscopy) has become widely used surgical procedure in the evaluation of thoracic trauma. Indications of VATS in thoracic trauma patients are signs of mild or moderate prolonged bleeding in haemodynamically stable and conscious patients, haemothorax, early treatment of fibrothorax, treatment of empyema in the initial stage of fibrin barrier formation, diaphragm injury (the advantage of VATS over laparoscopy is in fact that in laparoscopic procedure air may enter the pleural cavity and cause tension pneumothorax), traumatic chylotorax, removal of foreign bodies from the pleural cavity or the peripheral lung, evaluation of pericardium conditions, the heart and large vessels.

8. Monitoring of thoracic trauma

The surgeon must always have sufficient useful information about the patient's condition in order to be able to act in a timely way, monitoring the use of diagnostic and therapeutic procedures. Most reports deal with ideal conditions and well-equipped institutions providing optimal medical treatment and care. Of course, it is not always possible and therefore it is necessary to list the parameters applicable in most institutions. Minimal necessary parameters that are regularly monitored in all patients with thoracic trauma, immediately upon their admission in surgical unit and later, are the following: [23-27]

- Arterial pressure
- Arterial pulse and heart rate (obtained by electrocardiogram - ECG)
- Central venous pressure (in patients with shock and mechanical ventilation)
- Volume of urine (measured by urinary catheter in patients with shock)
- Cardiac index
- Arterial PO2, PCO2 and pH
- Haematocrit value

Monitoring of arterial pressure, pulse, haematocrit, and the volume of urine can be used as general parameters in the assessment of fluid replacement. Analysis of arterial blood gases is a very useful test of pulmonary function and in calculating the degree of metabolic acidosis, if occurs. In cases with permanent loss of circulating fluid (mostly due to bleeding), which is constantly replaced, it is necessary to insert a central venous catheter for pressure monitoring in order to calculate fluid volume replacement. Initial haematocrit values may be unreliable, especially in patients with excessive blood loss who receive crystalloid solutions. It is known that the restoration of circulating volume and haemodilution after a large amount of crystalloid solution is a slow process. Therefore, haematocrit value cannot be considered a parameter indicating the volume of blood loss or replacement in cases when acellular solutions are used in restoration of circulating volume. Haematocrit value can be accepted as a useful tool for determining the type of fluid rather than the fluid volume replacement. Thus, it cannot be accepted as a tool for estimating blood loss or for calculating fluid replacement and correction of fluids. Specific issues are control and blood pressure in patients who had greater blood loss and adequate compensation within a relatively short period of time (up to 2 hours). It is believed that the value of blood pressure in such patients after replacement should be lower if compared to the value before the injury. In other words, restoring blood pressure to normal values before the injury may result in hypervolaemia. It is satisfying to stabilize the systolic pressure at 90 mmHg or slightly above in order to correct hypovolemia and to prevent hypervolemia. Care must be taken in patients who had hypertension before the injury, because the pressure for lower values of 80 to 100 mmHg still may be a sign of hypovolemia and incomplete and inadequate volume replacement, regardless of the normal pressure that may be satisfying for the surgeon (90 mmHg or slightly above). Monitoring of patients cannot be exclusively based on physiological parameters, although it is desirable to conduct such monitoring for each of the injured patients. The benefits of such patient monitoring are particularly in careful interpretation of the obtained values in correlation with therapeutic procedures and the patient's recovery.

9. Shock in thoracic trauma

In a large number of casualties, shock is a consequence of hypovolemia, loss of circulating volume (haemorrhage) or loss of tissue fluids (burns). In the early stages of shock, venous flow to the heart (preload) is reduced due to the loss of circulating fluid, which decreases stretching of the cardiac muscle of the right and left ventricles resulting in decreased cardiac output and the development of hypotension and tissue hypoperfusion. The body strives to maintain a normal circulating volume by moving fluid from tissues into blood vessels, by increasing heart rate due to activation of the sympathetic nervous system and reduction the inhibitory effects of the parasympathetic nervous system, by vasoconstriction in the splanchnic bed and limb peripheries, and by fluid retention in the body due to the reduction of diuresis. In later stages of shock, at the cellular level hypoxia is compensated by anaerobic metabolism and lactic acid production, leading to the development of metabolic acidosis. If the shock is left untreated, tissues swell, oedema occurs and the cells lose functions. In order to prevent further cell damage, circulating fluid should be immediately compensated and adequate tissue oxygenation should be provided. It is believed that the average blood loss per fractured rib is approximately 150ml, and in haemothorax it can be 2-2.5L and above. In suspected case of shock, the condition of the injured should be quickly evaluated including: mental status (conscious people breathe spontaneously, they are able to communicate normally and adequate oxygenation and perfusion of the cortex are provided). Hypovolemia accompanied by subsequent hypoxia leads to changes in the level of consciousness, (from anxiety, through confusion and aggressiveness, to the development of coma and death), the colour of the skin and visible mucous membranes (hypovolemic patients are pale, their skin is cold and occasionally bedewed with sweat, with possible signs of cyanosis), the heart rate (the presence of a radial pulse implies that the systolic blood pressure is less than 90 mmHg, while the absence of radial pulse and the presence of femoral pulse imply systolic pressure of 80-90 mmHg; the pulse of carotis communis implies systolic pressure of 70 mmHg), and capillary charge and blood pressure control. Symptoms of shock can be easily identified, but they are not perceived before blood loss exceeds 30% of circulating volume. The first signs of hypovolemic shock are the symptoms of peripheral vasoconstriction and tachycardia and decreased pulse pressure. The goal of initial resuscitation is to achieve blood pressure, which ensures adequate tissue perfusion, i.e. blood pressure of 90 mmHg. In a state of shock, the priorities are ensuring the patient's airway, provision of supplemental oxygen (10-15 L/min) in case of respiratory distress using mask-balloon ventilation, and measures to stop both external and internal bleeding. A large-bore cannula should be inserted in the antecubital fossa in order to compensate the lost volume. If it is not possible, the cannula should be placed into the femoral vein or the central vein. Crystalloid solutions, colloids and blood transfusions are used to restore the volume. Crystalloids are saline-based fluids that remain only temporarily in the circulation (30 minutes) before passing into the intracellular space. They are useful for the immediate replacement of the circulating volume. Initially, two liters of crystalloid (Hartmann's solution or Ringer's lactate) should be infused. The advantages of crystalloids over other solutions are in their low cost, simple production, and long shelf life. Besides, they do not have allergenicity, do not cause coagulation problems and do not transmit transmissible diseases. Colloidal solutions are blood-derived, gelatin-derived or dextran-derived products. The advantages of these solutions are in their low cost, simple production, and long shelf life, as well as in lost volume replacement on a one-to-one basis, in their remaining in the circulation for long periods and avoiding disease transmission, while the disadvantages are in their occasional causing allergic reactions and coagulation disorders. The shock causes pain, so the injured should be given painkillers, fractures should be stabilized and immobilized. Distention of the stomach may be complicated by regurgitation and aspiration of gastric contents in the airway, and may be prevented by nasogastric suction. Endotracheal intubation and mechanical ventilation with high concentrations of inspired oxygen protect the airway from aspiration and ensure adequate ventilation and oxygenation. In patients with shock the following parameters should be monitored: heart rate and blood pressure, capillary refill time, respiration rate (frequency and symmetry of the chest) and neurological status. In addition to these basic parameters, it is desirable to monitor the following: pulse oximetry, diuresis (adults over 50 m/h, children 1-2 ml/kg/h), central venous pressure and blood gas analysis.

10. Acute respiratory distress syndrome (ARDS)

Acute respiratory distress syndrome (ARDS) is a life-threatening respiratory failure manifested by non-cardiogenic pulmonary oedema, hypoxemia, decreased lung compliance, high intrapulmonary shunt and progressive pulmonary fibrosis in the late stage of development. The American-European Consensus Conference of 1994 proposed new definitions:

1. Acute lung injury (acute lung injury – ALI)
2. Acute respiratory distress syndrome (ARDS)

In the first group are injured with mild hypoxemia (relation between the partial pressure of oxygen in arterial blood and fractional inspired oxygen concentration at the level of 300) (Pa02/Fi02). In the second group are injured with severe hypoxemia (relation between the partial pressure of oxygen in arterial blood and fractional inspired oxygen concentration at the level of 200) (Pa02/Fi02). The other three characteristics – their acuteness, bilateral infiltrates on chest radiography and pulmonary artery occlusion pressure of 18 mmHg – are common to both illnesses.

Predisposing risk factors for ARDS are classified into two groups. In the first group are pulmonary contusion, aspiration of gastric contents, pneumonia, inhalation injury and drowning. In the second group are: severe traumatic shock and need for repeated infusion/transfusion, head trauma, abdominal sepsis, burns, fat embolism, excessive volume replacement and disseminated intravascular coagulation. From a pathophysiological point of view, ARDS occurs as the consequence of the systemic inflammatory response of the injured. Neutrophil activation, aggregation and degranulation lead to the release of oxygen free radicals and proteases; monocytes/macrophages activation leads to the formation of arachidonic acid metabolites (prostaglandin, leukotrienes, prostacyclin); T-cells release cytokines (interleukins) inducing the damage of the capillary endothelium. Platelet activation and aggregation and fibrinolysis lead to microthrombosis causing further damage to microcirculation. Severe injury to type I pneumocytes and capillary endothelial cells leads to increased permeability of the alveolar membrane, so that the alveoli become progressively filled with exudate which is rich in plasma proteins, erythrocytes, platelets and leukocytes, which eventually leads to the development of interstitial and alveolar pulmonary oedema. Alveolar obliteration and surfactant dysfunction lead to numerous microatelectasis and increasing intrapulmonary shunt. Pulmonary circulation responds to hypoxemia with vasoconstriction, reducing blood flow to the unventilated alveoli, which is a strong risk factor for pulmonary hypertension and the load on the right heart, causing severe hypoxemia. The first exudative phase is followed by the second proliferative phase when type 2 pneumocytes proliferate and transform into pneumocite type 1, resulting in the regeneration of the alveolar membrane. In the third fibrotic phase large amounts of collagen accumulate in the lungs and pulmonary fibrosis is developed.

Clinical manifestation of ARDS depends on its causes. Very soon after the injury, during the first 12-24 hours, tachypnea and tachycardia occur. The patients use auxiliary respiratory muscles, and on auscultation they have high-pitched expiratory crackles. Arterial blood gas analysis indicates progressive hypoxia, hypercapnia, and acidosis. Chest X-ray shows diffuse spotty infiltrations becoming confluent with progressive clinical deterioration of ARDS. Prognosis of ARDS is uncertain and depends on the severity of the injury. Prevention of ARDS includes correction of disturbed ventilation and haemodynamics. The treatment of ARDS requires mechanical ventilation in order to achieve adequate oxygenation. The primary function of mechanical ventilation is to keep the alveoli open as long as possible, which is achieved by intermittent positive pressure ventilation with or without positive end-expiratory pressure. In the treatment of ARDS, fluid should be reduced in order to prevent pulmonary oedema. The intravascular volume should be maintained at the lowest level. Vasopressors and inotropes are used when the system is unable to maintain the perfusion by replacing of intravascular volume. Use of aerosolized surfactant was first appreciated while the nitric oxide, when inhaled, is a powerful pulmonary vasodilator. Glucocorticoids and other anti-inflammatory agents do not have significant effects on ARDS. Glucocorticoids are more efficient in preventing fibrosing alveolitis.

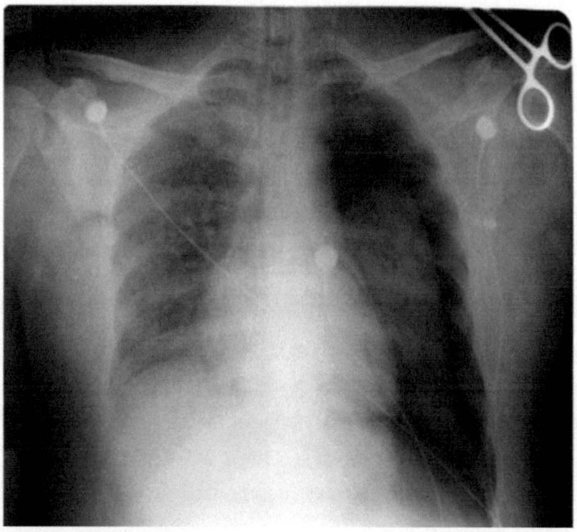

Figure 1. ARDS caused by left-sided pneumothorax

11. Blunt chest injuries

Blunt chest injuries are: contusions and haematoma in the chest wall, rib fractures, flail chest, broken sternum, blunt injury to the lung parenchyma, traumatic injuries to the trachea and major bronchi, traumatic pneumothorax, and traumatic haemothorax.

11.1. Contusions and haematomas of the chest wall

Chest wall contusion and haematoma are the most common thoracic injuries. As a result of blunt trauma to the chest wall massive bleeding may occur due to injured blood vessels in the skin, sub-cutaneous tissue, muscles, and intercostal blood vessels. Bleeding or extrapleural haematoma, manifested on X-ray as a semicircular model growing from the pleura, may appear in the chest wall, muscles of the chest wall, around the ribs and in the sub-pleural space. Most extrapleural haematomas do not require surgery because of the small amount of spilled blood. Only large haematomas or haematoma infection require surgical intervention

11.2. Rib fractures

Rib fractures are among the most common chest injuries, as a result of direct or indirect blunt force. Rib fractures occur in about 35% - 40% of thoracic injuries. Characteristics of rib injuries depend on the type of impact against the chest wall. Spontaneous rib fractures may be caused by a terrible cough (from rib VI to IX). Pathological rib fractures due to metastatic tumour or some other bone disease is very rare. In elderly patients, rib fractures may result from the chest injuries – after relatively low impact trauma. Even isolated rib fractures in elderly people can be a cause of death, with the range 10-20%. Rib fractures in children are rare, but when they occur they are clinical signs of thoracic injury, since the chest wall in children is very flexible, as opposed to adults. The mortality rate for rib fractures in children is about 5%. Lower chest wall injuries in children, but without rib fracture, is often associated with injuries to the diaphragm, spleen and liver. Discontinuity in the ribs without dislocation of sternal rib ends may be not revealed in the initial radiograph, but can be diagnosed as soon as callus begins forming. Rib cartilage fractures and fractures of the costochondral junctions cannot be seen on chest X-ray. They can be detected by careful physical examination, detection of crapitation and tenderness on palpation. Most common rib fractures are from rib IV - IX. In patients with serial rib fractures from IV-IX rib particular patience should be paid for possible intra-abdominal injuries. First, second and third ribs are relatively protected in blunt force trauma, supported by the strong back muscles and front pectoral muscles. The first and second ribs are further protected with the clavicle, scapula and shoulder harness. Only a severe traumatic force may break the first and second ribs. These fractures indicate possible associated injuries of large blood vessels in the aortic arch or injury to the tracheobronchial tree. In such cases, the mortality rate of up to 36% has been recorded. Anteroposterior compression of the chest causes the fractures of the lateral rib ends, which are then directed outwards. Injuries of the pleura or lungs rarely occur in such cases. Traumatic force may direct broken ribs to collapse inwards, leading to the subsequent lacerations of the intercostal vessels, pleura and lungs and may cause haemothorax, pneumothorax or haemopneumothorax. Specific symptom of rib fracture is pain. It increases with coughing, deep breathing or movement. The patient prevents the injured area from moving which consequently leads to hypoventilation. Decreased chest-wall movement and bad respiratory hygiene can cause atelectasis and pneumonia or the development of an infection. Oral/parenteral analgesics, intercostal nerve block, and intrapleural catheter analgesia or transcutaneous electrical nerve stimulation are used as methods of pain relief in chest trauma. Immobilization of the chest wall in order to achieve analgesia, especially thoracic cingulum, is not justified. However, in clinical practice, there is a relatively good

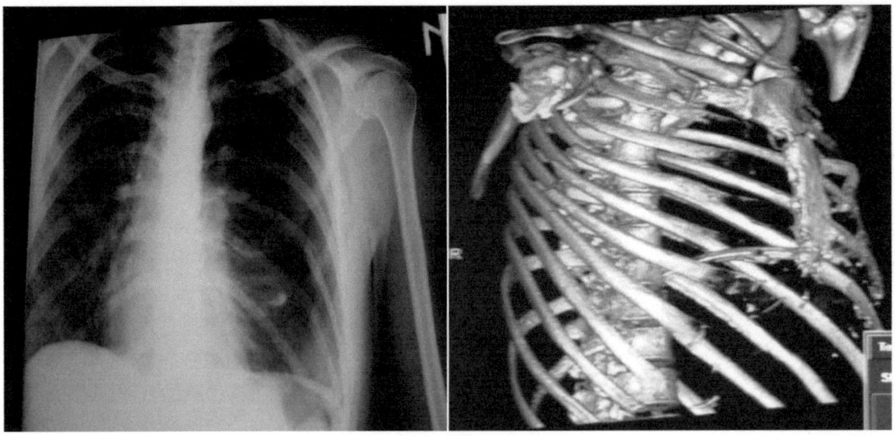

Figure 2. Serial fracture of ribs. Chest radiograph findings and MSCT

experience with unilateral fixation using adhesive materials (wide-strip leucoplast), in patients with individual rib fractures followed by severe pain. Fixation is performed during respiration in end-expirium by placing leucoplast between the edge of the sternum and the spine on the side of the fracture. Physical therapy is indicated in patients with serial rib fracture, and in more complex cases frequent bronchoaspiration is recommended for better hygiene of the tracheobronchial tree and prevention of atelectasis.

11.3. Flail chest

Flail chest is a medical condition when several adjacent ribs are double-broken unilaterally or bilateral fractures occur in the costochondral area associated with/without sternum fracture. The frequency of flail chest is about 5%, and road crashes account for most flail chest injuries. Pathophysiologically, the segment of the chest wall moves paradoxically, during the inspiratory phase it is drawn inward, while the expiratory phase it is drawn outward, preventing the air flow to the injured side. Firstly, deoxygenated air is retained within the injured side, but later it moves to the unharmed side, which leads to the disorders of ventilation and low vital capacity. According to the location, flail chest may be: anterior, lateral, bilateral and posterior. Anterolateral and posterolateral types also occur. Flail chest is diagnosed on the basis of physical examination of the injured, chest radiography and computed tomography of the chest. The treatment of flail chest can be divided into conservative and operative. In spontaneously breathing patients with posterior type or other types of flail chest where there are no difficult ventilation problems, analgesics and early physical therapy will help. In patients with severe disorders of ventilation, the application of mechanical ventilation with positive end-expiratory pressure (PEEP) will result in chest wall stabilization. Surgical treatment of the flail chest includes internal stabilization of the chest wall and can be early and late. Early internal stabilization is applied during the first 24 hours after injury, while late stabilization is performed 48-72 hours following injury.

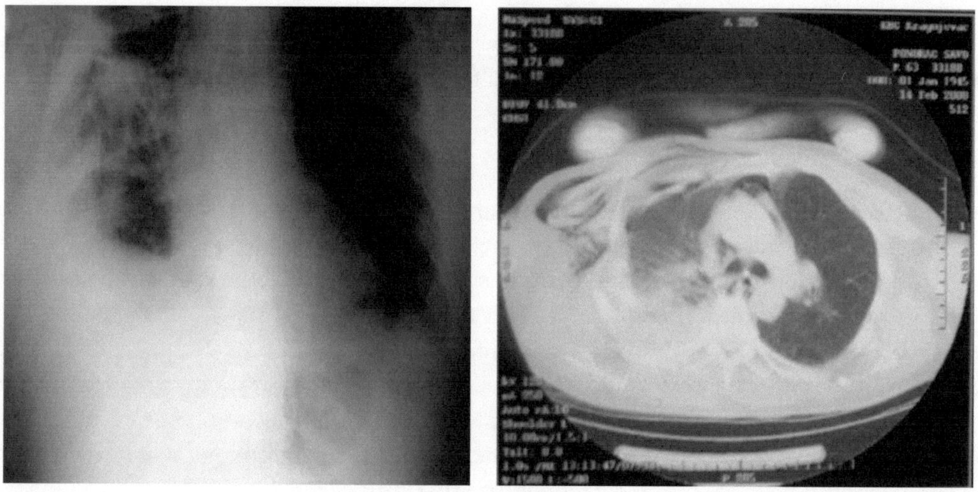

Figure 3. Right flail chest with right-sided pulmonary contusion. Chest radiograph findings and chest CT

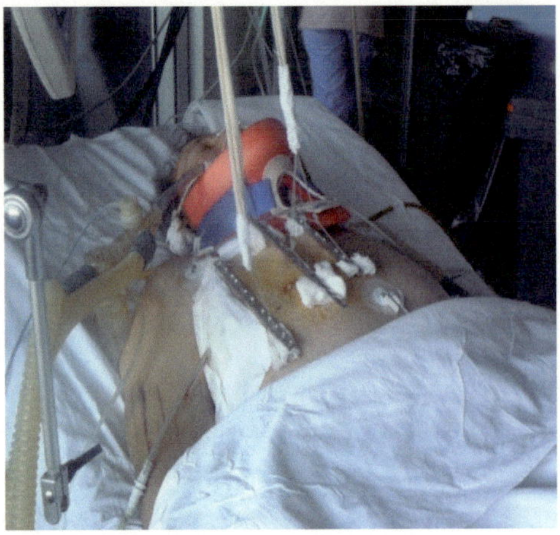

Figure 4. Anterior right-sided flail chest. Mechanically ventilated patient (internal stabilization). Right sided flail chest drainage and internal and external stabilization

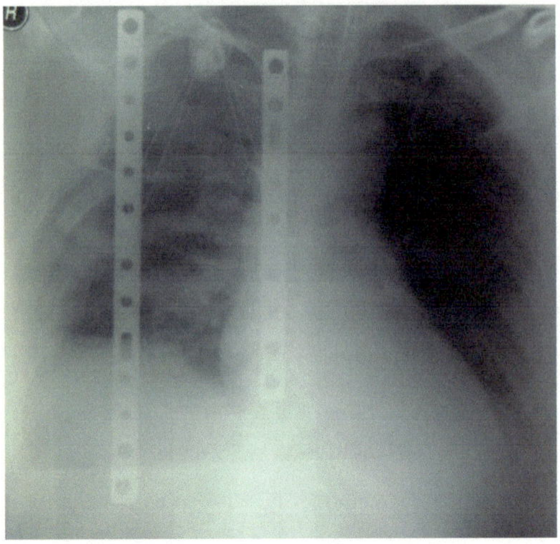

Figure 5. Patient's condition after the treatment of flail chest

11.4. Fractures of the sternum

Sternal fractures result from severe blunt trauma. They are often associated with multiple rib fractures. Sternal fracture is typically transverse and localized to the upper and middle parts of body of sternum. Mediastinal organs distortions may be expected with sternal fracture, primarily myocardial contusion (with typical precordial pain and dyspnoea). The fracture may be diagnosed on physical examination, detection of swelling, deformity and local tenderness. It can be confirmed with cephalometric chest radiographs, because the dislocations can be difficult to see in the anteroposterior projection. Sternal fracture is treated with rest, analgesics and airway hygiene. If the broken fragments were pushed over to the mediastinum because of the costochondral disruption, reduction surgery and internal fixation would be indicated.

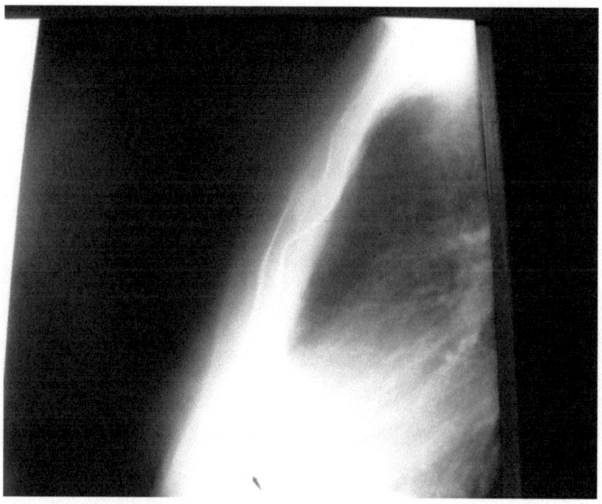

Figure 6. Sternal fracture

11.5. Lung parenchymal injuries

11.5.1. Lung contusion

Lung contusion is the most common manifestation of blunt chest trauma and represents parenchymal laceration accompanied by intra-alveolar haemorrhage. A pulmonary contusion is caused directly by blunt trauma to the chest wall, seriously damaging the parenchyma along with interstitial oedema and haemorrhage, and leading to hypoventilation in poorly ventilated parts of the lungs. Contusion may cause damage to a segment, several segments, or an entire lobe of the lung. Intrapulmonary haematoma occurs when larger blood vessels in the lung are injured. The diagnosis of pulmonary contusion is based on anamnesis, physical examination (gurgling sounds on auscultation), chest radiography and CT. Chest radiography may show irregular nodular infiltrates, homogeneous infiltrates and diffuse parenchymal infiltrates which disappear soon after the injury. Chest CT is much more detailed than standard radiography, and four types of lesions may be observed. Type I lesions are small parenchymal cavitary lesions or hydroaeric fluid collections. Type II lesions are hydroaeric and air cavitary lesions in parts of the lung in the paravertebral region. In type III besides hydroaeric and air cavity lesions in the peripheral lung fields there are always rib fractures. Type IV lesions result from the avulsion of pleuropulmonal adhesions, where the lung is drawn back due to a sharp blow to the chest wall. Complications of lung contusions may be immediate and secondary. Immediate complications include bronchopleural fistula, pneumothorax, haemothorax, subcutaneous emphysema, mediastinal emphysema, intrapulmonary haematoma, air embolism, haemoptysis, hypoxemia, arterio-venous shunt, and pulmonary hypertension. Secondary complications are atelectasis, pneumonia, empyema, sepsis, ARDS, lung abscess, and barotrauma. Pulmonary contusions require patient-specific treatment. Respiratory hygiene and pain relief are particularly important. A contusion involving more than 30% of lung parenchyma requires mechanical ventilation. Emergency surgery is needed in 5% of lung contusion cases, i.e. the injuries with a massive air leak, injuries with massive intra-thoracic haemorrhage (1500ml of blood on insertion of the thoracic drain and 200ml of blood every 3-4 hours, with continuous replacement), unilateral injuries with massive haemoptysis, and air embolism.

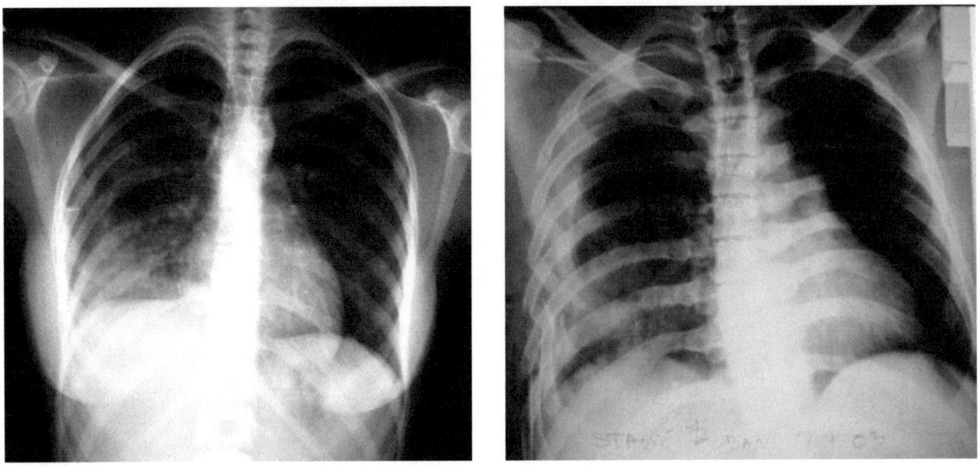

Figure 7. Lung contusion

11.5.2. Traumatic injuries of the trachea and bronchi

Traumatic injuries of the trachea and bronchi may occur as a result of blunt chest trauma, which is more often, or as a result of penetrating chest trauma in more rare cases. Blunt chest trauma may result in cleavage between the trachea and bronchi as a consequence of anteroposterior compression of the chest and the rapid increase in intraluminal pressure producing the airway rupture, or chest trauma may cause a sudden chest expansion with lung sliding laterally and, eventually, over-expansion and airway rupture. Traumatic ruptures of the bronchus are four times more likely than rupture of the trachea and usually occur within 1-2.5cm of the tracheal carina. The clinical manifestations of traumatic injuries to the trachea and bronchi are non-specific and variable. The clinical features may be divided into early and late symptoms and clinical signs. Early symptoms include haemoptysis, localized pain, neck contusion, subcutaneous emphysema, hoarseness, inspiratory stridor, progressive dyspnoea and auscultatory findings of "crackling" synchronized with the heartbeat and breathing (Hamman 's sign). Late signs and symptoms are dyspnoea and stridor (from scarring and stenosis) and distal infections of the lung parenchyma. Traumatic injuries of the trachea and bronchi are not often diagnosed immediately, but a few days, months or even years after the injury. Diagnosis is based on clinical findings, X-ray, CT and bronchoscopy. Acute injuries of the trachea and bronchi are amenable to surgical treatment, by means of suture, and chronic stenosis of the trachea and bronchi is treated with bronchoplastic reconstruction.

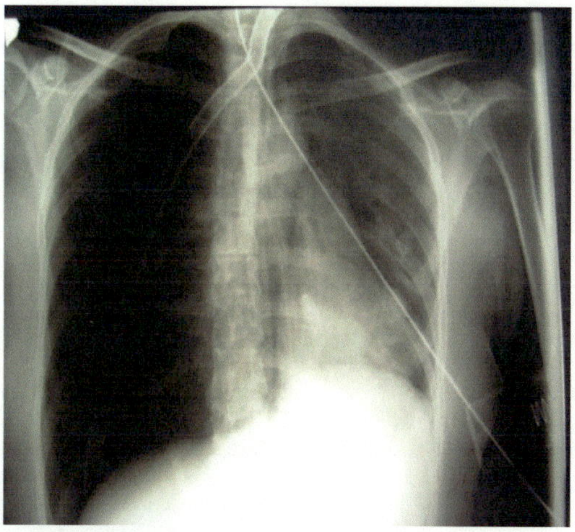

Figure 8. Rupture of the trachea - iatrogenic injury

11.5.3. Foreign bodies in the Tracheobronchial tree

Aspiration of the foreign body in the tracheobronchial tree is often seen at the injured with lost consciousness, at patients with the swallowing disorder, at intoxicated patients and small children. Clinical picture of the aspiration can be divided in three stages: first (acute) stage, second (asymptomatic) stage and third (late) stage. In the first stage, immediately after aspiration, symptoms of acute obstruction of the tracheobronchial tree occur in the form of a fit of coughing and cyanosis. After some time acute symptoms cease and there is an asymptomatic phase in duration of a few days, months or years. In the late stage the appearance of the high temperature, cough, wheezing – as well as the hemoptisis is present. Diagnosis is based on the standard radiography of the chest, in case of a radiosensitive foreign body, while the final diagnosis is made by the brochoscopy. Treatment includes

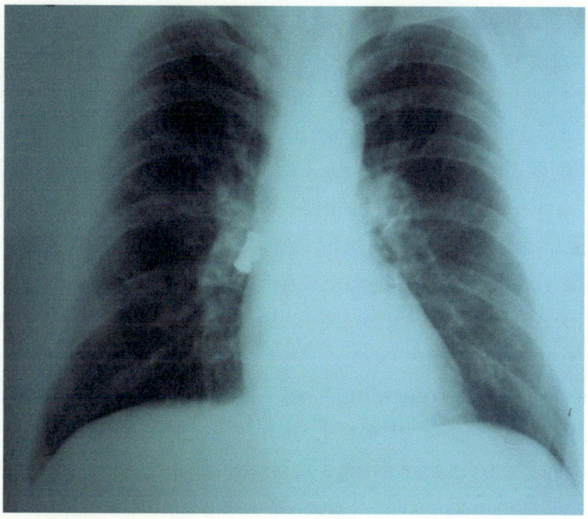

Figure 9. Foreign body in intermediate broncus

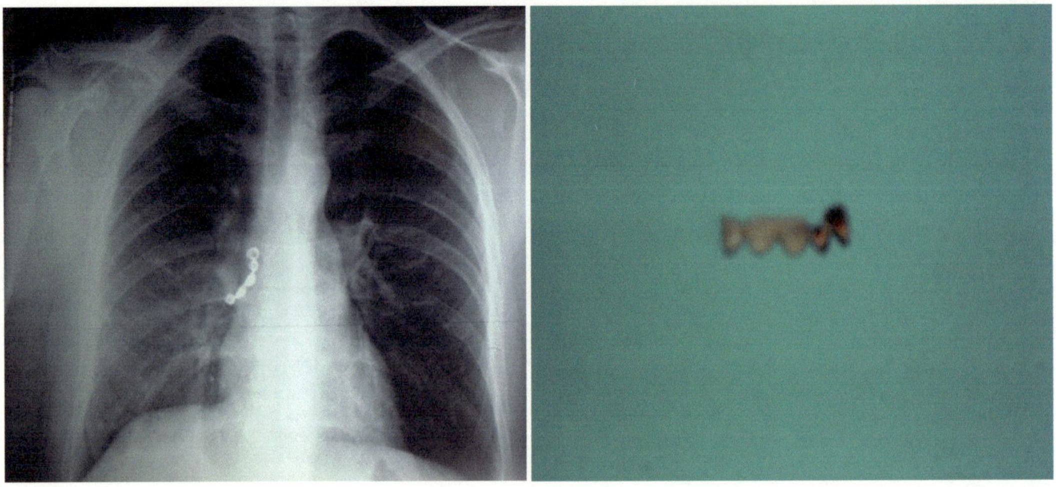

Figure 10. Foreign body in right main stem bronchus (dental prosthesis)

bronchoscopic extraction of the foreign body, specially in the case of fresh aspiration. At chronical foreign bodies, with developed granular tissue around the foreign body, the attempt of the bronchoscopic extraction can cause copious bleeding or perforation of the tracheobronchial tree, and in that cases mostly the operative treatment is applied, thoracotomy and brochotomy, or resection of lung parts distally from the area of obstruction.

11.5.4. Traumatic Injuries of Diaphragm

Traumatic injuries of diaphragm occur as a consequence of blunt and penetrating injuries of the chest, while the iatrogenec injuries of diaphragm are extremely rare. At blunt trauma around 1% to 4% of the injured occur, at penetrating injuries of the lower one third of the chest there are 15% of stab wounds and around 45% gunshot wounds. Mechanism of the diaphragm injury occurrence is explained by the deceleration. Injuries of the left diaphragm are more frequent due to the protective role of the liver toward the right diaphragm. In case of the left diaphragm injury, depending on the localization and rupture size, the stomach, omentum, small and large intestine, spleen, kidney can prolapse into the chest, while at the rupture of the right diaphragm the liver prolapses into the chest. Clinically the traumatic injury of diaphragm is manifested by early and late symptoms, when clinical picture may vary from the complete absence of symptoms to the stage which directly endanger the life of the injured. At the prolapse of intraabdominal organs into the chest, the combined respiratory and digestive symptoms occur. As the result of the prolapse of intraabdominal organs into the chest, most frequently of stomach, the paradoxal breathing with development of compressive gastrothorax, lungs collapse, hypoventilation and hypoxia occur. Late symptoms, that can occur after a few years or decades from the injury, are strong pain within the chest, dyspnea and signs of obstruction in small and large intestine. Diagnosis is made based on the clinical picture and radiographic findings. In some cases, by the auscultation the intestinal peristalsis can be heard in the chest. Final diagnosis is made by radiography methods. At these injuries, hydroaeric collection can be noticed on the native radiography, which must dyagnostically differ from the hydropneumothorax. Diagnosis of the stomach prolapse is made by the placement of nasogastric tube with contrast. Also, in diagnosis can be applied CT scan of the chest, MRI, liver scintigraphy and ultrasonographic examination of the thoracoabdomial region. Treatment of the traumatic rupture of diaphragm is surgical, it is adviced to treat fresh ruptures by the approach through laparotomy, while at old ruptures the adviced approach is through thoracotomy, due to adhesions in the chest.

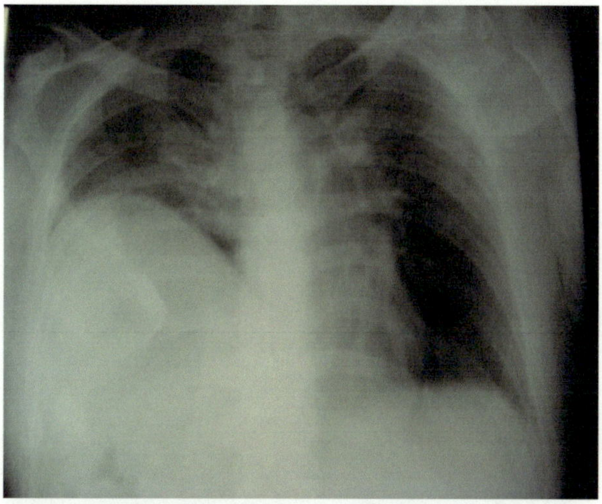

Figure 11. Traumatic rupture of the right diaphragm

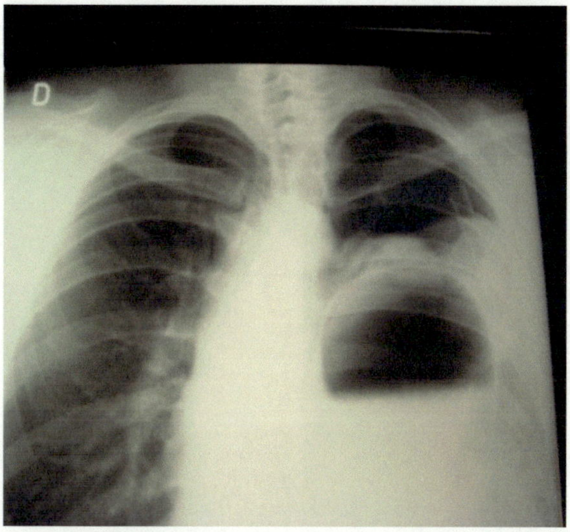

Figure 12. Traumatic rupture of the left diphragm, with the prolapse of stomach (visible after placement of left - sided thoracic drainage tube)

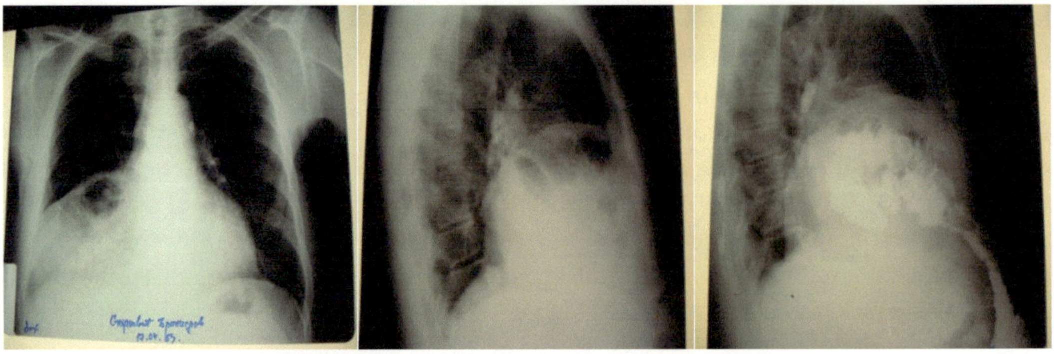

Figure 13. Posttraumatic right - sided diaphragmatic hernia (traffic accident)

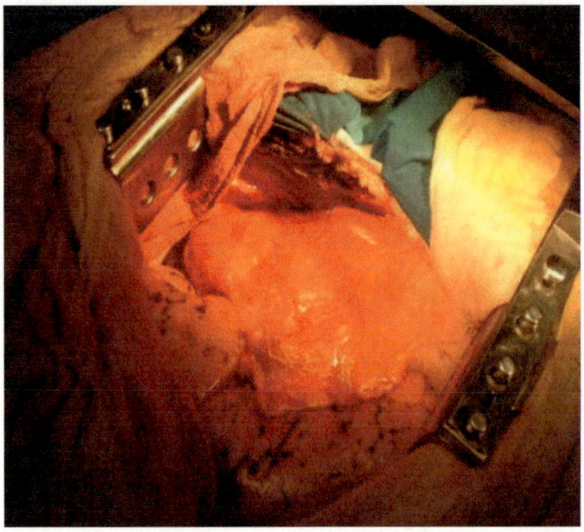

Figure 14. Post - traumatic right - sided diaphragmatic hernia (intraoperative findings)

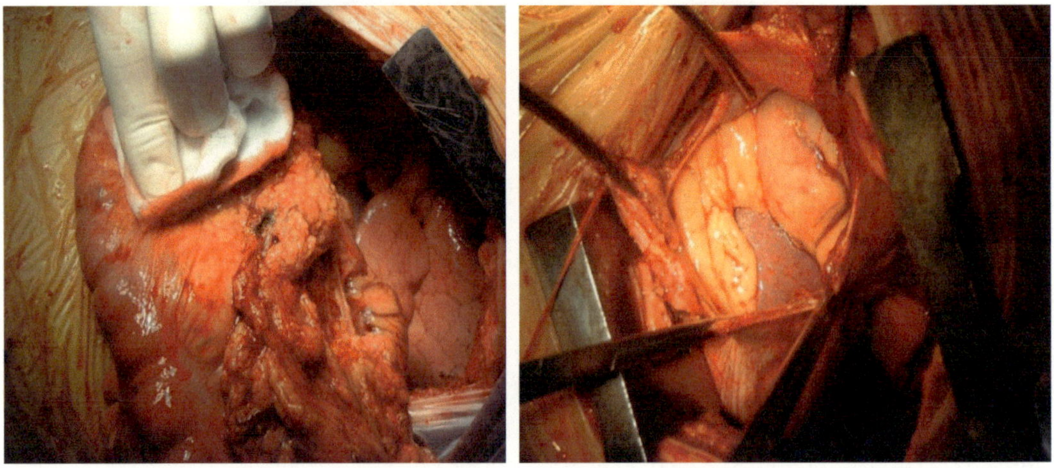

Figure 15. Traumatic rupture of the left diaphragm, with prolapse of intraabdominal organs

11.5.5. *Traumatic pneumothorax*

Pneumothorax marks the presence of air in the pleural space. Traumatic pneumothorax occurs as a consequence of blunt or penetrating injury of the chest, it can be developed at the time of injury, soon after injury or afterward. At the blunt injury of the chest, associated with the rib fracture, the laceration of the parietal and visceral pleura is most frequently caused by the fractured and/or dislocated rib ends. Laceration of visceral pleura and lung parenchyma has as the consequence the occurrence of pneumothorax, and the laceration of parietal pleura can contribute to the development of subcutaneous emphysema. However, at most injured with traumatic pneumothorax there is no the associated rib fracture. Mechanism of the pneumothorax occurrence in such cases can be explained on one of the following ways:

- During sudden chest compression, the increase of alveolar pressure occurs and it may cause the alveolus rupture. Air that comes out in the interstitial area by dissection toward the visceral pleura or mediastinum results in pneumothoracs or mediastal emphysema.
- Increase of pressure in the tracheobronchial tree, in the phase when the glottis is closed, has the impact on the increase of pressure especially in the level of the bifurcation of the trachea and/or bronchial tree, where lobar bronchi separate. Due to that the rupture of the trachea or bronchi may occur. Laceration of the lung tissue is rare, but possible.

Mechanism of the pneumothorax occurrence at the penetrating injury of the chest is easy to understand, for the wound in thoracic wall enables the communication with external surroundings and the air directly enters in the pleural space. In such cases the visceral pleura is often injured, enabling the entry of air from alveoli to the plural area. Blunt injuries of the chest in peacetime conditions often occur due to the traffic accidents. In traffic traumatology the five types of collisions are common: head - on, lateral, rare -end, rotating (turning around) and rollover. Each of mentioned types has its characteristics, but the mutual characteristic for all types is that they cause decelerational injuries. Mechanism that causes deceleration injuries is the same at falls from height (accidental or suicidal). During haulting of the object which moves with huge speed, the blow in the chest suddenly increases intrathoracic pressure, compresses lungs and with instinctive closed glottis, the disintergration of the lung parenchyma and central respiratory paths. Beside the chest injury in these situations injuries of thoracic wall structures are apparent, as other mediastinal organs (aorta, heart, trachea).

Penetrating injuries occur by the effect of firearms or cold weapons. Injuries' seriousness depend on the damage of interthoracic structures.

Penetrating wounds of thoracic wall may be classified in three groups:

1. « Blind » injuries without exit wound
2. Perforating wounds with the entrance and exit wound
3. Wounds where projectile passed through the whole intrathoracic area and stopped near the skin or in the extrathoracic soft tissues

At injuries of the chest by firearms the important fact is if the injury were developed by projectile of high or small speed. Mutual pathophisiological mechanism for penetrating injuries is creating of communication between pleural space and external surroundings. Immediate consequence of such communication is the occurrence of pneumothorax. Large defect on the chest wall as a consequence has the occurrence of open pneumotorax. Treatment of the broadly open wounds on the chest wall proceeds in two phases:

1. Operative debridement with removal of devitalized tissue and foreign bodies
2. Closing of the opening of thoracic wall

Pneumothorax is surgically treated by the thoracic drainage. Narrow penetrating wounds of the chest wall are often spontaneously closed, due to the muscle contraction or the tamponade occurs by blood coagulation. Air in the pleural space enters during the penetration or immediately after that. Penetrating injuries can provoke massive contamination of the pleural space, since in the moment of creating the communication with external surroundings it comes to the air suction with it, parts of the cloths and devitalized tissue. Presence of foreign bodies in the pleural space is favourable for development of a bacterial infection that can seriously complicate further course of the treatment. Pressure in the pleural space is negative in comperison with the atmospheric pressure during entire respiratory cycle. Negative pressure is a consequence of mutual relation between the lung tendency to collapse and thoracic wall to be expanded. Alveolar pressure is always higher than the pleural pressure. When communication arises between the alveolar and pleural spaces, the air passes from alveoli into pleural space, until there is a gradient of the pressure or until the communication is not closed. Air letting through into the pleural space is limited by the lung collapse and effect of closing the lung lesion. Most important pathophysiological consequence of the pneumotorax are decrease of the vital capacity and partial oxygen pressure in blood. Decrease of the vital capacity is well tolerated by the injured who were healthy before pneumotorax development. However, in case when the lung function is damaged by the previous lung diseases, any decrease of the vital capacity can cause the respiratory insufficiency with alveolar hypoventilation and respiratory acidosis. Lung collapse of 10% and less does not create more substantial ventilation disorders. Such collapse is marked as the minor pneumotorax. Moderate pneumotorax has the collapse of 10 - 60%, and large pneumotorax has over 60%. From pathophysiological point of view, the most important is the classification of traumatic pneumothorax to the following categories:

1. Simple or partial
2. Open or absorbing
3. Tension

Any injury of the chest can result with one of the mentioned types of pneumothorax. However, open pneumothorax is often associated with penetrating injury, while tension and simple pneumothorax are mainly seen at the blunt injury of the chest.

Simple pnemothorax often develops due to the laceration of the lung parenchyma fractured rib ends, or due to the gunshot wounds and stab wounds. Increase of the interalveolar pressure due to the effect of trauma causes rupture of alveoli and entry of the air into pleural space. Open pneumothorax appears due to the direct communication between pleural space and external surroundings. Disorder of the physiology of breathing in such a case depends on the size of perforation on the chest wall. Course and severity of pathophysiological changes depends on the age of the injured, state of respiratory system before injury, fixed condition of mediastinum, adhesions. Tension pneumothorax occurs when the pressure in the pleural space becomes positive in all phases of the respiratory cycle. Since the affected lung collapses, accumulation of an air from the external surroundings causes development of the positive pleural pressure that further pushes mediastinum toward healthy side. Positive pleural pressure can be so high to push or cause the inversion of ipsilateral diaphragm. Mechanism for development of the tension pneumothorax is connected with the specified type of a one-way-valve (valve mechanism). Valve is open during inspirium, so that the air enters into pleural space, and it is closed during expirium.

Traumatic pneumothorax occurs due to the entry of air in the pleural space, thus disintegrating the following structures:

- External part of thoracic wall
- Lung parenchyma
- Tracheobronchial tree out of the part covered by the mediastinal pleura
- Oesophagus and mediastinal pleura
- Diaphragm and associated perforations of intestines

At traumatic pneumothorax, the most frequent symptom is pain due to the chest wall injury. Occurrence of isolated traumatic pneumothorax apart from the pain may be followed by a certain degree of dyspnea which does not endanger the injured. Clinical picture of the open pneumothorax is significantly distinct, dyspnea and pain are dominant (specially locally in the area of wound on the chest wall). Often the sound of air suction through the wound can be heard during the inspirium. Locally, in the area of wound, a certain degree of subcutaneous emphysema is distinct. By inspection, decrease of respiratory mobility of affected hemithorax is noticiable. Percutaneously there is hypersonority, weaken or inaudible murmur is heard by auscultation. Pulse is accelerated, the fall of arterial pressure is present in case of distinct haemorrhage. Tension pneumothorax directly endangers the life of the injured and it belongs to the group of medical emergencies. Pathophysiology of the tension pneumothorax is not explained in its entirety, but it is considered that the basic disorders are related to the decrease of heart beat volume and progressive hypoxia. For diagnosis the clinical examination of the injured is often sufficient and only possible. Radiographic confirmation of the diagnosis requires a certain time, that is intolerable risk in some cases for the injured. Typical clinical picture of the tension pneumothorax shows a sever respiratory disorder of the ventilation, distinct tachypnea, cyanosis of the head and neck, tachycardia, hypotension, distension veins on the neck and profuse perspiration. By inspection it is obvious that affected hemithorax is significantly expanded in comparison with the opposite side, with distinct presence of subcutaneous emphysema. Percutaneously there is a tympanism, while auscultatory findings on lungs show an absence of breathing murmur on affected side. At atypical clinical picture, the tension pneumothorax may imitate the state of acute tamponade of the heart or massive hemothorax. Radiography is a basic additional diagnostical method in diagnosis of the chest trauma. Position of the injured during the imaging has the impact on the quality of the chest radiography and possibility for correct interpretation. General state of numerous injured, specially the polytraumatized patients, has the impact on the position for imaging. It is desirable that the imaging is performed in the standing position, when it is not possible, it can be the sitting position or semi-lying position. Correct interpretation of the chest radiography includs the assessment of the bony structure state of the chest, position and shape of the diaphragm and phrenicocostal sinuses, position of the mediastinum and trachea and the state of the lung parenchyma from the apex to the lung base. Radiographic diagnosis of the pneumothorax is made easily, when the line of visceral pleura is approved on the PA chest X - ray. Definitely radiological recognition of the pneumothorax depends on the lung collapse degree. Small pneumothorax is better presented on the standard radiography in the standing position during maximal expirium. In fact, in such a way radiological density of the collapsed lung parenchyma increases, while the density of air in the pleural space is not changed. Radiography of the chest in position of a lateral decubitus enables that the free air in the pleural space is lifted. Increased distance between the lungs and thoracic wall is present, for the easily identification of the visceral pleura line. When the air enters into the pleural space, lungs collapses, thoracic cavity is expanded. Radiographic air is presented as a zone of homogenous light with absence of the lung ornaments at the periphery. Collapsed lung is separated from this zone by the line of the visceral pleura.

At the side of pneumotorax, the pleural pressure gets to be less and less negative, i.e. it increases. Pleural pressure within the cotralateral pleural space is unchanged so that the mediastinum can be removed toward that side. Ipsilateral diaphragm is lowered due to decrease of the transdiaphragmaic pressure. Interpretation of radiographic imaging made in lying positions is more difficult. By initial radiological examination of the injured in lying position, the pnumothorax can be overlooked, in case of development of the tension pneumothorax can be fatal for the injured. Pain is a dominant symptom at the chest injury, causing the unproper ventilation presence and the standstill of the secretion in the tracheobronchial tree. For this fact it is necessary, during treatment and first aid administration of the injured, to realize proper analgesia with holding of passage for respiratory paths. Progressive dyspnea and cyanosis point to the development of the tension pneumothorax. First aid at the tension peumothorax is comprised of decompression, by the needle placement of the large diameter through second inter-rib area in the midclavicular line. Needle should stay « in situ » in the pleural space up to the definitive treatment of the pneumothorax. By procedure of needle placement, the tension pneumothorax becomes the open pnumothorax, easier to bear. At the open pneumothorax hermetisation of the wound is performed on the chest wall, taking into account to prevent development of the tension pneumothorax. Methods of treatment of traumatic pneumothorax are an observation, exsufflation (needle aspiration) and thoracic drainage. Observation is rarely applied.

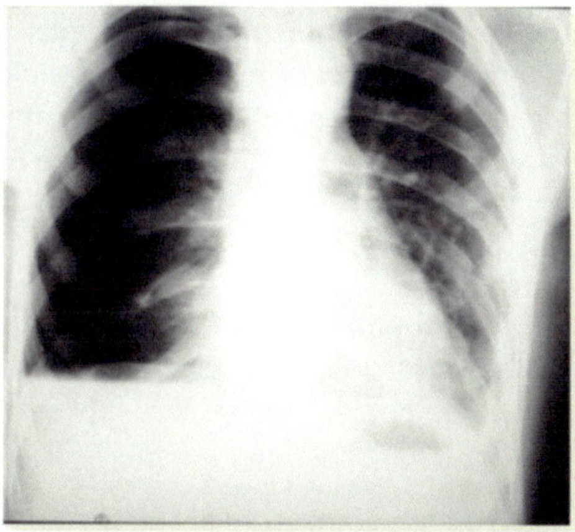

Figure 16. Traumatic right - sided hemopneumothorax

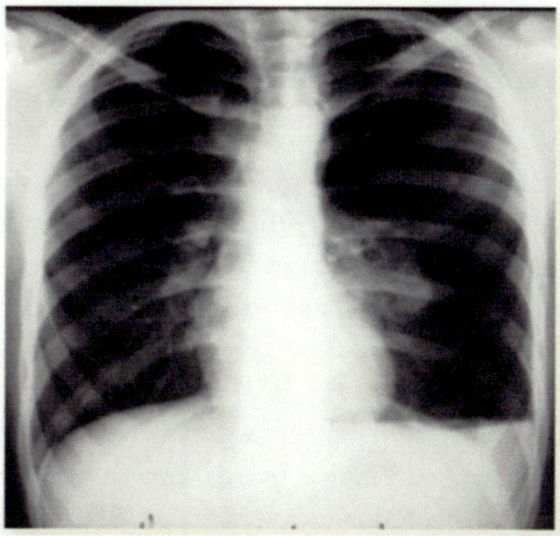

Figure 17. Traumatic left-sided hemopneumothorax

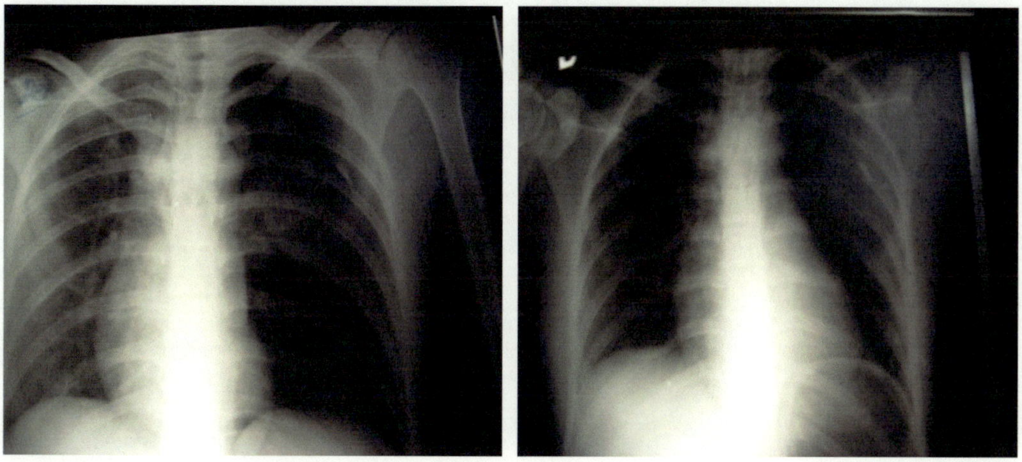

Figure 18. Tension left - sided pneumothorax and control radiography after left - sided thoracic drainage

Exsufflation is suitable for fine decompression of the pleural space at the tension pneumothorax, when it is not possible to perform thoracic drainage. However, a method is rarely applied as the definite procedure for solving of traumatic pneumothorax. Thoracic drainage is a method often used during definite treatment of the traumatic pneumothorax.

11.5.6. Subcutaneous emphysema

Subcutaneous emphysema defines the presence of the air within the subcutaneous tissue, and at traumatized patients it is most frequently, but not only, associated with the chest injury and occurrence of pneumothorax. Air in the subcutaneous tissue may be the consequence of:

- Wound that results in interruption of integrity of soft tissue of the chest wall
- Injuries of parietal and viscelar pleura enable that air from the chest or pleural space enters into subcutaneous tissue
- Mediastinal or retroperitoneal air which by dissection pass up to the chest wall, neck and face, or down toward loins and abdominal wall
- Infection at which occurs the gas formation.

Subcutanous emphysema may expend very quickly up to the neck and face or down to the scrotum. Clinical diagnosis of subcutaneous emphysema can be made palpably according to the characteristic sign of crepitation. At each injured patient with the subcutaneous emphysema, the radiography of the chest is necessary for the diagnosis of possible pneumothorax (often followed by such an occurrence). In terms of therapy the approach to the patient with subcutaneous emphysema is aimed to solving of basic leison, being the cause of the subcutaneous emphysema. In case when the emphysema occurs due to the injury of chest and parietal pleura and consequential pneumothorax, the thoracic drainage is identified. Wounds on the chest wall, through which the air can penetrate into subcutaneous tissue, must be treated according to surgical principles.

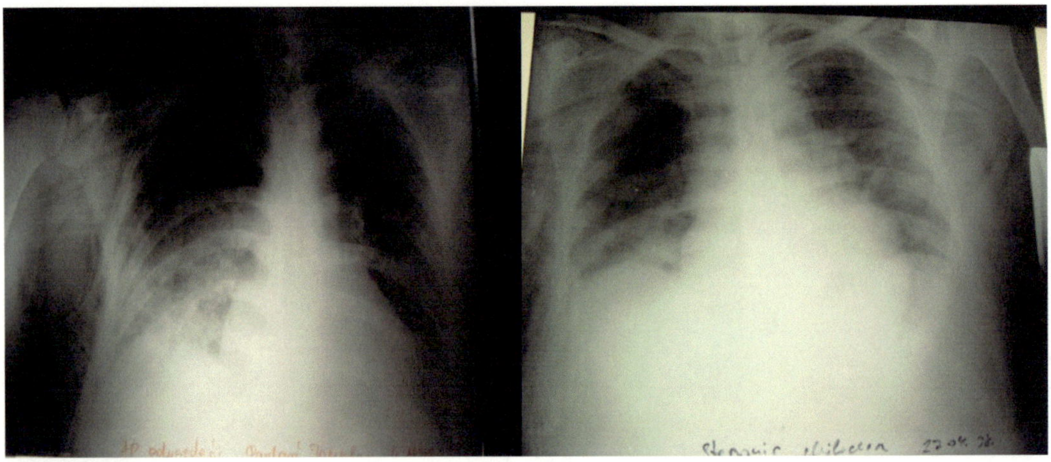

Figure 19. Subcutaneous emphysema – traffic accident

Pneumomediastinum marks the presence of the air in the mediastinum, and it can be caused by:

- Injuries of tracheobronchial tree or oesophagus
- Lung barotrauma with alveolar disruption
- Retroperitoneal air which by dissection enters mostly in mediastinum

11.5.7. Traumatic hemothorax

Hemothorax marks the presence of blood within the pleural space. Mostly hemothorax occurs as a consequence of the penetrating or blunt trauma of the chest. In rare cases, hemothorax can be a consequence of iatrogenic injury for example, during placement of catheter into the subclavian artery, or internal jugular vein or during translumbar aortography. Hemothorax is rarely a consequence of the pulmonary embolism or rupture of undiagnosed aneurysm of thoracic aorta. Blood can get to the pleural space after injury of the chest wall, diaphragm, lungs or mediastinum (in the first place of large blood vessels). After injury of thoracic spine, especially vertebrae at the level Th4 - Th6, the hemothorax can be developed, even a few days after the injury. Blood that gets into the pleural space quickly coagulates, but most frequent is an occurrence of the defibrinogenation of coagulation due to the heart and lungs movement, when the blood accumulation is slow and in smaller quantity. Localization, i.e. encapsulation of accumulated blood occurs relatively quickly and when the blood collection is not found and removed, the development of empyema is possible. In case that the bloody leak in the pleural space occurs related to a certain disease, diagnostical procedure, in terms of defining of the clean blood presence, is aimed at determining of haematocrits of pleural fluid. In most cases, however the pleural fluid is macroscopic with blood characteristics, the haematocrit of pleural fluid is under 5%. Hemothorax is diagnosed in such cases when the haematocrit of pleural fluid is at least 50% from the haematocrit in the peripheral blood. Traumatic hemothorax is the frequent findings within the surgical centers that treat the trauma. Incidence of the hemothorax is high at the blunt trauma, up to 37%, associated with the pneumothorax (hemopneumothorax) even up to 58%. Occurrence of the hemothorax is almost equally frequent without rib fracture (35%) or associated with rib fracture (38%). At patients with rib fracture, the occurrence of hemothorax is more frequent when the fractured rib-ends are dislocated.[29] When during the occurrence of hemothorax the arterial bleeding is diagnosed, there is no doubt that the thoracotomy will be applied as a therapy. Massive intrathoracic haemorrhage indicates an urgent thoracotomy and treatment of the bleeding place.[30] Hemothorax causes locally an atelectasis of lungs due to the compression causing that way, when the bleeding is massive, respiratory disorders. In some cases of massive hemothorax, the movement of mediastinum in opposite side is possible. Beside the local compressive effect, hemothorax causes hypovolemic problems which are expressed in a degree that depends on the quantity of lost blood in the pleural space.[32] Diagnosis of traumatic hemothorax must be taken into account at each blunt or penetrating chest injury. Hemothorax, after thoracic trauma, is often diagnosed by findings of pleural fluid at radiography of the chest. However, this method is not sufficient in all cases, or at least it is not proved to such a degree that it can be the only one during the examination of the injured. Smaller intrapleural collections can be hardly noticed at classical radiography, especially when the quantity of the discharged blood is small or when smaller leaks occur on both sides. Difficulties in such cases occur in the interpretation of radiography. When a patient is in the lying position, only slightly shadowing of hemithorax is recorded as a consequence of blood spillage along the back chest wall. Through such a shadow, the silhouette of the lung blood vessels can be obviously seen. Presence of a small hemothorax is hard to define in the lying position, especially when the noticeable contusion injuries of lungs are present and at subcutaneous emphysema, because it should be thought of the presence of a certain lung collapse. It is recommended to perform the radiography of the chest wall in standing position whenever it is possible, although hemothorax does not have to be found initially in that position. At imaging performed in standing posterioanterior (PA) or side position of a patient, free pleural fluid is collected by the effect of gravitation in the back costophrenic sinus, shadowing the costophrenic angle. In rare cases blood can be collected in the subpulmonary way between lungs and diaphragm when the costophrenic sinus is free, and the outline of diaphragm is partially changed. When the imagining is performed in PA position, the apex of diaphragmatic cupola is directed laterally toward the chest wall and the mistake in interpretation that it is the rupture of diaphragm is possible. However, at the side radiography the shadowing of the back costophrenic sinus is found and the angulation of the anterior shadow area of the alleged diaphragm, i.e. leak in the level of union with a large incision. Development of traumatic hemothorax can occur immediately after injury or the bleeding into thoracic cavity occurs later, i.e. after a few hours, even a few days later. Postponed occurrence of hemothorax is recorded after blunt and also after penetrating injury of the chest wall.[33,34] Patients with thoracic trauma, particularly those with assessment that it is potentially severe injury, should be followed by radiography in the period of at least -6 hours after the injury. In that period a small hemothorax and pneumothorax can be found. At penetrating injuries, with initially found hemothorax, development of pneumothorax can be found in over 80% cases.[35,36] Ultrasonography of the chest is an useful method in finding out of smaller pleural blood leaks, particularly at the lying patients and patients without consciousness. Computerized tomography (CT) is a very sensitive method for finding out even small intrapleural collections of fluid. It is proved method for differentiation of hydrothorax from hemothorax.[21] However, this method is rarely applied at the acute injured patients. CT of the chest can be used later for evaluation and differentiation of the lung atelectasis, rupture of diaphragm or finding out of extrapleural haematoma. Such states in the native radiography are manifested by shadowing hardly differentiated from the presence of the free fluid in the pleural cavity. CT of thorax is useful method and during the control of treatment effect, particularly in cases of the occurrence of encapsulation of hemothorax and ineffective drainage. Therapeutic approach of a surgeon toward each inury of the chest must be active, regardless of the known fact that in most cases may come to the spontaneous hemostasis. Such an attitude includs the constant observation of the injured, evacuation of collected blood, fight against atelectasis and follow up of effects of applied surgical treatment. Basic aims of the hemothorax therapy are: evacuation of collected blood from the pleural space, realization of the full reexpansion of lungs and realization of tamponade of the bleeding area by bringing lungs in an immediate contact with parietal pleura. Compensation od the lost blood is performed, in terms of therapy, parallelly with local treatment of hemothorax. It depends on the volum of lost blood.[36,37] Treatment of traumatic hemothorax depends on many parameters as: general state of the injured, state of the vital functions, character of the injury, i.e. is it the question of isolated thoracic injury or the injury is a part of politrauma, states of the injured part of the chest (unilateral, bilateral) and the occurance of bony structure fractures, combideness of many associated intrathoracic injuries, quantity of lost blood and possible area of bleeding, if the bleeding is recorded immediately after admission or it is determined a few hours or days after injury, if it is possible to apply conservative or it is necessary to apply immediately operative treatment, if there is associated pneumothorax with hemothorax, ect.[29,38,39] Most cases of traumatic hemothorax are treated without application of thoracotomy. By thoracentesis (pleural punction with application of large - bore needle) or thoracic drainage it is possible to solve hemothorax, i.e. evacuate entire quantity of blood from the pleural space. Attitudes related to the application of these therapeutical models are not clearly separated, particularly in relation to the thoracentesis. Thoracentesis is often applied at a uncomplicated hemothorax with smaller quantity of blood and at the injured where the shadow of the leak without the lung collapse is present during the clinical observation. In most cases they are patients with injuries caused by the effect of a weaker blunt stricking force and those with fractures of one to three ribs. Basic precondition for success of this method is that the blood in the pleural space is not coagulated. Some chest surgeons apply thoracentesis in diagnostical purposes as the first method for the recorded leak in order to orient themselves referring to the character of bleeding, i.e. to define if the obtained blood was immediately coagulated. Thoracic drainage is applied in most cases not only as the first therapeutic method but it is most frequently definitive therapeutic procedure. By thoracic drainage 85% of patients with chest injury are treated. At right diagnosed indications for thoracic drainage, the possibility of occurence of later complications is decreased.[40-42] Success of the thoracic drainage depends on several factors:

- General state of the injured
- Indication for drainage
- Choice of diameter and quality of thoracic drains and drainage systems
- Control of functioning of the entire drainage system, chest drains passing through and early detection of the problem in relation to that.

Indications for thoracic drainage are divided to absolute and relative.

Absolute indications for thoracic drainage at thoracic trauma are the following:

- Traumatic pneumothorax regardless of the degree of collapse
- Tension pneumothorax
- Pneumothorax on both sides regardless of the degree of lung collapse
- Massive hemothorax previously proved
- Associated collection of blood and air - hemopneumothorax, one - sided or on both sides.

In later clinical course of hemothorax, indications for drainage, i.e. re - drainage are related to the occurence of complication:

- At development of acute empyema of pleura
- Encapsulated hydroaeric collections
- Other collections of fluid and air.

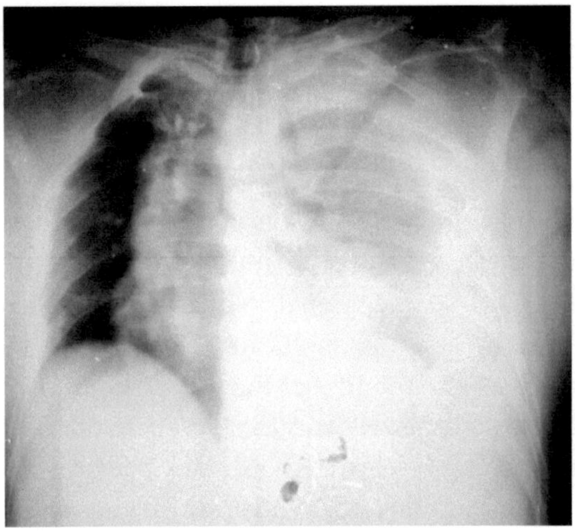

Figure 20. Left - sided traumatic hemothorax – Traffic accident

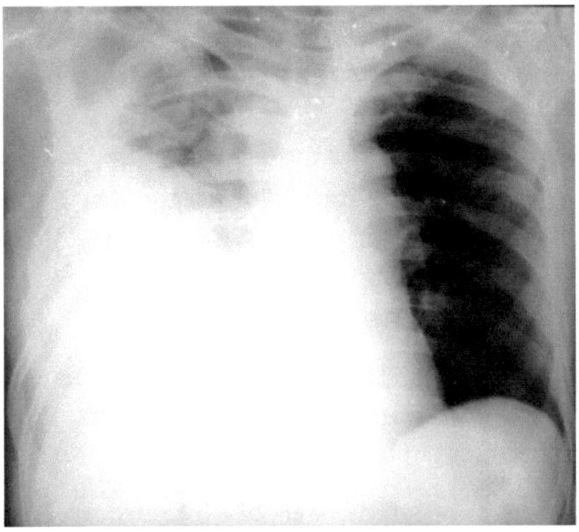

Figure 21. Right - sided traumatic hemothorax – Traffic accident

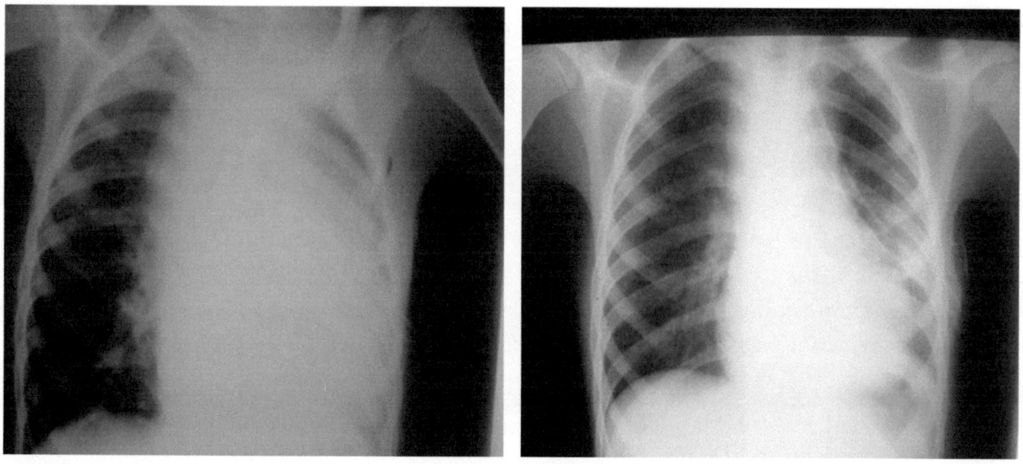

Figure 22. Fall from the height – traffic accident (child 8 years)

When the general endotracheal anaesthesia is planned for the surgery on the out thoracic organs at injured patients with the thoracic trauma or when the artificial ventilation by positive pressure is indicated, the attention should be paid to the possibility of development of the tension pneumothorax that in the aim of solving requires an urgent thoracic drainage. Preventive drainage of the thorax is not indicated when the obvious signs of pneumothorax are not present.

11.5.8. Types of drainage systems of pleura

There is more drainage systems used during thoracic drainage. In order to use in full the therapeutic effect of each system it is necessary to know the working principles each of them. Basic working principle of each drainage system is to: provide continued one-way evacuation, drainage of air and fluid from the pleural space into drainage collector, in the way that there is no possibility for an air circulation or fluid in the opposite direction, i.e. toward the pleural space. Basic aim of thoracic drainage is to evacuate the pleural content (air and fluid) and to achieve full reexpansion of lungs.

Classical drainage system is comprised of one bottle, which at the same time serves for collection of drainage content and as the water valve. Opening of the thoracic chest tube is connected to the rigid tube, passing through the stopper of sterile bottle. Top of the rigid tube is dived for around 2 cm under the surface of the physiological salt solution poured into the bottle. On the stopper of a bottle there is one more opening through which the tube is inserted, used for air egress (air valve). Top of the tube is above the fluid level. Such a system can be used for so-called submerged drainage, without active suction, or the tube of a valve is connected with the active suction, when the system is used for the active aspiration. Drainage system with two bottles is more reliable for the drainage of large quantity of fluid pleural content. Bottle which is closer to the patient serves as the collector of drainage fluid content, with second bottle the system of water valve is provided, similary to the system of one drainage bottle. Drainage system with three bottles is marked as the system for controlled suction of the pleura fluid content. Third bottle, added to the system of two bottles, serves for control of the active aspiration. It is connected to the second bottle that has the function of the water valve. Bottle for the pressure control for performance of the active suction has rigid tube, similar to the one on the second bottle, and on the stopper there is the connection linked with the source of active suction. System with three bottles is quite massive and it is not practical for patients who need transport. Commercial systems, for one-time usage, are designed according to the principle of functioning of the system with three bottles and they are considered to be fully proper for successful thoracic drainage. These systems are manufactured sterile and they are made of the plastic material, simple and practical for use. Most famous are Pleur-Evac and Argyl Double-Seal Units.

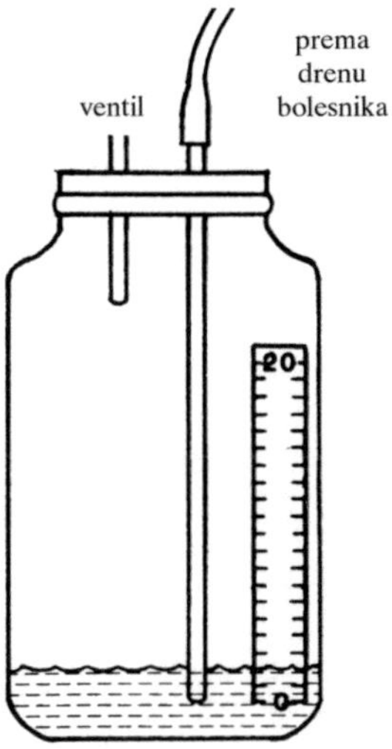

Figure 23. Drainage system one - bottle

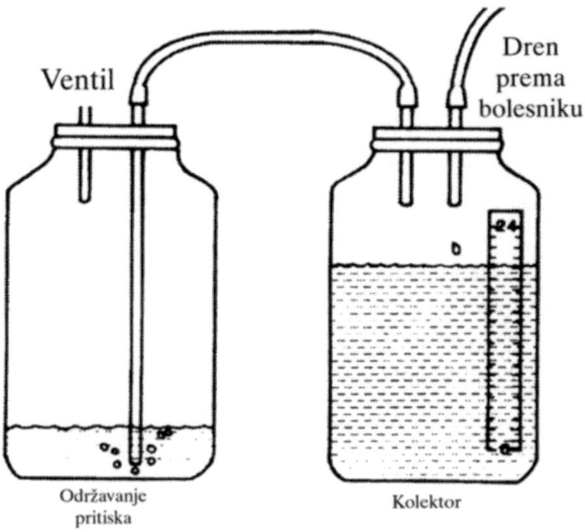

Figure 24. Drainage system two - bottles

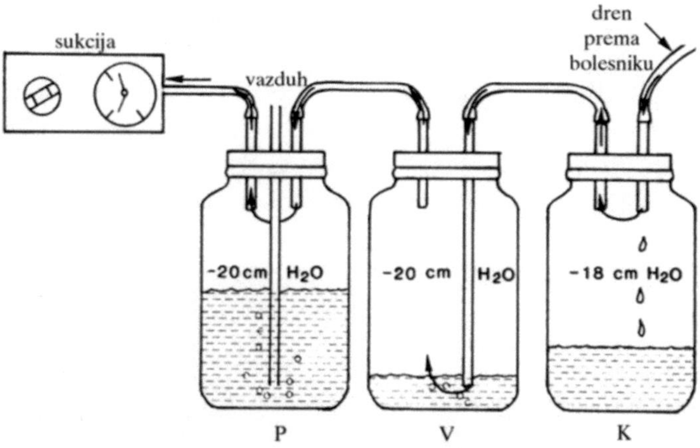

Figure 25. Drainage system three - bottles

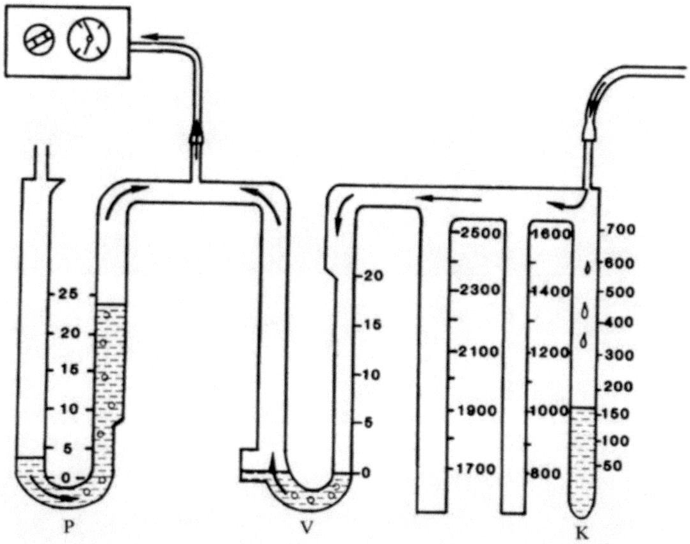

Figure 26. Commercial drainage system

11.5.9. Types of thoracic drainage

Practically, thoracic drainage can be performed in two different ways by:

- Operative thoracostomy – by classical incision of thorax in general or intravenous anesthesia, dissection and blunt preparation and placement of large-bore thoracic drain under finger control. Position of the patient is the lying, in decubitus on healthy side.
- Trocar thoracostomy – drainage is performed in local anesthesia by placemnt of the chest tube of narrow lumen through a metal thoracic trocar. Through previously performed incision on the chest wall, it is penetrated by sharp stiletto into the pleural space. During performance of drainage there is no possibility of digital control of the

lung parenchyma position in relation to the top of stiletto of the trocar. Variant of drainage by the trocar is the application of the commercial trocar catether, where the trocar is placed inside of thoracic drain. By trocar thoracostomy the chest wall is less damaged and the intervention is performed significantly more rapid, compered with the operative thoracostomy. Patient position is the sitting position with antebrachial region leaned against the backed chair or it is the lying position on the back.

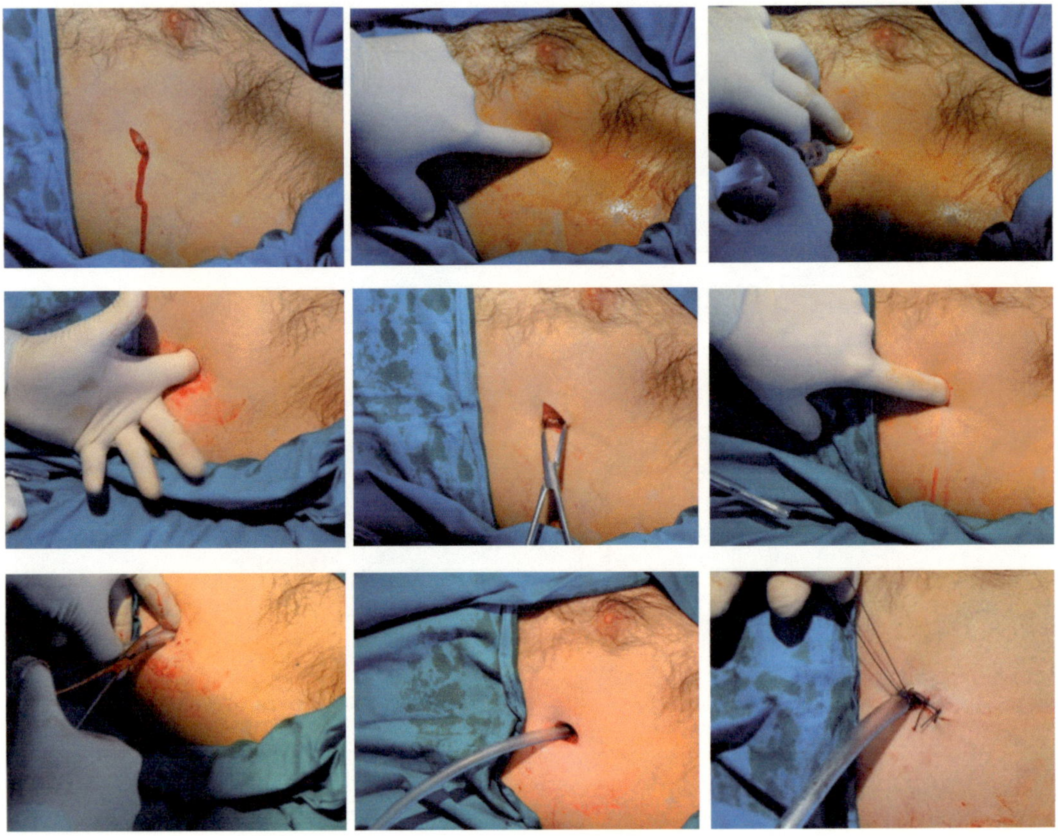

Figure 27. Operative thoracostomy

Proper premedication of a patient is obligatory regardless which of the mentioned ways is used by the suregeon. Position of the patient during performance of thoracic drainage is mostly defined by his general state.

By placement of thoracic chest tube, several favors are realized in hemothorax treatment:

- In most cases the complete evacuation of blood from the pleural space is possible
- It is possible to stop the bleeding completely that occurs due to the damage of pleural space
- Easy and simple control of the quantity of lost blood and assessment of the bleeding degree are possible, important for defining of the volume necessary for restoring

- Possibility for the occurence of bacteria infection is decreased due to the encapsulation of hematoma and development of empyema, i.e. fibrothorax
- Finally, in modern conditions there is a possibility of the blood autotransfusion, evacuated by the thoracic drain

Choice of thoracic chest tubes at fresh bleeding is mostly aimed in direction of placement of drains of a large-bore lumen (Fr 30 - 32, and according to some autors even Fr 36 - 40) for in that way the possibility of drains blockage with bloody coagulum is decreased. Recommendation for the massive hemothorax is to place a large - bore thoracic drain through IV and V interspace of ribs in the midiaxillary line. Drain is placed upward, for during drainage there is a possibility of the diaphragm damage due to its elevation caused by trauma, or within the thoracic cavity prolapsed intra-abdominal organs can be damaged at cases with the diaphragm rupture. Control of thoracic drain function is important and it is necessary to be constant. Passage of drains and quantity of evacuated content are controlled. It is necessary to control radiographic and roentgenoscopic states of extended lungs, diaphragm position and drain position. Control of functioning and efficiency of drains is important in order to prevent infection and development of empynema and if needed, when the thoracic drainage does not achieve a goal, to apply other models of treatment, i.e. thoractomy in the aim of haematoma removal and stopping of bleeding. Best way of prevention in infection development is an urgen and complete evacuation of blood from the pleural cavity. [29-31,33,40] It is useful to apply parenteral therapy of antibiotics. Indication for urgent thoracotomy is often connected with the occurence of massive hemothorax due to injuries of intrathoracic organs that can not be treated in a conservative way. Urgent thoracotomy is indicated at the hemothorax, complicated by a heart tamponade, injury of large intrathoracic blood vessels, primary pleural contamination, debridement of devitalized tissue, open thoracic wounds and at the tracheobronchial injuries.[41 – 44] Indications for urgent thoracotomy are special. After placement of thethoracic chest tube and assessment of the volume of continued pleural bleeding, i.e. quantity of lost blood in continuity through the thoracic drain. General rules include the rule that urgent thoracotomy is indicated in case if the constant loss at thoracic chest tube is 200ml per hour, in case that there is no indications to stop the bleeding. Of course, in order to make decision related to the thoracotomy and assess the state in the pleural cavity in such cases it is necessary to perform control by the radiography and radioscopy. When the continued loss of blood at the thoracic drain is determined and radiographic findings of hemothorax shadowing, the thoracotomi is necessary.[40,45] Indications for urgent thoracotomy are identical at the blunt and penetrating injuries. At each patient it is necessary to observe carefully all parameters, supposed for indication for surgical treatment, i.e. thoracotomy. Resectional lung surgery are rarely applied, mainly in cases of increased laceration of lung parenchyma and development of increased intrapulmonary haematoma, devitalization of lung parenchyma and injury of lung bood vessels.[43,44] It is proved that pneumonectomy should in any case be avoided, for the mortality rate after such an operation is almost 100%, i.e. such a resection should be performed only if there is no other choice. [46 – 48] Wedge - shaped resection is most often, resection of segments and lobectomy, it is possible to apply staplers. [43,44] At the presence of associated hemothorax and pneumothorax one should think of the possibility of injury of large respiratory paths, trachea and bronchi. When their fissure is determined, an urgent thoracotomy is indicated and the sutura of respiratory paths with caring for the site of bleeding. Thoracotomy is necessary at the traumatic hemothorax at around 20% of the injured. In medern conditions in cases of the occurence of hemothorax the video-assisted thorascopic surgery (VATS) can be applied, but up to recently experiences are still rather modest that it can be accepted that this surgical method belongs to the routine therapeutic methods.[49,50] Main pleural complications of traumatic hemothorax are: retention of blood coagulum in the pleural space, infection in the pleural space, effusion of the pleura and fibrothorax. In most cases surgical recommedation is to remove surgically the formed coagulum from the pleural area due to possible complications, in the first place the infection and development of empyema and fibrothorax.[51] Development of empyema can be expected at 1% - 4% cases. Application of antibiotics during the treatment of hemothorax by thoracic drainage is useful in the reduction of the occurence of empyema and pneumonia. If the thoracic trauma is combined with abdominal trauma, at extended thoracic drainage the possibility of the occurence and development of the pleural infection i.e. empyema is more definite. Complications of the pleural empyema are solved by the thoracotomy and decortication of the lung.[52,53] Occurence of the pleural effusion is possible after completed treatment and removal of thoracic drain. Development of leak is possible, regardless of the fact that residual hemothorax is present or not, but it is significantly more rare, when it is not present (at around 13% without residual hemothorax and around 34% of cases with the retention of the residual hemothorax, i.e. formed coagulum that can not be removed by thoracic drain).[54] Occurance of pleural leak is an indication for pleural punction (thoracocentesis), with the aim to determine the character of pleural fluid and to prevent development of the empyema. After completed treatment of the

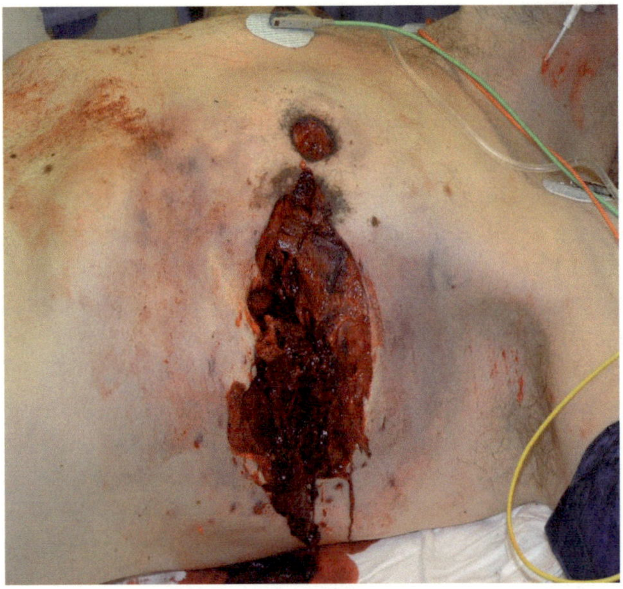

Figure 28. Penetrating injury – firearms

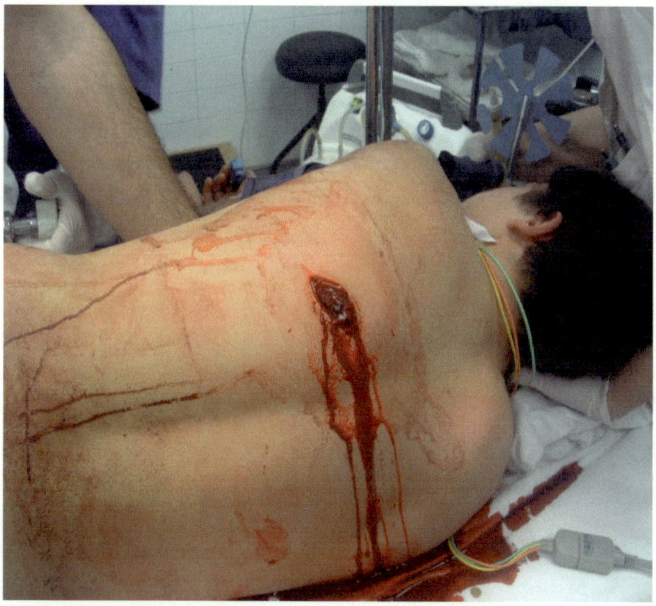

Figure 29. Penetrating injury – knife wound

hemothorax, in the period of a few weeks or months, due to the noticiable adhesions, the fibrothorax can be developed. Fibrothorax is developed at around 1% of treated patients from hemothorax and it is more frequent at patients with hemopnemotorax, or when in the early phase after injury the pleural infection appears. Complications due to the fibrothorax can be solved by the lung decortication.

Author details

Slobodan Milisavljević*, Marko Spasić and Miloš Arsenijević
Clinic for General and Thoracic Surgery, Clinical Center »Kragujevac«, Kragujevac, Serbia
Faculty of Medical Sciences, University of Kragujevac, Serbia

12. References

[1] LoCicero J, Mattox KL: Epidemiology of chest trauma, Surg Clin North Am 69:5,1989
[2] Shorr RM, et al: Blunt chest trauma in elderly. J Trauma 29:234,1989
[3] Besson A, Saegesser F: Color Atlas of Chest Trauma and Associated Injuries Vol.1 oradell.NJ:Medical Economics,1983,p.9.
[4] E. Q. Haxhija, H. Nöres, P. Schober and M. E. Höllwarth. Lung contusion-lacerations after blunt thoracic trauma in children Pediatric Surgery International 2004; 20(6): 412-414, DOI: 10.1007/s00383-004-1165-z

* Corresponding Author

[5] Shackford SR. : Blunt chest trauma: the intensivists's perspective. Intensive Care Med 1:125,1986
[6] MD R. Stephen Smith et al, Preliminary report on videothoracoscopy in the evaluation and treatment of thoracic injury The American Journal of Surgery 1993;166(6):690–695
[7] Hood-Boyd-Culliford: Thoracic Trauma, W.B Saunders Company, 1989
[8] Galan G,et al: Blunt chest injuries in 1696 patients, Eur J Cardiothorac Surg 6:284,1992
[9] Glinz W: Symposium paper: priorities in diagnosis and treatment of blunt chest injuries. Injury 17:318, 1986
[10] Kulshrestha P, et al: Chest injuries. A clinical and autopsy profile, Trauma 28:844,1988
[11] Serife Tuba Liman, Akin Kuzucu, Abdullah Irfan Tastepe, Gulay Neslihan Ulasan and Salih Topcu Chest injury due to blunt trauma Eur J Cardiothorac Surg 2003;23 (3): 374-378
[12] Glinz W: Causes of early death in thoracic trauma. In Webb WR, Besson A (eds): Thoracic Surgery: Surgical Management of Chest Injuries. Vol.7. St.Louis: Mosby-Year Book, 1991.
[13] Murray JA,et al: Penetrating left thoracoabdominal trauma: the incidence and clinical presentation of diaphragm injuries, J Trauma 43:624, 1997
[14] Campbell DB: Trauma to the chest wall, lung, and major airways. Semin Thorac Cardiovasc Surg 4:234, 1992
[15] Feliciano DV, Bitando CG, Mattox KL, et al: A 1 year experience with 450 vascular and cardiac injuries, Ann Surg 199:177, 1984
[16] Feliciano DV, Bitando CG, Cruse PA, et al: Liberal use of emergency center thoracotomy, Am J Surg 152:654, 1986
[17] Fisher RP, Jelense S, Perry ST Jr: Direct transfer to operating room improves care of trauma patients: A simple economically feasible plan for large hospital JAMA 240:1731, 1978
[18] Flynn TC, Ward RE, Miller PW: Emergency department thoracotomy Ann Emerg Med 11:413, 1982
[19] U. Obertacke , Th. Joka , M. Jochum , E . Kreuzfelder, W. Schönfeld und M. Kirschfink. Posttraumatische alveoläre Veränderungen nach Lungenkontusion Uniallchirurg 1991;94: 134-138
[20] Pearson FG, Deaslauriers J, Ginsberg RJ, Hiebert CA, McKneally MF, Urschel HC Jr (edts): Trauma, Pathophysiology and initial management, In Thoracic Surgery, Churchill Livingstone, p. 1532, 1995
[21] P Sinha and P Sarkar. Late clotted haemothorax after blunt chest trauma. J Accid Emerg Med. 1998; 15(3): 189–191
[22] Sisley AC, et al: Rapid detection of traumatic effusion using surgeon-performed ultrasonography J Trauma 44:291, 1998
[23] MD Hiram C. Polk Jr Factors influencing the risk of infection after trauma The American Journal of Surgery 1993;165(2):2S–7S
[24] Shorr RM, Crittenden M, Indeck M, et al: Blunt thoracic trauma, Ann Surg 206:200, 1987
[25] Valeri CR: Optimal use of blood products in the treatment of hemorrhagic schock. Surg Rounds 4:38, 1981

[26] J. Verheij,A. van Lingen, P. G. H. M. Raijmakers, E. R. Rijnsburger,D. P. Veerman W. Wisselink, A. R. J. Girbes and A. B. J. Groeneveld. Effect of fluid loading with saline or colloids on pulmonary permeability, oedema and lung injury score after cardiac and major vascular surgery. Br. J. Anaesth 2006; 96(1): 21-30
[27] West JG, Trunkey DD, Limm RC: Systems of trauma care Arch Surg 114:445, 1979
[28] Webb WR, A Besson: Thoracic Surgery: Surgical Management of Chest injuries. Vol 7. International Trends in General Thoracic Surgery
[29] Mattox KL, Allen MK: Systematic approach to pneumothorax, haemothorax, pneumomediastinum and subcutaneous emphysema, Injury 17:309, 1986
[30] Jordi Freixinet, Juan Beltrán, Pedro Miguel Rodríguez, Gabriel Juliá, Mohammed Hussein, Rita Gil, Jorge Herrero Indicators of Severity in Chest Trauma. Archivos de Bronconeumología ((English Edition)) 2008;44(5):257–262
[31] Weil PH, Margolis IB: Systematic approach to traumatic hemothorax, Am J Surg 142:692,1981
[32] Roy-Camille R, Beurier J, Maretingnon M et al: Les epanchements intra-thoraciques associes aux fractures due rachis dorsal. In Buff HU and Glinz W. editors: Respiratorische insuffizienz bei Mehrfachverletzten, Erlang, 1976
[33] Ross RM, Cordoba A: Delayed life-treatening hemothorax associated with rib fractures, J Trauma 26:576, 1986
[34] Kathirkamanathan Shanmuganathan, MD, Junichi Matsumoto, MD. Imaging of Penetrating Chest Trauma. Radiol Clin N Am 2006: 225-238
[35] Muckart DJ: delayed pneumothorax and haemothorax following observation for stab wounds of the chest, Injury 16:247, 1985
[36] Beal AC, Craword HW and DeBakey ME: Conditerations in the management of acute traumatic hemothorax, J Thorac Cardiovasc Surg 52:351, 1966
[37] Weil PH anb Margolis IB: Systematic approach to traumatic hemothorax, Am J Surg 142:692, 1981
[38] Cordice JWV and Cabezon J: Chest trauma with pneumothorax and hemothorax, J Thorac Cardiovasc Surg, 50:316, 1965
[39] Symbas PN: Acute traumatic hemothorax, Ann Thorac Surg 26:195, 1978
[40] MD Jeffrey R. MacDonald, MD Richard M. McDowell. Emergency department thoracotomies in a community hospital. Journal of the American College of Emergency Physicians 1978; 7(12): 423–428
[41] Glinz W: Symposium paper: priorities in diagnosis and treatment of blunt chest injuries, Injury 17:318, 1986
[42] Hood-Boyd-Culliford: Thoracic Trauma, W.B. Saunders Comp, 1989
[43] Asensio JA et al: Stapled pulmonary tractotomy: a rapid way to control hemorrhage in penetrating pulmonary injuries J Am Coll Surg 185:486, 1997
[44] Wall MJ et al: Pulmonary tractotomy as an abbreviated thoracotomy technique. J Trauma 45:1015,1998
[45] Sturm JT: Hemopneumothorax following blunt trauma of the thorax, Surg Gynecol Obstet 144:539, 1975

[46] Bowling R, et al: Emergency pneumonectomy for penetrating and blunt trauma, Am Surg 51:1365, 1985
[47] Moheb A. Rashid, Thore Wikström, Per Örtenwall. Outcome of lung trauma. European Journal of Surgery 2000;166(1):22–28
[48] Baumgartner F, et al: Survival after pneumonectomy: the pathophysiologic balance of shock resuscitation with right heart failure, Am Surg 62:967, 1996
[49] Meyer DM, et al: Early evacuation of traumatic retained hemothoraces using thoracoscopy: a perspective, randomized trial, Ann Thorac Surg 64:1396, 1997
[50] Heniford BT, et al: the role of thoracoscopy in the management of retained thoracic collections after trauma, Ann Thorac Surg 63:940, 1997
[51] A.V. Manlulu, T.W. Lee, K.H. Thung, R. Wong and A.P.C. Yim. Current indications and results of VATS in the evaluation and management of hemodynamically stable thoracic injuries. Eur J Cardiothorac Surg 2004;25 (6): 1048-1053.
[52] LeRoux BT, et al: Suppurative diseases of the lung and pleural space. Part I: Empyema thoracis and lung abscess. Curr Probl Surg 23:1, 1986
[53] Aguilar MM, et al: Posttraumatic empyema. Risk factor analysis Arch Surg 132:647, 1997
[54] Hanna JW, Reed JC, Choplin RH: Pleural infections: a clinical-radiologic review J Thorac Imaging 6:68, 1991

Chapter 12

Thoracic Vascular Trauma

Nicolas J. Mouawad, Christodoulos Kaoutzanis and Ajay Gupta

Additional information is available at the end of the chapter

http://dx.doi.org/10.5772/53060

1. Introduction

Traumatic injuries to the thoracic vasculature – the aorta and its brachiocephalic branches, the pulmonary arteries and veins, the superior vena cava and intrathoracic inferior vena cava, and the innominate and thoracic veins – occurs following both blunt and penetrating trauma. The primary cause of mortality remains acute exsanguinating hemorrhage. A high clinical index of suspicion along with prompt recognition and resuscitation are necessary components in the surgeon's armamentarium for dealing effectively with thoracic vascular trauma.

Thoracic injury is directly responsible for 25% of trauma deaths. Penetrating trauma accounts for the vast majority of thoracic great vessel injuries - over 90% - and is generally secondary to projectile missiles such as bullets and shrapnel as well as mechanical disruption by stab wounds and even therapeutic interventions. In fact, iatrogenic lacerations of the great vessels by rapid placement of percutaneous central venous catheter in the emergency department are frequently reported complications. Intercostal vessels and major pulmonary and mediastinal vasculature can be injured by the placement of smaller bore tube thoracostomies. More recently, self-expanding metal stents have been noted to produce perforations of the aorta and innominate artery following placement into the esophagus and trachea, respectively [1].

The sudden forceful deceleration following motor vehicle collisions is the primary mechanism regarding blunt trauma to the thoracic great vessels. The pulmonary veins, innominate artery, vena cava, and most commonly, the thoracic aorta are most susceptible to this kind of injury [2,3]. Thoracic aortic injuries generally involve the descending thoracic aorta in 54-65% of cases, the ascending aorta or transverse arch in 12% or multiple segments in 13-18% [4]. Mattox and colleagues hypothesized several mechanisms for blunt great vessel injury: (1) shear mechanical forces onto a relatively mobile segment of a vessel adjacent to a fixed portion – this is the postulated method for descending aortic tears due to its attachment at the ligamentum arteriosum distal to the left subclavian artery and the distal attachment at the diaphragm; (2) compression of a vessel between bony structures –

i.e. "the osseus pinch", such as that of the innominate artery between the sternum anteriorly and the vertebrae posteriorly during an anterior sternal impact; and (3) dramatic intraluminal hypertension during a profound traumatic event [4].

Importantly, isolated injury to the thorax and great vessels is the exception rather than the norm, particularly in blunt trauma. Patients with great vessel injury commonly have concomitant head, spine, abdominal, pelvic and extremity injury. It is imperative that the primary threat to the patient be rapidly analyzed and managed. Three distinctly different groups of patients with thoracic aortic trauma exist according to Mattox and Wall (Table 1).

Group	Description	Diagnostic Interval	Location of Death	Mortality	Cause of Death
1	Dead/dying at scene	<60min	Scene/EMS transport	100%	Hemorrhage/ exsanguinations
2	Unstable during transport	1-6hours	EMS/ED	>96%	Multisystem trauma
3	Stable	4-18hours	ICU	5-30%	CNS injury

Table 1. Mattox and Wall Patient Classification with Blunt Aortic Injury

The first group represents those with severe thoracic trauma. This is generally unsalvageable and patients are usually dead at the scene or die during transport from uncontrollable hemorrhage and exsanguination. Those that actually make it to the trauma center alive are divided into the second and third group. Unstable patients during transport that die in the emergency department, operating room, or intensive care unit usually succumb to hemorrhage from other sites secondary to multisystem trauma in the first few hours. The third group of patients that arrive in a relatively stable condition are usually found to have a thoracic aortic injury during trauma workup that is not immediately life-threatening; these patients usually suffer from a protracted course secondary to a major insult to the central nervous system.

2. Initial evaluation

2.1. Prehospital management

The initial evaluation of any trauma patient, whether with great vessel injury or not, should proceed along the Advanced Trauma Life Support (ATLS) protocol created by the American College of Surgeon's Committee on Trauma. The primary survey should be conducted with the priorities of airway, breathing and circulation, and basic life support interventions are usually already underway by paramedics who have responded to the scene.

Severe shock should be treated with blood transfusion; however, appropriate initial fluid management continues to be an ongoing debate. In general, judicious use of either blood or crystalloid fluids is the norm, especially in great vessel thoracic injury. The goal of increasing blood pressure to normal values has been shown to increase the incidence of acute respiratory distress syndrome (ARDS), postoperative complications, and mortality [5]. Permissive hypotension with mean arterial pressures of 65 mm Hg are an acceptable initial goal as aggressive fluid administration would be expected to increase ongoing hemorrhage by dislodging a soft perivascular clot if definitive surgical vascular control is not already achieved.

2.2. Clinical history

There is no substitution to a clear and comprehensive history of the event. Clearly, the mechanism of injury will yield the greatest amount of necessary data. Whenever possible, as much information should be gathered from the patient surrounding the events having had occurred. Many times, however, the patient has already been intubated in order to protect the airway and for analgesic control of traumatic injuries. Emergency Medical Service (EMS) personnel as well as law enforcement officers are trained in gathering and relaying the necessary information to medical providers. Noting the amount of external hemorrhage at the scene as well as hemodynamic instability during transport is imperative.

In cases of penetrating trauma, the type of firearm used as well as the number and caliber of the projectiles fired in addition to the distance the victim was from the weapon is important. If a knife is used, the length of the instrument and its design (e.g. serrated edges) should be noted.

Although blunt trauma to the thoracic great vessels has been reported with crush and blast injuries as well as falls from height (usually over 30 feet or more), overwhelmingly, the primary culprit is motor-vehicle collisions. Particular detail to the automobile damage, length of vehicular intrusion, starred or shattered windshields, bent steering wheels, front- or side-impact, airbag deployment, the number of passengers in the vehicle, and whether the passenger or others were wearing a seatbelt is important to ascertain.

2.3. Physical examination

A rapid comprehensive assessment should be performed as noted previously following ATLS protocol. Obvious external hemorrhage and other signs of blunt or penetrating trauma should be noted by inspection. Evidence of paradoxical thoracic wall movement can determine evidence of flail chest segments. Attention to the neck veins can help demonstrate concern of an intravascular pericardial injury with stigmata of pericardial tamponade or tension pneumothorax. Palpation of the chest wall can reveal disconnected rib segments. Although difficult to hear in a busy trauma bay, percussion of the thorax can reveal a classic "stony dullness" indicative of fluid, primarily a hemothorax.

Classic findings associated with great vessel injury include:

- External hemorrhage
- Hypotension
- Radio-radial pulse inequality secondary to innominate or subclavian injury
- Unequal blood pressure measurements between upper and lower limbs secondary to pseudocoarctation syndrome

- Expanding or pulsatile hematoma at the thoracic outlet
- Intrascapular murmur
- Palpable thoracic spine fractures or instability
- Palpable sternal fracture
- Left flail chest

3. Assessment and imaging modalities

3.1. Chest radiography

Although the formal "erect" postero-anterior chest radiograph has been shown to be much more valuable in detecting true-negative instances in patients suspected of aortic injury, it cannot be safely obtained in a patient with hemodynamic instability or suspected spinal injury[6]. As such, the supine antero-posterior chest radiograph is the initial screening imaging of choice in the trauma patient. Several findings seen on the chest x-ray should raise suspicion of thoracic great vessel injury although none are necessarily diagnostic.

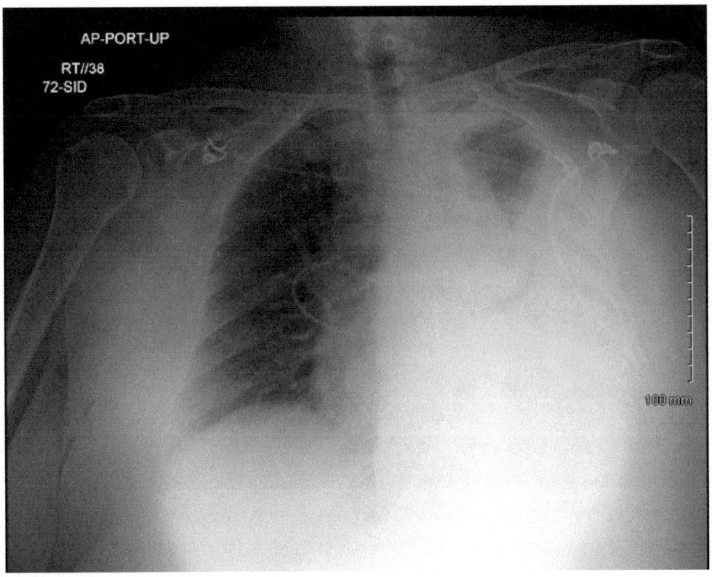

Figure 1. Left hemothorax secondary to significant blunt aortic injury

For blunt trauma, particular attention to the contour of the thoracic aorta is necessary. Evidence of mediastinal widening is the classic finding that represents a peri-aortic hematoma. Selective analysis of 16 radiographic signs by Mirvis and colleagues demonstrated that the most discriminating signs for traumatic aortic injury were loss of the aortopulmonary window, rightward deviation of the trachea, loss of the left paraspinal line without associated fracture, and abnormality in the contour of the aortic arch [6]. Other findings include an apical aortic or pleural cap, downward deviation of the left mainstem bronchus, and deviation of a nasogastric tube successfully placed in the esophagus. Of course, one needs to note any evidence of bony fractures such as the first rib, scapula and sternum, which generally require a large amount of force to cause such injury and should raise concern for underlying tissue and vascular structure damage.

In instances of penetrating trauma, radiographic findings that are suggestive of great vessel injury include a large hemothorax or a hemithoracic "white-out" (especially on the left), foreign bodies or missiles such as shrapnel or bullets, and an "out-of-focus" foreign body, which may indicate its intra-cardiac location.

3.2. Echocardiography and ultrasonography

As part of the Focused Assessment Sonography for Trauma (FAST) scan, a transthoracic approach with ultrasound should be routinely performed in both blunt and penetrating trauma to evaluate the pericardial space. In fact, FAST in rapidly becoming commonplace imaging in the initial assessment of trauma patients, expanding imaging to even assess the pleural space for hemothorax and pneumothorax following blunt and penetrating injury. There is an emerging role for the use of trans-esophageal echocardiography (TEE) and its application in acute and sub-acute trauma with suspicion of great vessel injury. Category 1 indications, or indications supported by strong evidence or expert opinion for the use of TEE in the trauma patient, include acute hemodynamic instability and the immediate evaluation of a patient suspected of thoracic aortic pathology such as a dissection, aneurysm or disruption [7]. TEE can rapidly diagnose such injuries by direct visualization of the aorta and a dissection, aortic wall thickening and the presence of a mural hematoma, evidence of an intimal or medial flap, and any intraluminal debris at the site of vessel injury [8].

In an evaluation of 101 trauma patients suspected of having aortic injury, Smith and colleagues conducted a prospective blinded study comparing conventional aortography and TEE. Imaging was performed sequentially by echocardiographic and angiographic personnel with the operators having had been blinded to the results of the previous evaluation. The sensitivity and specificity of TEE was calculated based on the results of aortography of the arch, surgery, and autopsy. The results demonstrated that TEE had a sensitivity of 100% and a specificity of 98%, with one false-positive TEE [9].

Although the use of TEE is safe, it is not without its risks and limitations [10]. Furthermore, as with most ultrasonography, it is operator dependent. TEE is not currently routine in the evaluation of a trauma patient suspected of great vessel injury, however, it remains a very useful adjunct in experienced hands.

3.3. Computed tomography

Contrasted, dynamic spiral computed tomography (CT) angiography is evolving into the imaging modality of choice in stable patients suspected of thoracic great vessel injury. It is of particular help in screening for great vessel injury in blunt trauma patients with a rapid deceleration mechanism. In addition to an evaluation of the aortic lumen and contour, it adds much information about the surrounding tissues and the presence of a mediastinal hematoma. It is also helpful for evaluating the trajectory of a missile in transmediastinal penetrating trauma.

Traditionally, the use of conventional CT was viewed as adding little extra knowledge to the clinical scenario. Surgeons, and even some radiologists, felt that obtaining a CT scan wastes valuable time, contrast administration would interfere and confound aortography, and that arteriography would still be necessary in a substantial number of cases [11,12]. However, with the use of helical CT technology, the aorta can be evaluated directly so that confusion of mediastinal hematomas and normal structures can be avoided. In addition, imaging of the aortic root with electrocardiographic gating can help minimize the pulsation and motion artifact that can leave concern about proximal aortic root injury that would traditionally require catheter-based angiography for definitive evaluation [13]. A study by Gavant and colleagues used helical scanning exclusively to screen over 1,500 patients with nontrivial blunt chest trauma. Those with abnormal CTs then underwent conventional aortography. Their evaluation yielded 100% sensitivity and 81.7% specificity for aortic injury [14].

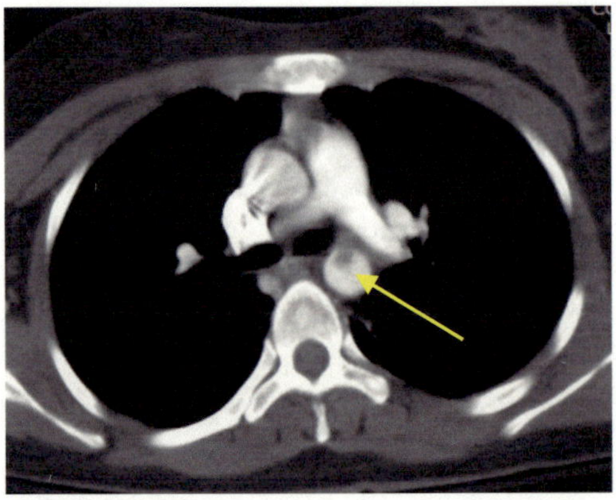

Figure 2. CT scan in axial section with aortic injury and intramural hematoma

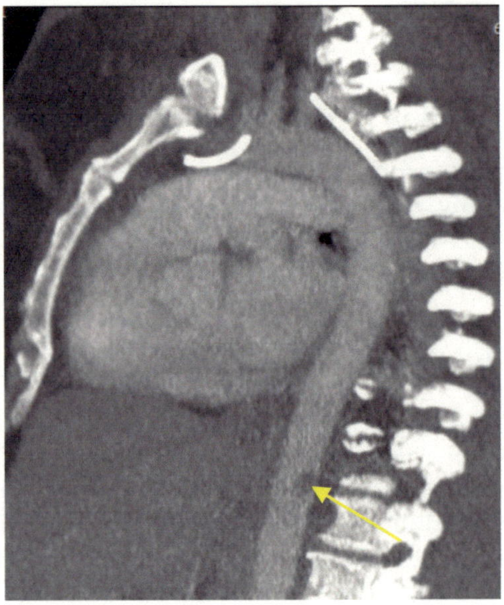

Figure 3. CT scan in sagittal section with intramural hematoma

Previously, the conventional CT scan was used as screening tool to guide further options. If no mediastinal blood is detected on CT, the probability of significant aortic injury is quite low and aortography is usually not needed [15]; efforts should be directed at the management of other injuries in the trauma patient. However, if the CT scan were positive for vascular injury, most surgeons would still proceed with aortography to help better delineate the exact location of the injury and possibly employ endovascular therapeutic options. With the advent of helical technology, however, CT angiography is considered a definitive diagnostic procedure that recognizes aortic injury and rupture.

3.4. Catheter-based thoracic angiography

Traditional teaching has placed conventional catheter-based angiography as the "gold standard" imaging modality when there is clinical or radiographic suspicion of a thoracic major vascular injury in the trauma patient. The information obtained from these studies help localize the injury and aid the surgeon in pre-operative planning and choice of incision as different thoracic approaches are needed for satisfactory anatomic exposure to obtain proximal and distal control of the affected vessels. Newer technology and better imaging resolution and capabilities are challenging this belief however.

In penetrating trauma, catheter arteriography is indicated for suspected aortic, innominate, carotid, or subclavian arterial injuries. Various film sequences have been used, including antero-posterior, lateral and oblique views. It is imperative that multiple views be obtained as more than one projection may be necessary to detect an aortic injury, especially if a small laceration has closed off or if a column of arterial contrast obscures a small extravasation in one view.

Indications for conventional angiography in patients presenting with blunt trauma include those with a rapid deceleration mechanism of injury, those with suggestive signs on chest radiograph – namely an obscure aortic knob or abnormal descending thoracic contour, a widened mediastinum – and those with a positive screening CT scan.

Angiography does have its limitations as well. It lacks spatial resolution, often requiring multiple injections in various different planes to demonstrate even minor lesions. In addition, it only provides luminal imaging and does not provide information on nearby parenchymal lesions and trauma as well as the integrity of adjacent venous structures. Furthermore, most institutions do not have an angiography team that remains "in-house" and as such, there is a time delay in assembling the necessary personnel to perform the imaging. Both false-positive and false-negative results have been reported [16]. These procedures are invasive and iatrogenic complications from catheter use such as arterial dissections, pseudoaneurysms, aortic lacerations, retroperitoneal hemorrhage as well as mortality have been reported [17]. Regardless, catheter-based thoracic angiography currently remains the frame of reference for the definitive diagnosis of thoracic vascular trauma.

3.5. Magnetic resonance angiography

For completeness, a note on magnetic resonance angiography is warranted. Although this modality can demonstrate evidence of acute or subacute mediastinal hemorrhage, its use in the acute trauma setting is not practical. Restricted access to a critically ill trauma patient while in the scanner is unsafe and the strong magnetic field can be severely limiting to those individuals requiring intensive monitoring and mechanical ventilator support.

4. Anatomy of the thoracic great vessels

Although a complete anatomic description of the thoracic vasculature is beyond the scope of this chapter, the relevant great vessel anatomy is described in the following subsections.

4.1. The aorta and its segments

The aorta is described in three different portions within the thoracic cavity; the ascending aorta, aortic arch and descending aorta.

The *ascending aorta* originates from the base of the left ventricle at the aortic orifice. Its origin and proximal aspect are contained within the pericardium. It courses anterosuperiorly and to the right where it becomes the aortic arch. Its total length is about 5 cm. Its only branches are the two coronary arteries, which arise immediately distal to the origin of the aorta just above the attached margins of the semilunar valves. Its location is central with respect to the other vascular structures. On the right side, it is in relation with the superior vena cava and right atrium. On the left side, it is in relation with the pulmonary artery. Posteriorly, it rests upon the right pulmonary artery and left atrium. It is separated from the sternum by the pericardium, the right pleura, the right lung anterior margin, some loose areolar tissue and the remains of the thymus.

The *aortic arch* runs at first posterosuperiorly and to the left, anterior to the right pulmonary artery and the carina of the trachea with its apex on the left of the distal trachea. It then courses downward posterior to the left hilum and becomes the descending aorta at the level of the lower border of the fourth thoracic vertebral body. Its branches, in order from right to left, include the brachiocephalic artery, the left common carotid artery and the left subclavian artery. All three branches arise from the convexity of the arch and are crossed close to their origins by the left brachiocephalic vein. Anteriorly, the vessel is covered by the lung pleura and the remains of the thymus. On the right side, it is in relation with the esophagus, the thoracic duct, the left recurrent laryngeal nerve and the deep part of the cardiac plexus. The trachea is also found on the right but posteriorly to the vessel. On the left side, the vessel is in contact with the left lung and pleura superiorly, and as it passes downward four nerves are encountered; the left phrenic, the lower of the superior cardiac branches of the left vagus, the superior cardiac branch of the left sympathetic, and the trunk of the left vagus. As the trunk of the vagus nerve crosses the aortic arch, it gives off its recurrent branch that wraps around the arch and then travels superiorly and to the right. Below the vessel are also the bifurcation of the pulmonary artery, the left bronchus, the superficial part of the cardiac plexus and the ligamentum arteriosum. The ligamentum arteriosum represents the remnant of the ductus arteriosus, connecting the inferior aspect of the aortic arch to the superior aspect of the pulmonary trunk.

The *descending thoracic aorta* is found in the posterior mediastinal cavity. It begins at the level of the fourth thoracic vertebra and descends on the left of the midline exiting the thorax through the aortic hiatus posterior to the diaphragm at the level of the twelfth thoracic vertebra. Its branches include the bronchial arteries, the posterior intercostal arteries as well as the pericardial, esophageal, mediastinal, superior phrenic and subcostal branches. On the anterior surface of the vessel, from above downward, are the root of the left lung, the pericardium, the esophagus and the diaphragm. Posteriorly, it is in relation with the hemiazygos veins and the vertebral column. On the left side of the vessel are the left pleura and lung, and on the right side are the azygos vein and thoracic duct. The esophagus lies on the right side of the descending aorta superiorly, then courses anteriorly and eventually to the left side of the vessel just above the diaphragm.

4.2. The great veins

The *brachiocephalic veins* are located on either side of the root of the neck and are devoid of valves. The right brachiocephalic vein is a short, about 2.5 cm long vessel and is formed by the confluence of the right subclavian and right jugular veins. Its origin is posterior to the medial aspect of the right clavicle. It runs vertically downwards and joins the left brachiocephalic vein just below the cartilage of the right first rib to form the superior vena cava. Its tributaries are the right vertebral vein, the right internal thoracic vein, the first posterior intercostal vein, the right inferior thyroid and thymic veins. The left brachiocephalic vein is about 6 cm long and is formed by the confluence of the left subclavian and left jugular veins. It begins behind the medial aspect of the left clavicle and travels obliquely downward and to the right posterior to the sternum to anastomose with the right brachiocephalic vein just below the cartilage of the right first rib. Its tributaries include the left vertebral vein, , the left internal thoracic vein, the left superior intercostal vein, the left inferior thyroid vein, and some thymic and pericardiac veins.

The *superior vena cava* is formed by the confluence of the right and left brachiocephalic veins. It has no valves. It measures about 7 cm in length and runs vertically downward posterior to the first two intercostal spaces to drain into the upper part of the right atrium The distal portion of the vessel is partially invested by pericardium. Its only tributary is the azygous vein. The inferior vena cava begins in the abdomen and enters the thorax through the caval hiatus in the diaphragm at the level of the eighth thoracic vertebra and immediately drains into the inferior aspect of the right atrium. It is partially invested by pericardium. It has no tributaries in the thorax.

The *azygous vein* begins in the abdomen and enters the thorax through the aortic hiatus in the diaphragm . It runs upward to the right side of the bodies of the thoracic vertebrae to the fourth thoracic vertebra, where it arches anteriorly over the right main bronchus and drains into the posterior aspect of the superior vena cava. It is found in the posterior mediastinum to the right of the esophagus and aorta, and to the left of the pleura and lung. Posteriorly, it is in relation to the lower right intercostal arteries and the thoracic vertebral bodies; anteriorly, to the root of the right lung and the pleura. Its tributaries include the hemiazygous vein, the right subcostal vein, some of the left intercostal veins and the nine lower intercostal veins on the right, the lower right superior intercostal vein, the right bronchial vein and several esophageal, mediastinal, and pericardial veins. The tributaries have complete valves, but the azygous vein itself only has a few imperfect valves.

5. Management options

With increases in technology and research, there are three mainstay treatments of blunt aortic injury: non-operative management, endovascular stent-graft methods, and traditional open repair (either immediate or delayed).

Azizzadeh and colleagues [18] initially proposed a classification system for blunt aortic injury based on the presence of an external aortic contour abnormality on computed tomography and/or the presence of free rupture noted on laparotomy.

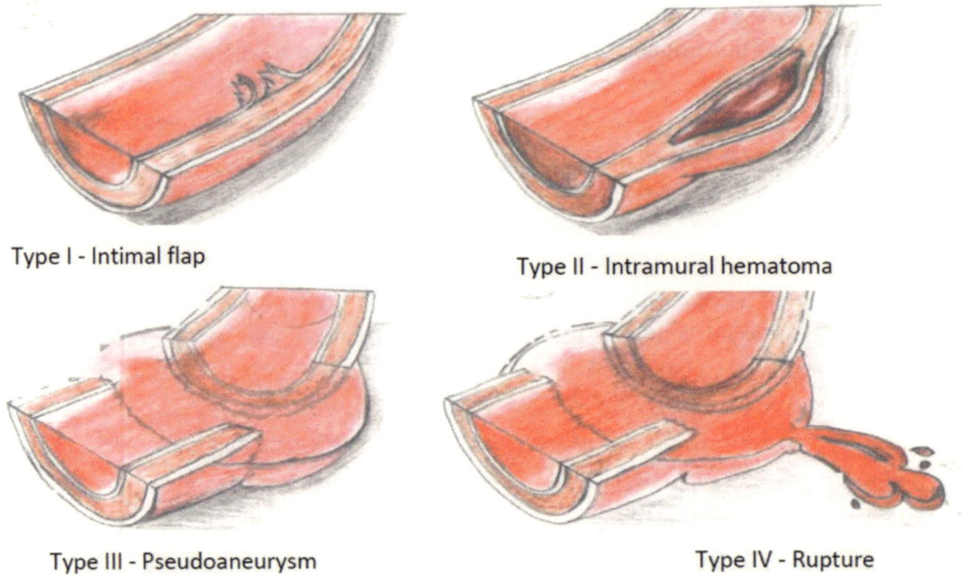

Figure 4. Schematic representation of blunt thoracic injury with implications for management

This classification system was further modified by Starnes and colleagues [19], as follows:

- Intimal tear: absence of aortic external contour abnormality and intimal defect and/or thrombus of <10mm in length or width
- Large intimal flap: absence of aortic external contour abnormality and intimal defect and/or thrombus of ≥10mm in length or width
- Pseudoaneurysm: external aortic contour abnormality and contained rupture
- Rupture: external aortic contour abnormality with free contrast extravasation noted on computed tomography or hemoperitoneum found on exploratory laparotomy

The Society for Vascular Surgery in 2011 has determined clinical practice guidelines for the repair of traumatic thoracic aortic injury [20]. Type I injuries can be managed expectantly with serial imaging; however, types II to IV should be repaired. Endovascular approaches are becoming the standard option in this regard if amenable.

5.1. Non-operative management

The advent of multi-detector CT and TEE has resulted in the identification of subtle injuries that were previously beyond the resolution of traditional imaging techniques. This has resulted in a dilemma of which particular injuries require immediate treatment and which ones can be safely observed. Some practitioners withhold intervention for minor aortic injuries such as minor intimal defects of 1 cm with no or minimal periaortic hematoma [21]. Complete resolution of such injuries has been noted but complications have also been documented from such non-operative management, even many years later. The natural history of these injuries is unknown but such complications include delayed rupture of pseudoaneurysms or even fistulization with profound hemorrhage [22]. Those patients that are treated non-operatively for blunt aortic injuries should undergo careful follow-up with imaging to observe and document injury resolution.

Patients that should not undergo immediate repair of blunt aortic injury include:

- Severe hemodynamic instability from concomitant injuries within the abdomen or pelvis
- Severe head injury
- Prohibitive medical co-morbidities
- Severe pulmonary injury
- Patients with progressive coagulopathy, acidosis and hypothermia
- Severe burns
- Profoundly contaminated wounds
- Severe sepsis
- Patients not in a trauma center capable of definitive repair

The mainstay of non-operative management involves aggressive pharmacological control of blood pressure with beta-blockers and critical care in an effort to delay the physiological insult of surgical intervention until the patient is adequately resuscitated and optimized. Avoiding hypertension is recommended to minimize intraluminal stress on the injured vessel from increased systolic blood pressure.

5.2. Endovascular stent-graft interventions

The advancement of endovascular techniques and device technology has truly revolutionized the treatment of blunt aortic injury over the last few years. In fact, at many centers, the use of thoracic endovascular repair (TEVAR) has become an attractive approach whereas initially it was only used in highly selected patients deemed too high risk for conventional open repair.

There are multiple advantages to the use of TEVAR, especially in the high-risk patient population. By nature, endovascular treatment is less invasive than open surgery, and if successful, averts the need for a traditional thoracotomy. It is associated with decreased morbidity and mortality, as has been noted in several studies [23-25]. Blood loss is minimal. Placement of a stent-graft does not require aortic cross clamping, which reduces the risk of distal visceral and spinal ischemia. In addition, such cross-clamping and unclamping complicate resuscitation and anesthesiologist management in patients with circulatory collapse and hemodynamic instability. Respiratory compromise from lung and thoracic wall injuries is magnified by thoracotomy, and single ventilation in such patients may be quite problematic. Furthermore, appropriate positioning for open surgery may compound neurologic deficits in patients with spinal fractures. Although systemic heparinization is usually employed during routine stent-grafting procedures, in cases of polytrauma with concomitant visceral organ injuries and fractures of the pelvis and long bones, heparin is withheld. Importantly with TEVAR, the absence of circulatory assistance with bypass and the need for high systemic doses of heparin, limit the feared hemorrhagic complications. Xenos et al. performed a meta-analysis of seventeen retrospective cohort studies evaluating 589 patients, and indicated that endovascular management of descending thoracic aortic injuries is a viable alternative to traditional open repair; it is associated with decreased ischemic spinal cord complication rates and lower postoperative mortality [23].

Successful use of endovascular stents in this patient population requires a sophisticated multidisciplinary and experienced team approach. Strict evaluation of the patient's anatomy is imperative. Current devices were primarily designed to treat aneurysmal disease, which is more prevalent in an aging population. Trauma patients have a considerable young demographic. As such, appropriate "fitting" of commercial devices is not always possible, rendering the use of stent-grafts difficult. Some young patients have aortic diameters less than 20 mm, which are too small for standard devices, even if oversizing the device diameter by the recommended 10-15% is employed. Adolescents and young teens also commonly have an aortic arch with a tight radius of curvature making sufficient apposition suboptimal due to inflexibility of devices. Most importantly, most reports of the use of stent-grafts demonstrate great short- and mid-term results. However, the data is lacking on long-term results, a concern for young patients expected to have a considerable life expectancy following the incident. Such patients will need close follow-up and continued surveillance imaging; the associated cost for the continued evaluation and the radiation burden is a concern [26].

It should be noted that endovascular options such a balloon occlusion, arterial embolization, and stenting or stent-grafting are viable endovascular options for the management of other great vessel trauma, such as the carotid, vertebral, subclavian, and axillary arteries.

5.3. Surgical repair

The standard of care for treating blunt aortic trauma has been emergent thoracotomy with interposition prosthetic graft or direct aortic repair with either a "clamp and sew" technique or with some variation of circulatory assistance and bypass. The rationale for treating blunt aortic injury is to essentially prevent early rupture from the acute injury and to prevent late aneurysm formation and subsequent rupture. The traditional approach is through a left thoracotomy with single lung ventilation, however, as noted previously, patients with pulmonary injuries and thoracic wall trauma may not tolerate single-lung ventilation [26-28].

Despite the many advances in peri-operative management and operative techniques, there continues to be a high morbidity and mortality with these injuries. The risk of paraplegia varies from 2.3% with active distal aortic perfusion to over 19% with the "clamp and sew" approach [26]. Mortality rates have been reported between 5% and 28% [28].

The indications for urgent thoracotomy remain hemodynamic instability, continued and significant hemorrhage from an adequately place tube thoracostomy, and rapidly expanding mediastinal hematoma noted on imaging. Certain pre-operative considerations are necessary prior to operative intervention, and include adequate pre-operative preparation, pharmacologic control, choice of incisions, availability of prosthetic material, and surgical repair techniques.

5.3.1. *Pre-operative preparation*

After confirmation of great vessel injury, the patient should expeditiously be prepared for immediate transport to the operating room for definitive surgical vascular control. While in the trauma bay, however, intravenous access should be obtained and cross-matched blood should be sent for; O negative blood should be used for immediate resuscitation efforts along with crystalloid fluids in the judicious manner described previously. Large bore central venous catheters should be placed on the side contralateral to the injury, above and below the diaphragm. It should be noted again, however, that no efforts should delay transport.

In the operating suite, close collaboration with the anesthesiologists is imperative. A double-lumen endotracheal tube should be placed (or converted to from the single-lumen endotracheal tube), if possible. Induction anesthetic agents can cause a precipitous decline in blood pressure that should be avoided, and artificial elevation of the blood pressure with vaso-active agents is also undesirable, especially when vascular control is not yet achieved. A nasogastric tube should also be inserted if not already done so. An arterial radial line will help with real-time hemodynamic monitoring. Perfusionists and full cardio-pulmonary bypass capabilities and circulatory assistance must be readily available in addition to an auto-transfusion device. A urinary catheter should also be placed. Prophylactic antibiotics are administered and tetanus prophylaxis should be ensured.

Although all efforts are moving at a fast pace to transport the patient to the operating room, it is essential that the surgeon be forthcoming about the seriousness of the situation and the high potential for post-operative complications with the patient and family whenever possible. The possibility of neurological damage, paraplegia, myocardial infarction, cerebrovascular accidents, renal failure and death must be discussed.

5.3.2. *Pharmacologic control*

Use of beta-blockers has become quite commonplace. The goal is to reduce the pressure on the injured aortic wall in order to avoid fatal rupture while maintaining cerebral perfusion.

Pate and colleagues demonstrated that the use of antihypertensive strategies in the management of acute traumatic aortic injuries eliminated in-hospital rupture of blunt aortic trauma when a delay in operative intervention was necessary [29]. In fact, the EAST Practice Management Guidelines Work Group recommends the use of vasodilators such as sodium nitroprusside or beta-blockade when non-operative or delayed management of blunt aortic injuries is considered [30].

5.3.3. *Choice of incision*

Adequate anatomic exposure is clearly imperative to visualize the injury and achieve appropriate proximal and distal vascular control. Injury detection through imaging greatly aids the surgeon in selecting the best incision to manage thoracic great vessel injuries.

Injured Vessel	Recommended Incision
Unidentified vessel in hemodynamically unstable patient	Left anterolateral thoracotomy ± transverse sternotomy ± right anterolateral thoracotomy (clamshell incision)
Ascending aorta	Median sternotomy
Transverse aortic arch	Median sternotomy
Descending thoracic aorta	Left posterolateral thoractomy
Brachiocephalic (innominate) artery	Median sternotomy with right cervical extension
Right subclavian artery or vein	Median sternotomy with right cervical extension
Right common carotid artery	Right cervical incision
Left common carotid artery	Median sternotomy with left cervical extension
Left subclavian artery or vein	Left anterolateral thoracotomy and separate left supraclavicular incision ±vertical sternotomy (book thoracotomy)
Pulmonary artery (main segment)	Median sternotomy
Pulmonary artery (intrapericardial segment)	Median sternotomy
Pulmonary artery (right or left hilar segment)	Ipsilateral posterolateral thoracotomy
Superior vena cava	Median sternotomy
Intrathoracic inferior vena cava	Median sternotomy
Innominate vein	Median sternotomy
Pulmonary vein	Ipsilateral posterolateral thoracotomy

Table 2. Recommended incisions for thoracic vascular injuries. Adapted from Feliciano, Mattox, and Moore, Thoracic Great Vessel Injury, 2008, p. 597.

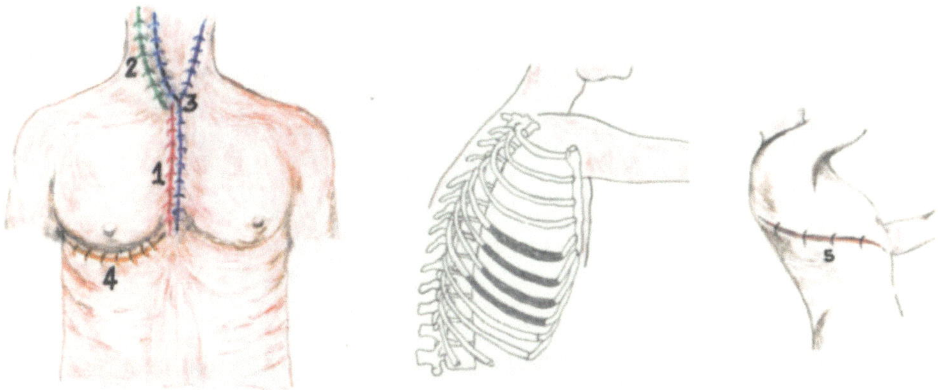

Figure 5. Incisional choices to approach the thoracic great vessels. (1) Median sternotomy; (2) Right cervical extension; (3) Median sternotomy with left cervical extension; (4) Ipsilateral anterolateral thoracotomy; (5) Ipsilateral posterolateral thoracotomy

In the unstable patient, the classic left anterolateral thoracotomy is performed with appropriate extensions as needed for adequate vascular control. It is important that the patient be prepped and draped from the neck down to the knee to allow for any and all possibilities. In stable patients, pre-operative radiography will allow specific identification of injuries and the incisions are tailored to the particular site.

5.3.4. Prosthetic materials

Availability of appropriate prosthetic material is important in emergency situations where aortic reconstruction is necessary. For vessels larger than 5 mm, a prosthetic material (either Dacron or PTFE) is generally used. For smaller thoracic vessels that are injured, some would advocate the use of autogenous conduits, such as the saphenous vein, for concerns of long-term patency. Prosthetic graft material soaked in antibiotic solution may theoretically prevent infection and bacterial seeding.

6. Great vessel injuries

6.1. Arterial injuries

6.1.1. Ascending aorta

Blunt trauma to the ascending aorta is relatively rare and patients rarely survive transportation to the hospital. Open repair is indicated and usually involves placement of an interposition prosthetic Dacron graft with total cardiopulmonary bypass. The injury is approached through a median sternotomy.

Penetrating injuries are equally uncommon secondary to protection from the sternum. If anterior injuries are encountered, they may be repaired directly without cardiopulmonary bypass, however, circulatory assistance is usually necessary if concomitant posterior injuries are noted.

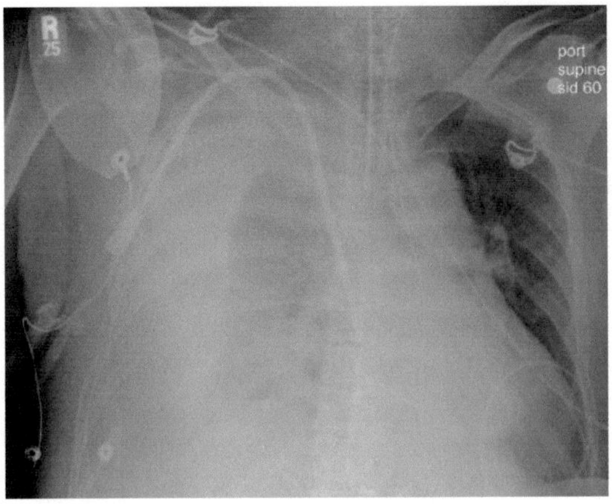

Figure 6. Unusual presentation of a patient with a right hemothorax after a retrograde dissection of the descending thoracic aorta into the transverse aortic arch and ascending aorta

6.1.2. Transverse aortic arch

Injuries to the transverse aortic arch pose a challenge as control of initial massive hemorrhage is difficult and usually the cause of surgical failure. Such injuries are exposed with a median sternotomy and commonly with a neck extension to allow for satisfactory distal control of the arch vessels. A variety of surgical methods such as tangential incomplete or intermittent complete aortic occlusion, vena caval occlusion, the use of temporary shunts, and even ventricular fibrillation have been used to help control hemorrhage during repair [31-33].

Deep hypothermia and circulatory arrest are recommended during the repair of these injuries to allow for optimal exposure, especially when posterior arch injuries are detected or suspected. Anterior injuries can be directly repaired.

6.1.3. Descending thoracic aorta

The descending thoracic aorta is the most commonly affected segment of the great vessel. In blunt mechanisms, it is usually just distal to the ligamentum arteriousum that the aorta is injured. Evaluation of the aorta at the aortic hiatus in the diaphragm should also be conducted because the vessel is tethered at this location and therefore susceptible to rapid deceleration forces.

It is important to note that trauma patients presenting to the hospital with blunt aortic injury usually have multiple other injuries. If the aortic injury is stable without evidence of an expanding hematoma and the patient continues to demonstrate hemodynamic instability, an expeditious search for other major trauma, primarily to the abdomen or pelvis, should be performed and addressed first. This may in fact necessitate laparotomy and control of intra-abdominal hemorrhage prior to managing the great vessel injury, which can be conducted in a delayed fashion. Contemporarily, the use of intraluminal stents and TEVAR can be performed immediately following laparotomy.

Open surgical repair methods include either a primary direct repair of the aortic injury with either the "clamp and sew" approach or via circulatory assistance, or with placement of an interposition graft. The descending thoracic aorta is approached through a posterolateral thoracotomy, usually through the 4th intercostal space.

With the so called "clamp and sew" technique, the aorta is clamped distal to the left subclavian artery take-off, if possible, in order to allow cephalad perfusion; if not, the transverse aortic arch is clamped just distal to the left common carotid artery take-off with a second clamp placed on the left subclavian artery. A distal clamp is then placed as proximal as possible on the descending thoracic aorta to allow spinal cord perfusion while maximizing anatomic exposure for repair. If feasible, the clamps should be moved closer to the injury when identified. Care should be taken to not debride the aorta. This technique is particularly useful in the polytrauma patient as the additional risks of systemic heparinization are avoided as circulatory assistance is generally not used; however, this comes with the increased risk of paraplegia. This most feared complication – paraplegia – has an incidence of 0% to 19% [34] and is thought to be directly due to spinal cord ischemia from aortic cross clamping. The lowest reported rates of paraplegia have been noted with cross-clamp times less than 30 minutes [34]. Eighty-five percent of blunt aortic injuries are repaired with a soft interposition graft, however, if less than 50% of the aortic diameter is injured, primary repair may be employed. In addition, care should be taken not to sacrifice intercostals vessels – only those that compromise exposure due to continued bleeding should be ligated.

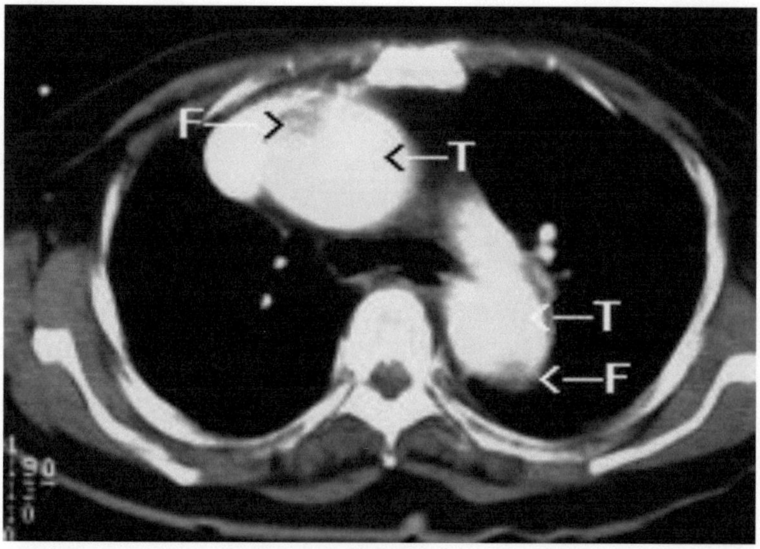

Figure 7. Aortic injury with secondary dissection from an intimal flap. (T) – true lumen; (F) – false lumen

The other alternative is to perform the repair while the distal thoracic aorta is perfused with extracorporeal circulation. This can be either via temporary, passive bypass shunts such as left ventricle to aorta or ascending to descending aortic shunts, or with active pump assisted left atrial to femoral bypass in a traditional format which requires heparin or a centrifugal pump mechanism. This method has been associated with decreased rates of paraplegia due to continued perfusion of the distal thoracic aorta, and as such, the spinal cord, during aortic repair. Some series even note no post-operative paraplegia with this technique [36].

Clearly, it is important to note that endovascular stent-grafts offer a particular advantage in these patients, if the anatomy is favorable, as morbidity and mortality are decreased.The paraplegia rate with this method is essentially close to zero. These interventional techniques have become quite commonplace in many trauma centers with such capabilities, and when possible should be considered.

6.1.4. Brachiocephalic artery

The brachiocephalic (or innominate) artery is approached via a median sternotomy to achieve proximal control at its origin from the aortic arch, with the incision extending into the right neck depending on how distal control is necessary. Exclusion and bypass via the "bypass principle" is the most common method of repairing a brachiocephalic injury, which occurs mostly at its origin.

The areas for bypass are from the ascending aorta to the distal brachiocephalic artery, just proximal to its bifurcation into the right common carotid and right subclavian. The brachiocephalic artery is clamped proximal to the injury while allowing continuous perfusion to the remainder of the body through the aorta. Distally, the brachiocephalic artery is clamped proximal to its bifurcation. A prosthetic Dacron graft is used for bypass. A side-biting clamp is placed onto the ascending aorta at the point for the proximal anastomosis, and an end-to-end anastomosis is performed distally. The native brachiocephalic origin is oversewn to complete the repair. Circulatory arrest and cardiopulmonary bypass is not necessary [36].

6.1.5. Subclavian artery

The right subclavian artery can be approached through a median sternotomy and right cervical extension. The left is approached through a left anterolateral thoracotomy for proximal control and a separate left neck incision for distal control. Pre-operative imaging with computed tomography or angiography is extremely helpful in delineating the exact location of the injury. The relation to the scalene muscles is also beneficial – if the injury is medial to the muscle, then a mid-sternotomy alone with extension should suffice, however, a supraclavicular approach will generally be satisfactory with a lateral injury.

Injuries are usually repaired either by lateral arteriorraphy or by placement of an interposition graft. When a graft is employed, the anastomosis is usually created in an end-to-side fashion as end-to-end can be quite difficult. Clearly, it is important to avoid the brachial plexus roots and the phrenic nerve during exposure.

The use of endovascular options is attractive for these injuries in particular. White et al. have noted one year primary patency and exclusion rates of 86% and 90%, respectively [37]. Complications are much less severe than with open surgical repair with stenoses and occlusions predominating however.

6.1.6. *Left common carotid artery*

The approach to the left common carotid artery mirrors that of its contralateral companion. A median sternotomy is employed with a left neck cervical extension when necessary. Small injuries can be repaired with primary arteriorraphy or with a patch; however, more severe injuries are preferentially repaired with bypass grafts.

6.1.7. *Internal mammary artery*

Internal mammary artery (IMA) injuries are more common with penetrating injuries rather than blunt injuries, however, the disruption of the IMA during latter has been described. It may follow relatively minor trauma resulting in a self-limited hematoma either in an extra-pleural setting or in between parietal pleura and the transversus thoracic muscle, or worse leading to a mediastinal hematoma with cardiac compression and/or hemodynamic instability.

The standard approach to repair involves a thoracotomy for adequate exposure. Small injuries in this setting may be repaired with primary arteriorraphy or via a patch. As with other thoracic injuries, more severe vessel trauma will require a bypass graft. It should also be noted that an endovascular approach with selective embolization using coils has been reported.

6.1.8. *Pulmonary artery*

Pulmonary artery injuries are very lethal and fortunately quite uncommon. Their management depends on where along the course the trauma has occurred. Proximal pulmonary and intrapericardial portions are approached through a median sternotomy. As with most other thoracic great vessel trauma, anterior injuries can usually be repaired directly, however, posterior injuries usually require total cardiopulmonary bypass to allow for satisfactory exposure.

The repair of distal or hilar pulmonary artery injuries is made difficult by the presence of the lung. These injuries are approached via an ipsilateral posterolateral thoracotomy. The need to perform a trauma pneumonectomy should be in the surgeon's armamentarium in cases of rapid hemorrhage so as to facilitate the necessary exposure to a major distal hilar injury.

6.2. Venous injuries

6.2.1. *Thoracic vena cavae*

Injury to the superior vena cava or intrathoracic inferior vena cava is infrequent due to the short length of these vessels within the thorax. Hemopericardium with pericardial tamponade physiology is usually found with such injuries. The surgical approach is through a median sternotomy. Superior vena cava injuries can usually be repaired via lateral venorrhaphy. The main difficulty with repair of caval injuries, however, is obtaining adequate exposure because of hemorrhage. Vascular isolation techniques such as atrio-caval shunting have been proposed to limit bleeding in pursuit of the strategy of direct repair of these venous injuries. However, mortality rates are fairly high, which has made many surgeons question the reliability of these approaches. As such, total cardiopulmonary bypass can be used as an alternative technique in order to decrease the blood return to the surgical field while maintaining perfusion of the body. Using circulatory assistance, an abdominal inferior vena caval to right atrial cannulation circuit should be used. The vena cava is repaired from within the lumen via access through a right atriotomy. Short inflow occlusion can be used if necessary.

Several surgical techniques have been used for reconstruction of the IVC including patch angioplasty and saphenous vein grafting. For extensive injuries, however, PTFE interposition grafts are preferred based on their superior patency rates and rapidity of the repair [38,39]. It is also important to exclude any other injuries that may preclude the use of systemic anticoagulation prior to total cardiopulmonary bypass.

Of note, thoracic inferior vena cava injuries that extend into the abdominal segment or that even include the retrohepatic veins can be repaired in a manner similar to the above description of cardiopulmonary bypass and total hypothermic circulatory arrest, if a completely bloodless surgical field is required. [40].

6.2.2. Pulmonary veins

Approach to the pulmonary veins is employed through an ipsilateral posterolateral thoracotomy. Repair with lateral venorraphy is preferred but technically difficult. If ligation is necessary, the respective lobe must also be resected.

6.2.3. Subclavian veins

Exposure for subclavian vein injuries is similar to the exposure necessary for subclavian artery injuries. Repair is either performed via a lateral venorraphy or suture ligation of the vessel.

7. Post-operative considerations and critical care

Patients suffering from thoracic great vessel injury clearly require critical care management in an intensive care unit setting. Hemodynamic monitoring and strict measurement of fluid inputs and outputs is necessary. Measures should be taken to avoid significant variability in blood pressure by judicious use of fluids and pharmacologic agents.

A tertiary survey will be required to evaluate for any further suspicion of injuries and commonly, repeat imaging is employed. Patients with multi-trauma will have an exaggerated systemic inflammatory response syndrome and hemodynamic support should be carefully instituted. Care must be taken to avoid attributing hypotension due to this exaggerated response – continued hemorrhage from unrecognized injuries or technical surgical failure must be excluded immediately.

Although the operation, revascularization, and reconstruction may be successful, patients are still susceptible to the many postoperative complications following major surgery, including pneumonia, urinary tract infections, wound disruption, adult respiratory distress syndrome, transfusion reactions, and coagulopathy. Management of these patients should be performed in an interdisciplinary approach with critical care physicians and the trauma surgeon playing a lead role in directing care.

Author details

Nicolas J. Mouawad*
Clinical Fellow, Division of Cardiovascular Diseases and Surgery, The Ohio State University Wexner Medical Center, Columbus, OH, USA

Christodoulos Kaoutzanis
Resident, Michigan Heart and Vascular Institute, Saint Joseph Mercy Health System, Ann Arbor, MI, USA

Ajay Gupta
Attending Surgeon, Division of Cardiothoracic Surgery, Michigan Heart and Vascular Institute, Saint Joseph Mercy Health System, Ann Arbor, MI, USA

Acknowledgement

We would like to thank Doros Polydorou, MD, for producing the schematic illustrations for Figure 4 and 5.

8. References

[1] Alfaro J, Varela G, DeMiguel E, de Nicilas M (1993) Successful management of a traceho-innominate artery fistula following placement of a wire self-expandable tracheal Gianturco stent. Eur J Cardio-ThoracSurg 7:615.

[2] Horton TG, Cohn SM, Heid MP, Augenstein JS, Bowen JC, McKenney MG, Duncan RC (2000) Identification of trauma patients at risk of thoracic aortic tear by mechanism of injury. J Trauma 48: 1008-1013.

[3] Katyal D, McLellan BA, Brenneman FD, Boulanger BR, Sharkey PW, Waddell JP (1997) Lateral impact motor vehicle collisions: significant cause of blunt traumatic rupture of the thoracic aorta. J Trauma 42:769-772.

[4] Mattox KL, Wall MJ, Lemaire S (2008) Thoracic Great Vessel Injury. In: Feliciano DV, Mattox KL, Moore EE, editors. Trauma: McGraw-Hill. pp 589-603.

* Corresponding Author

[5] Bickell WH, Wall MJ, Pepe PE, Martin RR, Ginger VF, Allen MK, Mattox KL (1994) Immediate versus delayed fluid resuscitation for hypotensive patients with penetrating torso injuries. N Engl J Med 331:1105-1109.

[6] Mirvis SE, Bidwell K, Buddemeyer EU, Diaconis JN, Pais SO, Whitley JE, Goldstein LD (1987) Value of chest radiography in excluding traumatic aortic rupture. Radiology 163:487-493.

[7] Shanewise JS, Cheung AT, Aronson S, Stewart WJ, Weiss RL, Mark JB, Savage RM, Sears-Rogan P, Mathew JP, Quinones MA, Cahalan MK, Savino JS (199). ASE/SCA guidelines for performing a comprehensive intraoperative multiplane transesophageal echocardiography examination: recommendations of the American Society of Echocardiography Council for Intraoperative Echocardiography and the Society of Cardiovascular Anesthesiologists Task Force for Certification in Perioperative Transesophageal Echocardiography. Anesth Analg 89:870-84.

[8] Marciniak D, Smith CD (2010) Pros and Cons of Transesophageal Echocardiography in Trauma Care. The Internet Journal of Anesthesiology 23: 2.

[9] Smith MK, Cassidy JM, Souther S, Morris EJ, Sapin PM, Johnson SB, Kearney PA (1995) Transesophageal echocardiography in the diagnosis of traumatic rupture of the aorta. N Engl J Med 332:356-362.

[10] Vignon P, Ostyn E, Francios B, Jojeij J, Gastinne H, Lang RM (1997) Limitations of transesophageal echocardiography for the diagnosis of traumatic injuries to aortic branches. J Trauma 42:960-963.

[11] Wills JS, Lally JF (1991) Use of CT for evaluation of possible traumatic aortic injury (letter). AJR 157:1123-1 124.

[12] Groshkin SA (1992) Selected topics in chest trauma. Radiology 183:605-617.

[13] Schertler T, Glucker T, Wildermuth S, Jungius KP, Marincek B, Boehm T (2005) Comparison of retrospectively ECG-gated and nongated MDCT of the chest in an emergency setting regarding workflow, image quality, and diagnostic certainty. Emerg Radiol 12:19-29.

[14] Gavant ML, Menke PG, Fabian T, Flick P. Graney MJ, Gold RE (1995) Helical CT of the chest to detect blunt traumatic aortic rupture. Radiology 197:125-133.

[15] Scaglione M, Pinto A, Pinto F, Romano L, Ragozzino A, Grassi R (2001) Role of contrast-enhanced helical CT in the evaluation of acute thoracic aortic injuries after blunt chest trauma. Eur Radiol 11:2444-2448.

[16] Fenner MN, Fisher KS, Sergel NL, Porter DB, Metzmaker CO (1990). Evaluation of possible traumatic thoracic aortic injury using aortography and CT. Am Surg 56:497-499.

[17] LaBerge JM, Jeffrey RB (1987). Aortic lacerations: fatal complications of thoracic aortography. Radiology 165:367-369.

[18] Azizzadeh A, Keyhani K, Miller CC III, Coogan SM, Safi HJ, Estrera AL (2009) Blunt traumatic aortic injury: intial experience with endovascular repair. J Vasc Surg 49:1403-8.

[19] Starnes BW, Lundgren RS, Gunn M, Quade S, Hatsukami TS, Tran NT, Mokadam N, Algea G (2012) A new classification scheme for treating blunt aortic injury. J Vasc Surg 55:47-54.

[20] Lee WA, Matsumura JS, Mitchell RS, Farber MA, Greenberg RK, Azizzadeh A, Murad MH, Fairman RM (2011) Endovascular repair of traumatic thoracic aortic injury: clinical practice guidelines of the Society for Vascular Surgery. J Vasc Surg 53:187-92.

[21] Rousseau H, Dambtin C, Marcheix B, Richeux L, Mazerolles M, Cron C, Watkinson A, Mugniot A, Soula P, Chabbert V, Canevet G, Roux D, Massabuau P, Meites, Tran Van T, Otal P (2005) Acute traumatic aortic rupture: a comparison of surgical and stent-graft repair. J Thorac Cardiovasc Surg 129:1050-1055.

[22] Hirose H, Inderjit S, Malangoni M (2006) Nonoperative management of traumatic aortic injury. J Trauma 60:597-601.

[23] Xenos ES, Abedi NN, Davenport DL, Minion DJ, Hamdallah O, Sorial EE, Endean ED (2008) Meta-analysis of endovascular vs open repair for traumatic descending thoracic aortic rupture. J Vasc Surg 48:1343-1351.

[24] Amabile P, Collart F, Gariboldi V, Rollet G, Bartoli JM, Piquet P (2004) Surgical versus endovascular treatment of traumatic thoracic aortic rupture. J Vasc Surg 40:873-879.

[25] Rousseau H, Elaassar O, Marcheix B, Cron C, Chabbert V, Combelles S, Dambrin C, Leobon B, Moreno R, Otal P, Auriol J (2012) The role of stent-grafts in the management of aortic trauma. Cardiovasc Intervent Radiol 35:2-14.

[26] McPherson SJ (2007) Thoracic aortic and great vessel trauma and its management. Semin Intervent Radiol 24:180-196.

[27] Kasirajan K, Heffernan D, Langeld M (2003) Acute thoracic aortic trauma: a comparison of endoluminal stent grafts with open repair and non-operative management. Ann Vasc Surg 17:589-595.

[28] Peterson BG, Matsumura JS, Morasch MD, West MA, Eskandari MK (2005) Percutaneous endovascular repair of blunt thoracic aortic transaction. J Trauma 59:1062-1065.

[29] Pate JW, Fabian TC, Walker W (1995) Traumatic rupture of the aortic isthmus: an emergency? World J Surg 19: 119-126.

[30] Nagy K, Fabian T, Rodman G, Fulda G, Rodriguez A, Mirvis S (2000) Guidelines for the diagnosis and management of blunt aortic injury: an EAST Practice Management Guidelines Work Group. J Trauma 48:1128-1143.

[31] Pate JW, Cole FH, Walker WA, Fabian TC (1993) Penetrating injuries the aortic arch and its branches. Ann Thorac Surg 55:586-592.

[32] Buchan K., Robbs J (1995) Surgical management of penetrating mediastinal arterial trauma. Eur J Cardiothorac Surg 9:90-94.

[33] Fulton JO, De Groot MK, von Oppell UO (1996) Stab wounds of the innominate artery. Ann Thorac Surg 61:851-853.

[34] Simeone A, Freitas M, Frankel HL (2006) Management options in blunt aortic injury: a case series and literature review. Am Surg 72:25-30.

[35] Attar S, Cardarelli MG, Downing SW, Rodriguez A, Wallace DC, West RS, McLaughlin JS (1999) Traumatic aortic rupture: recent outcome with regard to neurologic deficit. Ann Thorac Surg 67:959-964.

[36] Wall MJ, Tsai PI, Gilani R, Mattox KL (2010) Open and endovascular approaches to aortic trauma. Tex Heart Inst J 37:675-677.

[37] White R, Krajcer Z, Johnson M, Williams D, Bacharach M, O'Malley E (1999) Results of a multicenter trial for the treatment of traumatic vascular injury with a covered stent. J Trauma 60:1189-1196.

[38] Lam Bk, Pettersson GB, Vogt DP (2003) Urgent inferior vena cava replacement with an autologous pericardium tube graft. J Thorac Cardiovasc Surg 126:2101-2103.

[39] Gloviczki P, Pairolero PC, Toomey BJ, Bower TC, Rooke TW, Stanson AW, Hallett JW Jr, Cherry KJ Jr (1992) Reconstruction of large veins for nonmalignant venous occlusive disease. J Vasc Surg 16:750-761.

[40] Kaoutzanis C, Evangelakis E, Kokkinos C, Kaoutzanis G (2011) Successful repair of injured hepatic veins and inferior vena cava following blunt traumatic injury, by using cardiopulmonary bypass and hypothermic circulatory arrest. Interact Cardiovasc Thorac Surg 12:84-86.

Chapter 13

Endoscopic Clipping and Application of Fibrin Glue for an Esophago-Mediastinal Fistula

Hiroshi Makino, Hiroshi Yoshida and Eiji Uchida

Additional information is available at the end of the chapter

http://dx.doi.org/10.5772/46872

1. Introduction

Anastomotic leakage is one of the most serious complications following surgery of the esophagus. Post-surgical fistula and anastomotic leakage are major causes of morbidity and mortality. The reported incidence of anastomotic leakage after an esophagectomy is between 2.3 % and 5.9 % [1,2]. It is associated with a high rate of mortality. Conservative treatment with nutritional support and antibiotic therapy is usually adopted at first, but this is sometimes insufficient to obliterate leakage or can take 20-30 days, even if it is successful. Anastomotic leakage is usually improved simply by draining the anastomotic site [3], but sometimes an esophago-respiratory fistula occurs due to penetration by the abscess to the trachea or main bronchus [4-6]. This causes a very serious clinical condition, predisposing the patient to life-threatening pneumonia.

If conservative therapy fails, re-surgery remains as a final option. These surgical operations are invasive. The cases in which it is impossible to accomplish primary closure require another operation that is selected on consideration of the patient's general status and prognosis. There are reports of the use of a muscle flap in the pectoralis major to repair a tracheomediastinal fistula after esophagectomy [3]. Surgical intervention such as suturing and covering with omentum or muscle flap and esophageal bypass is indicated for mediastinitis, widespread graft necrosis and abscesses due to leakage [7] and is thought to be necessary if the fistula leads to a respiratory tract because repetitive pneumonia would result in poor physical condition [8,9]. But occasionally it would have been invasive and then no surgical attempt to treat the fistula was considered.

Currently, there are a various endoscopic techniques for the management of anastomotic leakage. Endoscopic techniques are useful and technically feasible in chronic fistulas. This procedure is a less invasive alternative to traditional surgical revision.

There are reports of closing a gastrointestinal fistula or anastomotic leakage using fibrin glue, but fibrin glue is sometimes insufficient and is used with growth hormone or a clip. Several investigators reported a failure to close the fistula with this technique.

A clip is used firstly for hemostasis and applied for spontaneous closure of a perforation or endoscopic mucosal resection and sub-mucosal dissection. Rodella reported that endoscopic clipping to close an anastomotic leakage after a gastrectomy was effective and required only a short hospital day [10]. There are hardly any reports of endoscopic clipping for anastomotic leakage after an esophagectomy, although this technique has been performed on rare occasions for anastomotic leakage of duodenal stump or colorectal surgery.

Esophageal stenting at the anastomotic site is an effective method for treating anastomotic leakage after an esophagectomy, but when the anastomotic site is not stenotic and located near the neck, so it was predicted that migration and odynophagia would occur after stenting.

In this chapter, the treatment process using endoscopic clipping with fibrin glue after an operation that leads to a favorable outcome in which an esophago-mediastinal fistula is successfully repaired is discussed.

2. The treatment method for esophago-mediastinal fistula and anastomotic leakage

2.1. Conservative management

Conservative treatment excludes surgical treatment.

Leakage and fistula of the esophagus often lead to a localised infection and systemic sepsis. In particular, mediastinitis is a serious complication of esophageal surgery. The use of broad-spectrum antibiotics is initiated.

Total parenteral or enteral nutrition is provided. Leakages and fistula are associated with malnutrition, due to protein loss, lack of food intake and hypercatabolism, often associated with sepsis. Malnutrition causes hypoproteinaemia with an increased risk of wound dehiscence and infection and decreases muscle bulk and function. In this situation fibroblastic activity is reduced and leads to failure of scar contraction, leading to fistula formation with a delayed healing time.

Nasogastric decompression is performed, and the infected area is cleaned by orally administered saline. The region of the leak is drained and perianastomotic drainage is applied to the patients.

Cervical anastomotic leaks are successfully treated with conservative approaches. Thoracic anastomotic leaks, in the past, were related to high mortality rates [11]. When the abscess was limited to the pleural cavity, a chest tube could achieve adequate drainage. However previous studies had revealed that most of the contained leaks were limited to the mediastinum [4, 5]. It is difficult to deal with this type of leakage because abscess cavities close to the mediastinum are difficult to reach with a conventional chest tube. Thoracic drainage inserted through trans-nasal route may be a helpful treatment for this type of leak. Moreover endoluminal application of a vacuum-assisted wound closure (EVAC) system is reported as an available method for the leak of colon, gastric and esophageal anastomosis.

2.1.1. Thoracic drainage inserted using interventional radiology (CT-guided)

Anastomotic leakage and a thoracic abscess are sometimes detected after the esophagectomy. Established options for sealing intrathoracic anastomotic leaks after esophagectomy include surgical revision and conservative treatments, such as percutaneous chest tube drainage (the traditional "three-tube method"). The traditional "three-tube method" was the most widely applied method. However, it is difficult to insert a drain into a cavity that is very close to the trachea or aorta. (Fig.1. A) Percutaneous CT-guided abscess drainage is associated with high technical and clinical success rates. This minimally invasive form of therapy may have a role in the management of patients with potentially life-threatening mediastinal abscesses [12].

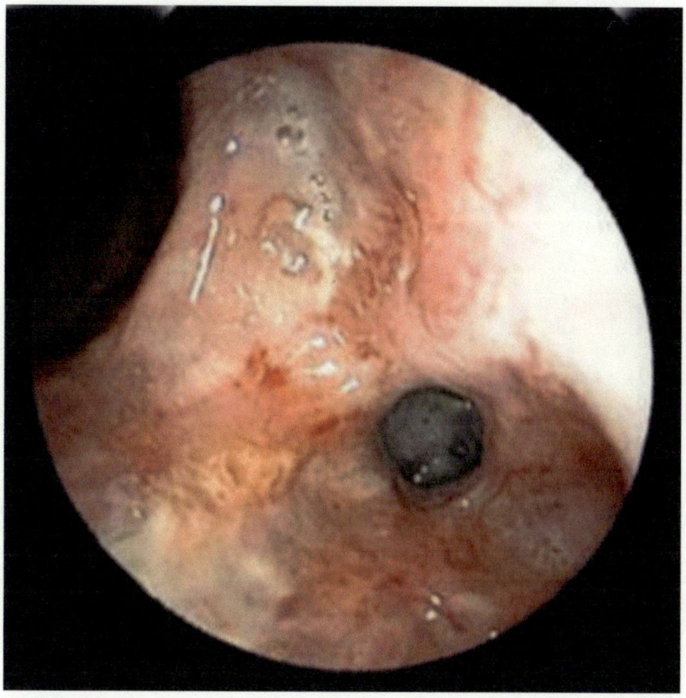

(A)

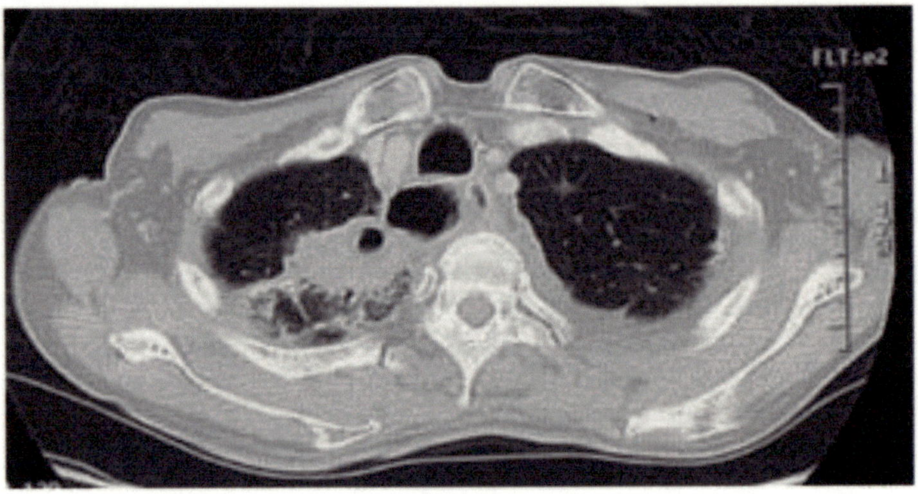

(B)

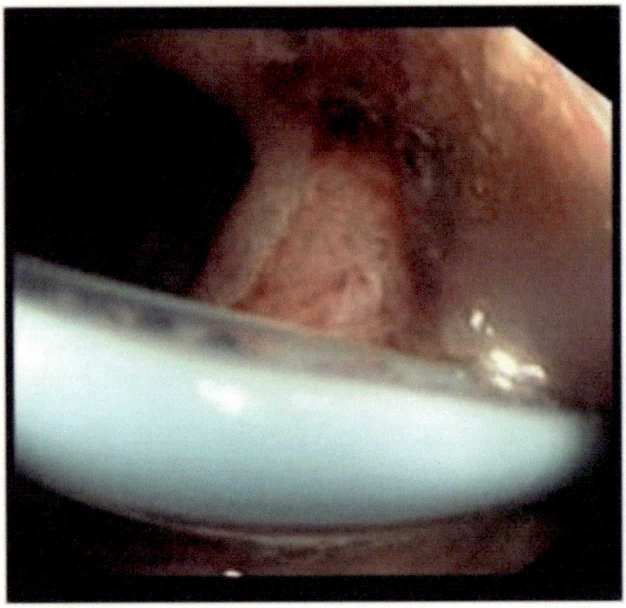

(C)

Figure 1. A. The esophagomediastinal fistula had not closed after surgery. B. The abscess is located in the site surrounding lung tissue and close to the trachea and inferior subclavian artery and then thoracic drainage is difficult. C. A trans-nasal-gastric tube is inserted into the esophagomediastinal fistula.

2.1.2. Thoracic drainage inserted through trans-nasal route

Thoracic drainage through the rans-nasal route is performed, when it is difficult to insert a drain into the cavity. This technique appears to be an effective, technically feasible, and minimally invasive treatment option for intrathoracic esophagogastric anastomotic leak [13]. We performed trans-nasal drainage at the site of intrathoracic esophagogastric anastomotic leak. (Fig.1. A,B,C) Recently, the endoluminal application of a vacuum-assisted wound closure (EVAC) system for the closure of esophagogastric anastomotic fistulas has been reported [14]. The sponge results in formation of granulation tissue, and the vacuum removes wound secretions, reduces edema, and improves blood flow, leading to wound closure. EVAC is available and recommended for cases refractory to established endoscopic treatment options [15].

2.2. Endoscopic management

A leakage or fistula will close with basic conservative treatment and local irrigation of between 50 and 80%. The rate of spontaneous closure diminishes rapidly. Fistulae or leakages of anastomotic junctions of the gastrointestinal tract used to be an indication for surgery. However, patients are often severely ill and endoscopic therapeutic options have been suggested to avoid surgical intervention. When it fails to close the cavity of the esophago-mediastinal fistula (Fig.2. A), additional treatment is necessary, so endoscopic techniques are performed. The aim of the endoscopic treatment is also to shorten the closure time of the leakage.

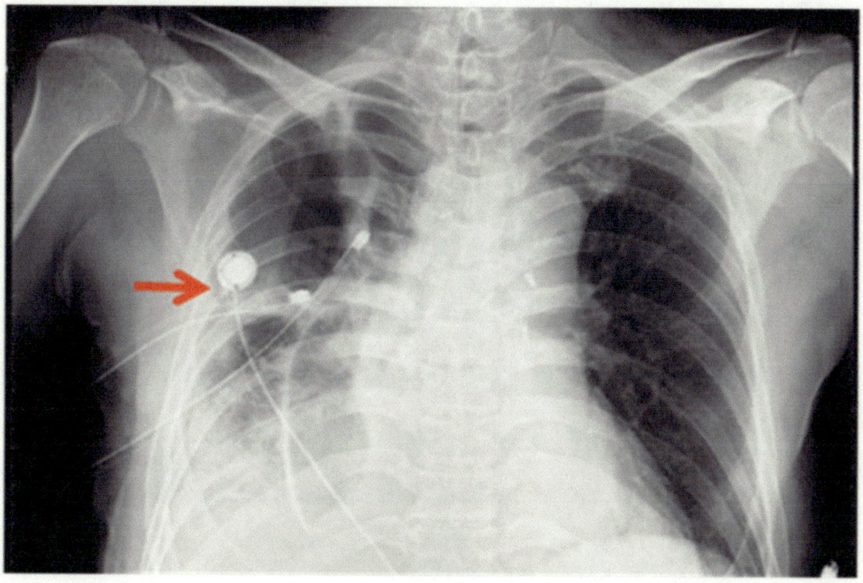

(A)

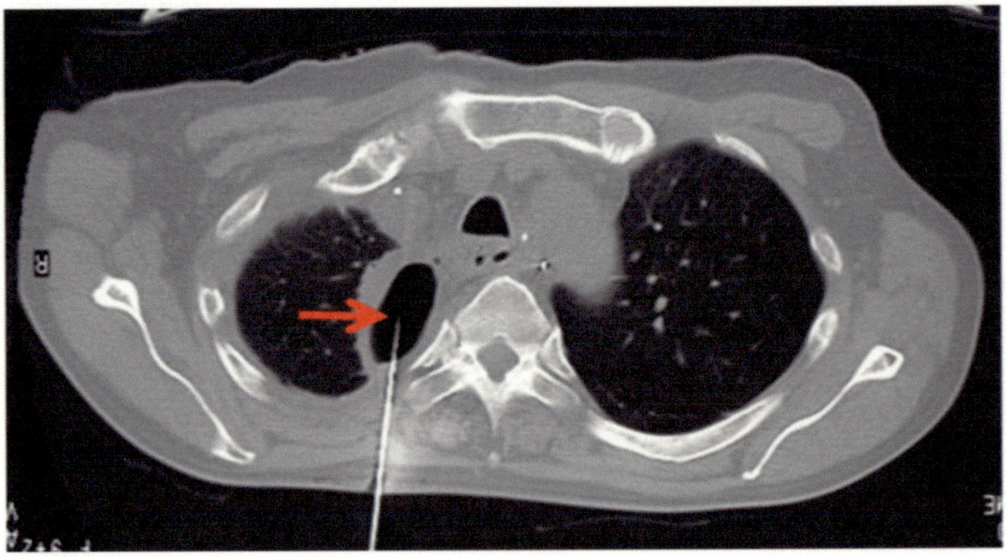

(B)

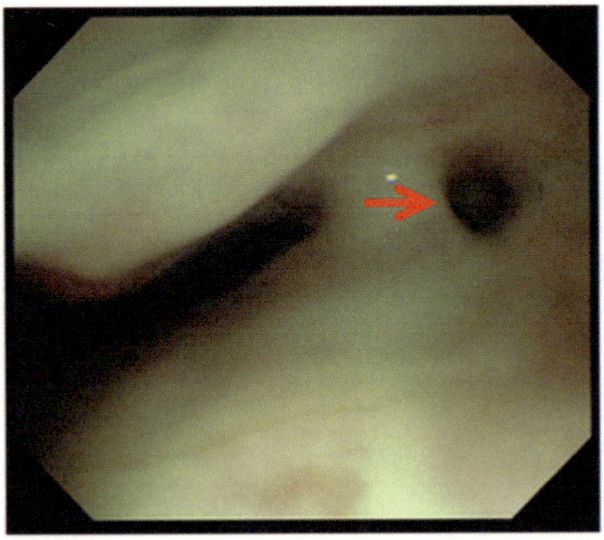

(C)

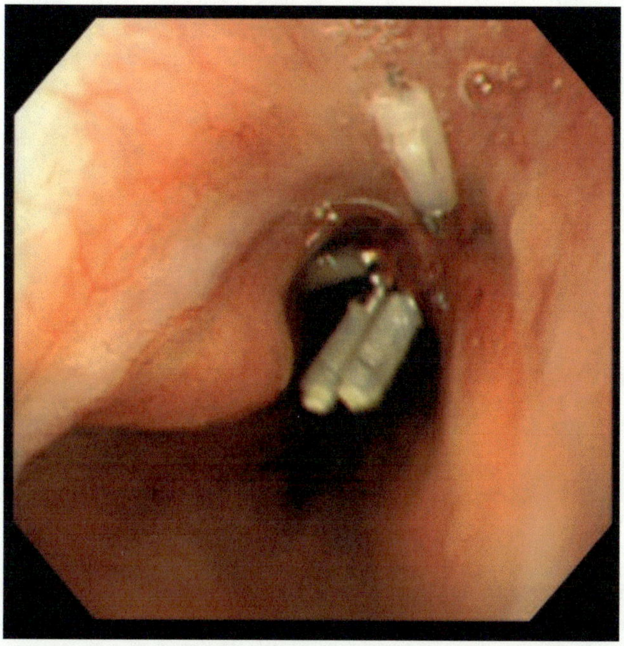

(D)

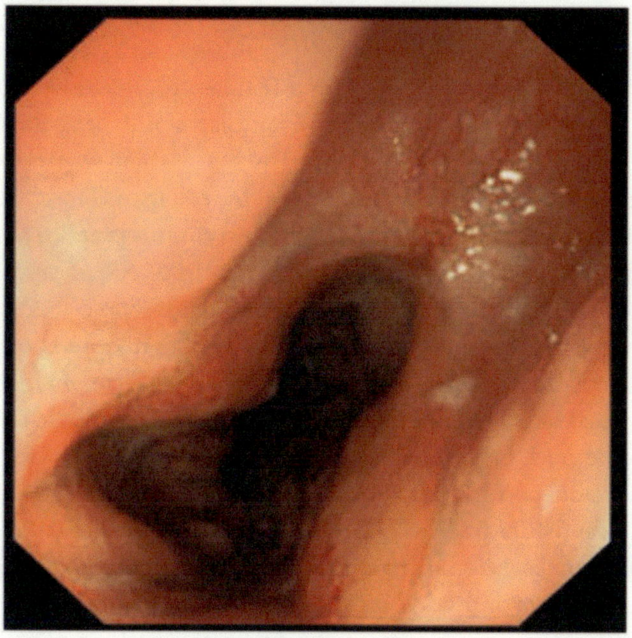

(E)

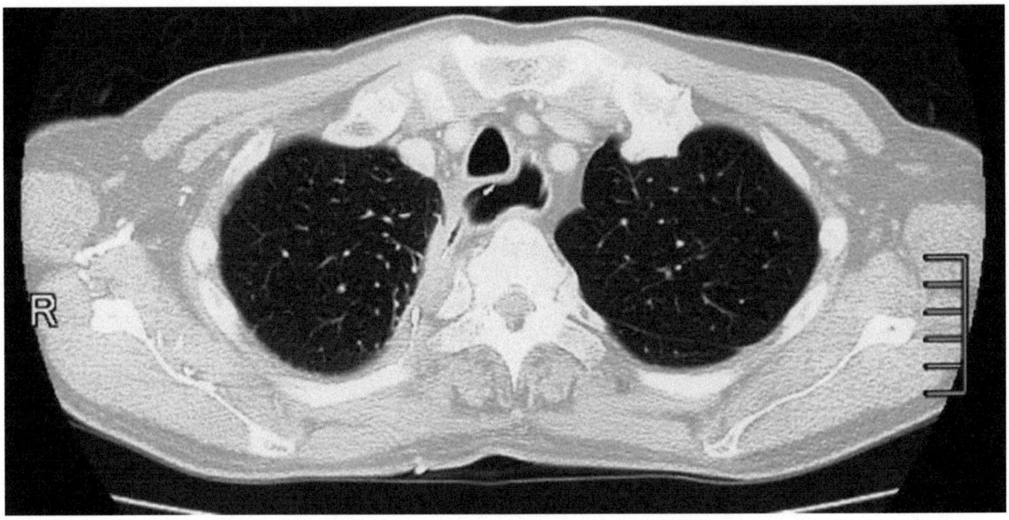

(F)

Figure 2. A. The drain is inserted into the mediastinal fistula and abscess cavity after operation showed by X-ray film. B. CT detects anastomotic leakage and a thoracic abscess cavity. C. An endoscopy revealsthat the fistula has failed to close after the operation. D. Endoscopic clipping with fibrin glue. E. An endoscopy indicates that we succeeded in closing the fistula. F. CT revealed no cavity or fistula.

2.2.1. Endoscopic management of anastomotic leakage using fibrin glue

Fibrin glue is used to support the growth of fibroblasts, stimulated from fibrin, thrombin and factor XIII. The Basic principle of sealing a fistula with fibrin is that the mixture of the two components (fibrinogen and thrombin) simulates the coagulation cascade in the fistulous tract while forming a matrix of fibrin. The scar formation process is stimulated and in the process the fibrin will be replaced slowly by collagen. Fibrin glue application has become an alternative and relatively novel method in clinical practice to avoid surgery after different kinds of leakages within the last few years. In 36.5% of cases, treatment success was reached with fibrin glue application as the sole endoscopic therapy [16]. Endoscopic fibrin glue-based interventions are a valuable option in the treatment of leakages or fistulae of the gastrointestinal tract [17]. The endoscopist can perform this treatment easily and safely; and it is not necessary to be very experienced in this technique because it is based on the use of the needle injector [18]. H. Messmann reported that 1–4 ml of fibrin sealant is applied per session and performed an additional sub-mucosal injection of fibrin near the orifice after filling the fistula tract with fibrin if the orifice was small because the swelling induced by the sub-mucosal depot may contribute an additional closure effect. They also mentioned that this additional fluid volume may lead to washing part of the sealant into the gastrointestinal-tract. After application of the fibrin the endoscopist should refrain from using the suction system of the scope. Endoscopic sealing has to be repeated, in most cases, in intervals of a few days until closure achieved.

However, severe infection complications are associated with a poor success rate. Moreover, the cost of fibrin glue is high but the advantage of a shorter hospital stay is significant in reducing global costs [17]. Treatment success with further endoscopic procedures was seen. Vicryl plug or clipping are reported as additional endoscopic procedures because endoscopic treatment failure with consecutive surgical intervention became necessary [15,19-22].

2.2.2. Endoscopic management of anastomotic leakage using clipping

The use of metallic clips has been reported for hemostasis and closure of a perforation caused by various matter. Endoscopic closure by clipping was found to be effective for idiopathic or iatrogenic esophageal perforation.

Application of an endoclip is a relatively simple procedure and recently reported as a method for closing anastomotic leakage of gastrointestinal tract [10,23-28] (Table.1.). The clip fixing device with a loaded clip can be passed through the forceps channel of a standard endoscope. As soon as the Teflon coating is in endoscopic sight the clip can be pushed forward out of the coating. Stepwise pulling on the handle of the fixing device leads to opening of the prongs. Through manipulation of the tip of the endoscope the clip can be brought into position to grasp the tissue flanks of the leakage. It may be helpful to apply suction during this manoeuvre so that leaks that have a larger diameter than the total span of the clip can be treated. A further pull on the handle mechanism closes the endoclip and detaches the whole clip from the fixing device. Usually several clips are applied, positioning the first clips to the extremities of the leak or even outside the leakage borders to obtain a kind of 'zipper' effect while grabbing tissue step by step from the outside to the centre of the defect. With this method leaks up to 2 cm in diameter can be closed; larger leaks need more than one session. Exact data on clipping for therapy of post-surgical leakage are rare; most articles relate to endoscopic clipping of perforations following endoscopic procedures.

Author /year	Organ of Surgery	Aditional Treatment	Jounal, Year
Rodella L. et al.	Stomach		Endoscopy. 1998
Familiari P. et al.	Colon		Dig Liver Dis. 2003
Messmann H. et al.	Esophagus	fibrin glue	Best Practice & Research Clinical Gastroenterology., (2004)
Teitelbaum JE. et al.	Stomach		Gastrointest Endosc. 2005.
Merrifield BF. et al.	Stomach		Gastrointest Endosc .2005
Dolay K. et al.	Rectum	fibrin glue	J Endourol., 2007
Grupka MJ. et al.	Stomach		J Dig Dis. 2008
Ibis M.et al.	Rectum		Am J Gastroenterol. 2010
Makino H. et al.	Esophagus	fibrin glue	Esophagus. 2011

Table 1. Endoscopic clipping to close the anastomotic leakage of gastrointestinal tract

2.2.3. Endoscopic clipping with fibrin glue

A contrast instillation and radiological visualisation of the fistula system or cavity was performed during the endoscopic procedure of every therapeutic closure, both with fibrin and clips. H. Messmann reported that a double-lumen catheter can be placed over the guide wire into the fistula [18]. If a single-lumen catheter is used instead of a double-lumen probe for sealing, the catheter lumen has to be flushed between the instillation of fibrinogen and thrombin. The sealing of the fistula begins as far as possible away from the orifice; thus the risk of fluid retention can be minimised.

Metallic endoclips were applied, controlling the closure of the leakage by endoscopy.

A combination of clipping and fibrin sealing is probably more effective, especially in treatment of larger leakages [10,28,29]. H. Messmann et al. applied several careful injections into the tissue using a double-lumen needle between the placed clips and also mentioned that their own experience with clips alone is not as positive as it is mentioned. Clips are used to close the fistula while suction is applied to reduce the size of the fistula hole after filling the fistula with fibrin glue. Application only of synthetic glues via endoscopy or clipping is not available.

2.2.4. Endoscopic stenting

Esophageal stenting at the anastomotic site is reported as an effective method for treating anastomotic leakage after an esophagectomy and is one of the most popular endoscopic treatments. The use of a removable covered stent in the setting of anastomotic leak or spontaneous perforation, alone or as an adjunct to conventional surgical management, is feasible in sealing the leak, resolving sepsis, and expediting return to enteral nutrition [30]. Stent migration is a commonly observed complication in other reported series occurring in up to 50% of patients and frequently requires restenting to regain control of a leak [31]. We had a case of stent migration after leak closure. (Fig.3.A,B) The rate of distal stent migration is possibly even higher following stenting of malignant stenoses due to the lack of a stricture. The patients who had the stent sutured, all required operative intervention for debridement of the necrotic and contaminated tissue so the stent and suture were placed at the time of this surgery. It is also predicted that odynophagia would occur after stenting if the anastomotic site is close to the neck. However new plastic stents are easy to remove, very effective and might have therapeutic potential to replace fibrin glue application and clipping.

2.2.5. Other endoscopic therapy

To reduce the necessity of another surgical intervention and enhance natural healing other endoscopy-based therapeutic options are available.

Endoscopic suturing seems to be a promising new treatment.

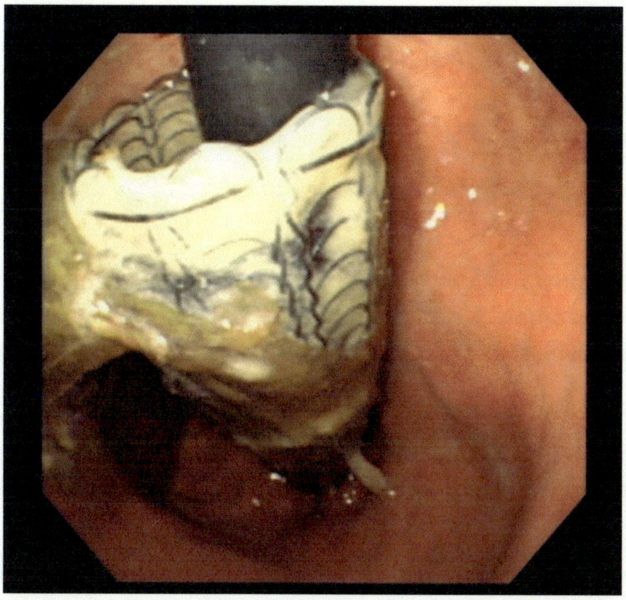

(A)

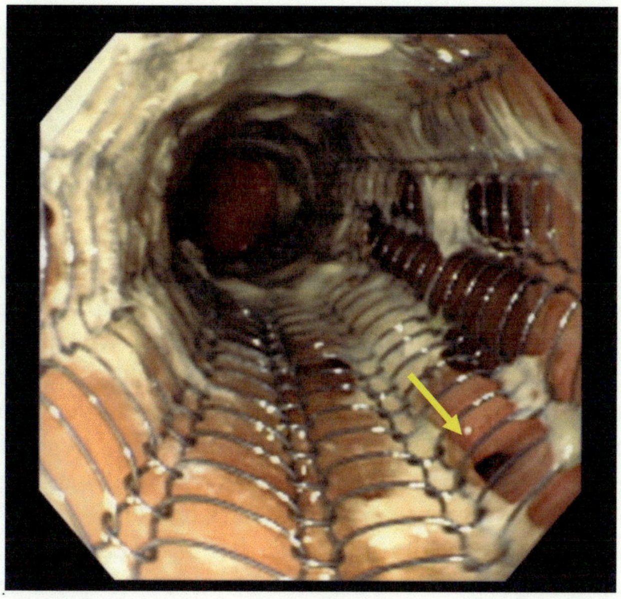

(B)

Figure 3. A. Endoscopy indicated distal covered metallic stent migrated to the stomach. B. A fistula is observed in the non-covered part of a migrated metallic stent.

Pross et al. presented a successful closure method with a resorbable vicryl cylinder used as a plug [21]. The plug was inserted into the defect after repeated fibrin therapy. Little data has been published regarding these methods and is still lacking .

2.3. The treatment process

2.3.1. Thoracic drainage inserted using interventional radiology or through trans-nasal route

A chest X-P revealed pneumothorax, and anastomotic leakage and a thoracic abscess were detected after the operation via CT (Fig. 2B). For approximately one month, thoracic drainages, and the nasogastric placement of sump tube through the leak were performed and conservative therapy with total enteral nutrition was continued. The cavity of the thoracic abscess caused by the leakage reduced in size, but the esophago-mediastinal fistula and the air cavity were still present 33 days after the operation. An additional thin drain was inserted using interventional radiology, but it failed to close the fistula 68 days after the operation (Fig. 2C).

Additional treatment to the thoracic drainages was necessary, so we decided to perform other endoscopic techniques.

2.3.2. Endoscopic clipping with fibrin glue

First we applied synthetic glues via endoscopy. The nasogastric placement of tube through the leak is already performed. We flushed the fistula system with physiological sodium chloride solution. And then fibrin was applied through the nasogastric tube located at the lowest position of the anastomosis. In the next step we usually insert a standard sump tube and apply thrombin into the fistula; a guide wire can be helpful to advance the probe to the distal end of the fistula with complicated or very long fistulae. A contrast medium was used through the endoscope we could confirm no leakage after filling with fibrin glues. However, an X-P taken three days after this technique indicated air leakage. Next we applied clipping to close the fistula twice, but within one week after clipping a clip had dropped out. We use metallic endoclips (MD 850,Olympus Corp., Tokyo, Japan) which have a fully opened distance between the clip prongs of 12 mm long and 6 mm wide. In our case a clip dropped out a few days after clipping at the first and second sessions, and we expected that a single clip would not allow a successful closure. Esophageal pressure in swallowing at the neck site is high and the movement of air entering a gap in the fistula appeared to dislodge the clip. Finally, we succeeded in closing the fistula using three clips with fibrin glue because we eliminated the gap in the fistula (Fig. 2D). It was important to apply suction by endoscope when we attempted to close the fistula by clipping as the suction reduced the size of the fistula and facilitated the clipping. At the third treatment, we also filled with fibrin glue at the right lateral position where the fistula was located at the lowest position of the anastomosis and then followed this with endoscopic closure. An endoscopy indicated that we had succeeded in closing the fistula (Fig. 2E). A gastrographin swallow showed no leakage (data not shown) and CT revealed no cavity or fistula 7-10 days after clipping (Fig. 2F). We had succeeded in closing the fistula with clip and fibrin glue in our case [29].

3. Conclusion

Several investigators reported a failure to close a fistula with only fibrin glue. Rodella reported that endoscopic clipping to close an anastomotic leakage after a gastrectomy was effective [10]. Endoscopic closure by clipping was found to be effective for idiopathic or iatrogenic esophageal perforation. Clipping alone also sometimes fails to close an anastomotic leak or fistula. Esophageal pressure in swallowing at the neck site is high and the movement of air entering a gap in the fistula appeared to dislodge the clip. It is important to apply suction by endoscope when we attempt to close the fistula by clipping as the suction reduced the size of the fistula and facilitated the clipping. Endoscopic clipping is recommended by Rodella et al. to treat leakages less than 2 cm in diameter.

The endoscopic clipping with fibrin glue treatment is effective and not invasive. Fibrin sealant and clipping are effective and probably established methods. It results in a steady improvement of the patient's condition and minimized surgical stress, so it should be started earlier.

Furthermore a reduced hospital stay will obviously decrease the costs of treatment.

The cost of fibrin glue is high but the advantage of a shorter hospital stay is significant in reducing global costs. In conclusion, the endoscopic use of fibrin glue and clip are easy, safe and can shorten the time of closure of fistula, in selected cases, with an apparent reduction of global costs.

Author details

Hiroshi Makino and Hiroshi Yoshida
Department of Surgery, Nippon Medical School, Tama-Nagayama Hospital, Japan

Eiji Uchida
Department of Surgery, Nippon Medical School, Japan

Acknowledgement

The authors want to acknowledge Dr.Tsutomu Nomura and Dr.Nobutoshi Hagiwara for their clinical support.

4. References

[1] Page, R.D., Shackcloth, M.J., Russell GN, Pennefather, S.H. Surgical treatment of anastomotic leaks after oesophagectomy, *Eur J Cardiothorac Surg.* Vol. 27, (2005), pp. 337-343,

[2] Liu, J.F., Wang, Q.Z., Ping, Y.M., Zhang, Y.D. Complications after esophagectomy for cancer: 53-year experience with 20,796 patients. *World J Surg.*, Vol. 32,(2008), pp. 395-400,

[3] Baulieux, J., Adham, M., Roche, E., Meziat-Burdin, A., Poupart, M., Ducerf, C. Carcinoma of the oesophagus. Anastomotic leaks after manual sutures--incidence and treatment. *Int Surg.* Vol. 83, (1998), pp. 277-279,

[4] Bamba, T., Kosugi, S., Kanda, T., Koyama, Y., Suzuki, T., Hatakeyama, K. Successful treatment for a benign esophagorespiratory fistula with perioperative nutritional management and multistep esophageal bypass operation: a case report. *Esophagus*, Vol. 5,(2008), pp. 93-97,

[5] Koga, T., Morita, M., Nishida, K., Oki, E., Kakeji, Y., Maehara, Y. Successful treatment of tracheomediastinal fistula after tracheal injury obtained during esophagectomy using the pectoralis major muscle: a case report. *Esophagus*, Vol. 5, (2008), pp. 41–44,

[6] Morishima, Y., Toyoda, Y., Fukada, T., Suzuki, I., Aoki, Y., Tazawa, Y., Kobayashi, J., Tashiro, T.: Successful esophageal bypass operation for esophagobronchial fistula following chemotherapy for malignant lymphoma: a case report. *Esophagus*, Vol. 2 , (2005), pp. 165-168,

[7] Salo, J.A., Isolauri, J.O., Heikkila, L.J., Markkula, H.T., Heikkinen, L.O., Kivilaakso, E.O., Mattila, S.P. Management of delayed esophageal perforation with mediastinal sepsis. Esophagectomy or primary repair?, *J Thorac Cardiovasc Surg*, Vol. 106, (1993), pp. 1088-1091,

[8] Suzuki, T., Narisawa, T., Tanaka, H., Hirai, Y., Sanada, Y., Chiba, M. Closure of a cervical H-type tracheoesophageal fistula, *Thorac Cardiovasc Surg*, Vol. 52, (2004), pp. 57-59,

[9] Thakur, B., Zhang, C.S., Cao, F.M. Use of greater omentum in thoracic onco-surgery, *Kathmandu Univ Med J (KUMJ)*, Vol. 5, (2007). pp. 129-132,

[10] Rodella, L., Laterza, E., De Manzoni, G., Kind, R., Lombardo, F., Catalano, F., Ricci, F., Cordiano, C. Endoscopic clipping of anastomotic leakages in esophagogastric surgery. *Endoscopy*, Vol. 30, (1998), pp. 453-456,

[11] Turkyilmaz, A., Eroglu, A., Aydin, Y., Tekinbas, C., Muharrem Erol, M., Karaoglanoglu, N. The management of esophagogastric anastomotic leak after esophagectomy for esophageal carcinoma., *Diseases of the Esophagus* ., Vol. 22 , (2009), pp. 119–126 ,

[12] Arellano, R.S., Gervais, D.A., Mueller, P.R., Computed Tomography–guided Drainage of Mediastinal Abscesses: Clinical Experience with 23 Patients. *J Vasc Interv Radiol.* Vol. 22, (2011), pp. 673–677,

[13] Jiang, F., Yu, M. F., Ren, B. H., Yin, G. W., Zhang, Q., Xu, L. Nasogastric Placement of Sump Tube Through the Leak for the Treatment of Esophagogastric Anastomotic Leak After Esophagectomy for Esophageal Carcinoma., *Journal of Surgical Research* ., Vol. 171, (2011), pp. 448–451,

[14] Wedemeyer, J., Brangewitz, M., Kubicka, S., Jackobs, S., Winkler, M., Neipp, M., Klempnauer, J., Manns, M.P., Schneider, A.S., Management of major post-surgical gastroesophageal intrathoracic leaks with an endoscopic vacuum-assisted closure system. *GASTROINTESTINAL ENDOSCOPY* ., Vol. 71, (2010), pp. 382- 386,

[15] Ahrens, M., Schulte, T., Egberts, J., Schafmayer, C., Hampe, J., Fritscher-Ravens, A., Broering, D.C., Schniewind, B. Drainage of esophageal leakage using endoscopic vacuum therapy: a prospective pilot study. *Endoscopy*, Vol. 42, (2010), pp 693–698,

[16] Lippert, E., Klebl, F.H. , Schweller, F., Ott, C., Gelbmann, C.M. , Schölmerich, J., Endlicher, E., Kullmann, F., Fibrin glue in the endoscopic treatment of fistulae and anastomotic leakages of the gastrointestinal tract. *Int J Colorectal Dis.*, Vol.26, (2011), pp. 303–311,

[17] Groitl, H., Scheele, J. Initial experience with the endoscopic application of fibrin tissue adhesive in the upper gastrointestinal tract., *Surg Endosc.*, Vol. 1, (1987), pp. 93-97,

[18] Messmann, H., Schmidbaur, W., Ja¨ckle, J., Fu¨rst, A., Iesalnieks, I.,Endoscopic and surgical management of leakage and mediastinitis after esophageal surgery. *Best Practice & Research Clinical Gastroenterology.*, Vol. 18, (2004), pp. 809–827,

[19] Rio, P.D., Abtae, P.D., Soliani, P., Ziegler, S., Arcuri, M., Sianesi, M., Endoscopic treatment of esophageal and colo-rectal fistulas with fibrin glue. *ACTA BIOMED.*, Vol.76, (2005), pp. 95-98,

[20] Böhm, A.G., Mossdorf, A., Klink, C., Klinge, U., Jansen, M., Schumpelick,V., Truong,S., Treatment algorithm for postoperative upper gastrointestinal fistulas and leaks using combined Vicryl plug and fibrin glue. *Endoscopy.*, Vol. 42, (2010), pp. 599–602,

[21] Pross, M., Manger, T., Reinheckel, T., Mirow, L., Kunz, D., Lippert, H., Endoscopic treatment of clinically symptomatic leaks of thoracic esophageal anastomoses. GASTROINTESTINAL ENDOSCOPY. Vol.51, (2000), pp. 73-76

[22] Truong, S., Bo¨hm, G., Klinge, U., Stumpf, M., Schumpelick, V., Results after endoscopic treatment of postoperative upper gastrointestinal fistulas and leaks using combined Vicryl plug and fibrin glue. *Surg Endosc.*, Vol. 18, (2004), pp. 1105–1108,

[23] Familiari, P., Macri, A., Consolo, P., Angio, L., Scaffidi, M.G., Famulari, C., Familiari, L., Endoscopic clipping of a colocutaneous fistula following necrotizing pancreatitis: case report., *Dig Liver Dis.*, Vol. 35, (2003), pp. 907-910,

[24] Grupka, M.J., Benson, J., Endoscopic clipping, *J Dig Dis.*, Vol. 9, (2008), pp. 72-78,

[25] Lee, J.Y., Ryu, K.W., Cho, S.J., Kim, C. G., Choi,I.J., Kim, M.J., Lee, J.S., Kim, H.B., Lee , J.H., Kim, Y.W., Endoscopic Clipping of Duodenal Stump Leakage After Billroth II Gastrectomy in Gastric Cancer Patient. *Journal of Surgical Oncology.* Vol. 100, (2009), pp. 80–81

[26] Teitelbaum, J.E, Gorcey, S.A., Fox, V.L., Combined endoscopic cautery and clip closure of chronic gastrocutaneous fistulas. *Gastrointest Endosc.* Vol. 62, (2005), pp.432-435,

[27] Ibis M, Beyazit Y, Onal, I.K., Kurt, M., Parlak, E., Successful Endoscopic Closure of Anastomotic Leakage Following Anterior Resection of the Rectum by Endoclip Application. *The American Journal of Gastroenterology.* Vol. 105, (2010), pp.1447-1448,

[28] Dolay, K., Aras, B., Tugcu, V., Ozbay, B., Aygun, E., Tasci, A.I. Combined treatment of iatrogenic rectourethral fistula with endoscopic fibrin glue application and clipping, *J Endourol.*, Vol. 21, (2007). pp. 433-436,

[29] Makino, H., Miyashita, M., Nomura, T., Hagiwara, N., Takahashi, K., Matsuno, K., Sumiyoshi, H., Iwamoto, M., Yokoi, K., Uchida, E. Successful endoscopic clipping and

application of fibrin glue for an esophago-mediastinal fistula after an esophagectomy. Esophagus, Vol. 8, (2011), pp. 113-117,

[30] Babor, R., Talbot, M., Tyndal, A., Treatment of Upper Gastrointestinal Leaks With a Removable, Covered, Self-expanding Metallic Stent. *Surg Laparosc Endosc Percutan Tech.* Vol.19, (2009), pp. e1-e4,

[31] Nguyen, N.T., Rudersdorf, P.D., Smith, B.R., & Reavis, K., Nguyen, X.T., Stamos, M.J., Management of Gastrointestinal Leaks After Minimally Invasive Esophagectomy: Conventional Treatments vs. Endoscopic Stenting. *J Gastrointest Surg*. Vol. 15, (2011), pp. 1952–1960

Chapter 14

Localized Drug Delivery for Cardiothoracic Surgery

Christopher Rolfes, Stephen Howard, Ryan Goff and Paul A. Iaizzo

Additional information is available at the end of the chapter

http://dx.doi.org/10.5772/48577

1. Introduction

It is noteworthy to consider that extensive bioavailability and bioequivalence studies are typically required before new drug therapies can be approved [1]. These studies include pharmacokinetic studies that take into account: 1) dosing, absorption, and elimination rates of the drug and its active metabolites, as well as 2) the potential effects of multiple doses, drug interactions, and the differences whether medications are taken with or without food. A major therapeutic factor that compounds the variations often seen from patient to patient is individual differences in absorption and elimination rates. This will also cause variations in the amount of drug that reaches the desired targeted tissue when used as a clinical therapy.

While oral administrations are common and the easiest means to deliver outside of a hospital or clinical setting, intravenous (IV) delivery can eliminate some of the aforementioned patient to patient variability by bypassing the ingestion and absorption into a patient's bloodstream. However, a major obstacle with either of these delivery methods is that once a drug is in the blood plasma, the medication will circulate throughout the patient's body, not only reaching the intended site, but unintended sites as well. Hence, this will greatly increase the possibility of causing unwanted side effects. Thus, it is required that side effects on each and every tissue be well described when therapeutic levels of the medication are administered.

Importantly, many drugs have described narrow therapeutic ranges. Slight increases in levels could cause severe undesired effects, whereas slight decreases often eliminate any therapeutic benefit. We describe in detail here how the targeted and local delivery of medications may overcome many of these obstacles in traditional delivery methods by simplifying the pharmacokinetics, reducing variability, and allowing higher doses to reach the intended target.

1.1. Targeted drug delivery

"Targeted drug delivery" is a general term that describes a variety of methods that can be used to increase the concentrations of a given drug at a primary location within the body relative to other body tissues. Often called "smart therapies," targeted delivery includes methods such as antibody labeling, ultrasonic release, and/or localized delivery that can increase drug concentrations at the desired tissue. The primary intent is to increase the intended beneficial effects while reducing side effects.

Developments in targeted drug delivery were commonly pioneered with anti-cancer drugs. These treatments are often highly toxic and have undesirable side effects, which in turn can greatly reduce quality of life and limit the dose levels that can be administered. Therefore, if the levels of these drugs can be increased specifically at the site of a tumor relative to the rest of the body, the same or reduced dose levels will have much greater effects at the site of the cancerous tumor.

One commonly described method for accomplishing this is creating or adding components to cancer drugs that preferentially bind within the tumors. More specifically, the identification of differences in endothelial surfaces in growing tumors has led to the development of cancer medications that preferentially adhere to the endothelial surfaces within the vasculature of the tumor, thus increasing the desired effects. This results in lower exposures of non-target tissues to the drug than were previously possible. In a similar manner, numerous biomarkers have been identified that become upregulated in diseased cardiac tissue, and therefore have become targets in emerging therapies [2], [3]. Alternatively, drug treatments can be encapsulated in such a way that they are released at the desired location, such as where triggered by high frequency ultrasound, causing focal increases in drug concentrations [4–6]. Table 1 summarizes many currently used and investigated targeted therapies, several of which are described in greater detail throughout this chapter.

1.2. Localized delivery

"Localized drug delivery" is defined as a specific form of targeted delivery where the medication is given at a certain site which allows for reduced movement and subsequent absorption into the bloodstream. Localized delivery is often provided to a naturally enclosed space, such as the bladder or into the vitreous humor of the eye, but other techniques can limit movement such as a gel or patch. In general, by delivering a given pharmacological treatment to a specific target tissue site via an implantable pump or acute access, localized therapy will reduce systemic effects on peripheral tissue thereby limiting side effects, while maintaining increased control.

Just as IV delivery increases control and decreases variability compared to oral delivery by eliminating the gastrointestinal tract, local delivery increases control and decreases variability by eliminating reliance on patient circulation for distribution. Thus localized drug delivery carries the potential for increased effectiveness of treatments, while reducing the quantities needed (Figure 1). These reductions have important applied implications when one employs either drug pumps or impregnated gels to delivery therapies, as they can only hold limited volumes.

Delivery Method	**Advantages**	**Disadvantages**
Targeted Drug Delivery		
Ultrasound or heat disrupted carriers	non-invasive focal treatment to potential asymmetric areas	equipment intensive, potential buildup within liver and spleen
Biomarker targeted	simple administration	designer molecules need to be created, approved
Localized Drug Delivery		
Pericardial delivery	entire epicardium treated, well contained, easy access in surgery	invasive, pericardium often left open after surgery
Direct myocardial/tissue injection	increases myocardial concentrations, long lasting	invasive/minimally invasive
Drug eluting wafers	long or short lasting, tunable degradation	minimal migration small doses, reliant on resorbable wafer or must be explanted
Implantable pump	local drug delivery on demand, larger continuous dosing possible	invasive, needs refilling, shortcomings associated with implantable devices
Coronary injection	increases myocardial concentrations	invasive/minimally invasive, treatment still enters blood

Table 1. Various targeted therapies and their advantages and disadvantages.

Finally, an additional benefit often seen with localized delivery is a relative increase in the therapeutic drug half-lives. For example, since localized treatments typically have minimal crossover with the patients' circulation, there is limited exposure to their livers and kidneys, which are typical sites for drug metabolism. Thus the relative therapeutic half-lives of many pharmaceuticals will be increased, creating another mechanism to decrease the amount of a given agent required to achieve sustained therapeutic dose levels [7].

While targeted drug delivery is the focus of broad research, it is our intent with this chapter to narrow the focus more specifically on localized therapy and the unique opportunities provided by the access obtained during thoracic surgery. For instance the pericardium surrounds the heart and provides a unique enclosed volume in which one can target the epicardial surfaces. In other words, the localized drug delivery to the pericardial space will allow the agent to diffuse into the myocardium while reducing those amounts present in the circulating blood. During cardiothoracic surgery one has unique access to this otherwise difficult to reach space where subsequent therapy can be delivered throughout the perioperative period. Therefore, as therapies emerge to treat heart failure, local delivery during thoracic surgery is positioned to be a viable therapeutic option that can be delivered with minimal added time, as well as few complications or complexities. At the same time it has the potential to reduce ischemic damage and arrhythmias, and holds great potential for improved outcomes, reduced morbidity, and increased cardiac health.

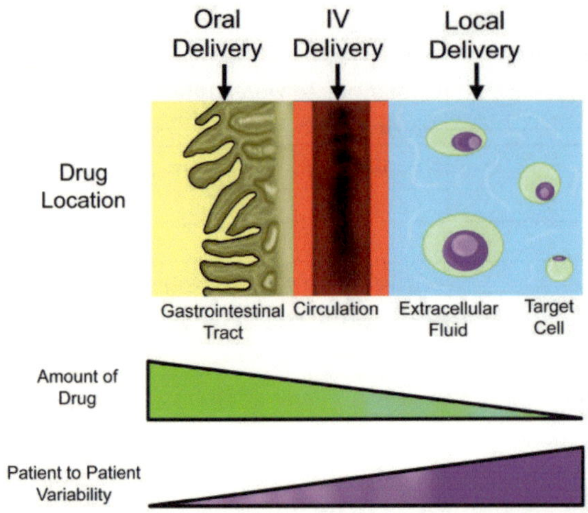

Figure 1. Schematic of differences in drug delivery by oral, IV or local delivery modalities. Increasing the number of transport steps increases the amount of drug necessary and patient to patient variability increases at each step.

2. Known procedural complications and potential therapeutic opportunities

Cardiac surgery is typically defined by a broad class of surgeries intended to correct heart problems. They can be broken down into several categories that include: 1) valve repair and replacements, 2) structural heart repairs, 3) implantations of devices for either the maintenance of rhythm or mechanical performance, and 4) heart transplants. Today, the most common cardiac surgery is coronary artery bypass grafting (CABG) [8]. Despite the recent trend towards minimally invasive cardiac procedures, there still remains a significant need for open surgical techniques. Due to the invasive, and many times emergent, nature of these procedures they are also excellent candidates for targeted delivery (it should also be noted that many minimally invasive and scheduled procedures could also take advantage of target therapeutic delivery of various agents).

It is generally accepted that open cardiac surgery is not without potential complications. On the other hand, the occurrences of such complications can be viewed as unique opportunities for introduction of localized drug delivery to improve patient outcomes. It is important to note that complication rates and outcomes can only be truly assessed on both procedural and patient population bases; yet there are often common complications across all classes of cardiac surgery. Statistics on the following procedural complications and proposed treatments using targeted delivery will be discussed: neurologic, arrhythmic, gastrointestinal, bleeding, and infection. These complications when present will impact both short- and long-term morbidity and mortality, i.e., influence length of hospital stays, quality of life, as well as financial burdens on both patients and healthcare providers.

To begin with, neurologic complications such as stroke, post-operative cognitive deficit, encephalopathy, and transient ischemic attack are of particular concern because of their much feared, potential long-lasting effects. Due to the nature of cardiac surgery and cardiopulmonary bypass, it can be foreseen that thrombosis or air emboli may occur from time to time, potentially causing these aforementioned complications. Poor neurological outcomes may also be caused by or related to arrhythmias, bleeding, or other complications. For example, prospective studies on the outcome of CABG patients show that the expected stroke rates vary from 1.5% [9] to 5.2% [8]. A broad range of disorders fall under the umbrella of post-surgical encephalopathy, a syndrome stemming from many causes. Its prevalence has been described to vary based on the definition, with as many as one third of patients eliciting an encephalopathy post-operatively [10], but prospective studies show that by day four the number is reduced to 11.6% [11] indicating a transient nature. Expectedly, these complications occur more frequently in combined procedures and/or more technically challenging cases.

It should be mentioned that numerous modern surgical techniques, such as the no-touch aorta technique, have attempted to mitigate such neurologic complications. However, it will likely remain that current advances in surgical techniques may only reduce, but not totally eliminate, these undesired events. Nevertheless, one can envision the added use of tailored drug cocktails with various procedures that could directly target the heart (pericardial space) or mix within the blood returning from cardiopulmonary bypass. To date, potential therapeutic agents which have been shown to be effective include: 1) oxide scavengers, 2) nitric oxide inhibitors [12], 3) agents to inhibit glutamate related neural excitotoxicity [13], and 4) the administration of aprotinin, a serine protease inhibitor [14]. It is possible that prior to patient rewarming, agents similar to tissue plasminogen activator could be administered in a manner that targets or localizes only the cerebral circulation and potentially destroys clots that were formed, thus mitigating negative effects prior to rewarming.

It is generally considered that atrial fibrillation (AF) is the most common complication to occur after cardiac surgery, occurring in up to 30% of cases [15]. A recent meta-analysis of 94 trials by Burgess and colleagues has shown that the five most common interventions were all effective at reducing the incidence of AF, but to varying degrees. These treatments included beta-blockers, sotalol, amiodarone, magnesium, and atrial pacing. It should be noted that amiodarone was the only intervention that was reported to reduce stroke on its own. Nevertheless due to the well documented negative systemic effects of such antiarrhythmics, several studies have begun to investigate the use of localized delivery to the pericardial space, discussed in more detail below. On the other hand, it should be noted that the systemic administration of modified agents could also prove effective and avoid side effects if targeting functionality was incorporated into the drug molecule. For example, this could be done by adding cardiac specific antibodies or ligands to therapeutic molecules. Nevertheless, such newly developed drug isoforms will require additional regulatory approval, perhaps only after clinical studies prove them safe and effective.

Gastrointestinal complications after cardiac surgery are less common, but importantly are associated with high rates of morbidity and mortality. Reported incidences are in range of <1%, but mortality associated with this complication is approximately 25% versus approximately 3% without gastrointestinal complications [16], [17]. The most common of these complications include: upper intestinal bleeding, intestinal ischemia, acute pancreatitis, and perforations.

Despite the use of modern day antibiotics, infection still remains a prevalent problem in cardiac surgery, as does administration of blood products. The two are commonly interrelated and it has been shown that transfusions of packed red blood cells (PRBCs) are significantly associated with post-operative infections [18]. However, this correlation does not necessarily imply causation, and the use of PRBCs may be related to procedural difficulties, which may be the real underlying causation of such infection rates. It should also be considered that stored red blood cells also do not function normally, and therefore PRBCs may contain inflammatory and immuno-mediating substances. It was reported in a CABG patient series study at Duke University that as many as 39.5% of patients received PRBCs [18]. Furthermore, out of the entire series, the post-operative infection rate was found to be 6.2%; specifically, patients that received PRBCs elicited infection rates ranging from 6-8.1% versus 5.1% for those who received no PRBCs [18]. Additionally, in a recent five-year study on long-term survival following transfusion for CABG procedures, it was observed that patients not transfused have approximately 2.5-fold better survival rates than those that did [19].

Interestingly, it has been proposed that actively targeted treatments could possibly restore normality to the RBCs prior to administration; such treatments could also incorporate anti-infection components. As mentioned above, RBCs can change drastically and immediately upon storage. It is considered that due to the low oxygen environment within the blood collection bag, RBCs switch to anaerobic metabolism, which in turn leads to lactic acid buildup and an overall reduction in blood pH. Furthermore, it is known the RBCs lose their signature bi-concave shape and become more spherical with storage; recall that it is this bi-concavity that is necessary for the cells to efficiently travel through capillary networks. Stored RBCs will also form aggregates due to activated surface proteins by crosslinking fibrinogen between GPIIb/IIIa binding sites [20]. This crosslinking increases the longer PRBCs are stored, and potentially could contribute to neurologic complications and thus post-operative cognitive deficits. Therefore, one could consider that prior to infusion of PRBCs, a targeted drug cocktail could be added to prevent or break these fibrinogen crosslinks and/or suppress immuno- and inflammatory effects.

Finally, one should also consider that infection rates could potentially be reduced by localized drug delivery at the end of a given cardiothoracic surgical procedure. For example, one such method might take the form of an antibiotic that could be sprayed on or within the thoracic cavity immediately prior to and after closure of the surgical entrance site. Such an application method may also have the potential to reach interstitial areas that are at risk for infections, specifically those with inherently minimal blood flows; in other words, these tissue areas would otherwise receive minimal amounts of orally or intravenously administered antibiotics.

2.1. Other drug targets

With recent advances in microfabrication, it is feasible to locally deliver drugs in ways that were previously not possible. The field capsule endoscopy is a good example of these technologies and also one that may be further miniaturized and exploited for drug delivery. "Capsule endoscopy" is the swallowing of a pill with a video camera inside. The pill travels through the gastrointestinal system and records its journey. Even more sophisticated versions of these devices are being developed to be actively propelled by magnetic energy [21] or flagella type [22] propellers. It should also be noted that magnetic pills for drug delivery are currently under development [23]. One should consider that these novel technologies may also be exploited for cardiac use. For example, a patient could have a magnetic pill guided endovascularly to the heart and anchored to the endocardial surface where therapeutic (biologics or drugs) agents are released. Furthermore, one could even envision that the administration of these therapeutics could be controlled wirelessly and facilitated by micropumps and valves.

In the near future, it is considered that drug eluting microfabricated devices with incorporated biosensors could be implanted locally such that they release drugs in response to given physiological stimuli. For example, a small sphere, capsule, or micelle containing insulin producing cells could be implanted in the pancreas, subdermally, or intramuscularly. The cells could then respond to fluctuations in glucose levels automatically. Extensive research has gone into such closed loop systems for insulin delivery for diabetes patients, with the eventual goal of developing an artificial pancreas [24–27]. In the more distant future, genetically engineered cells could be programmed to produce other drugs as needed and subsequently deliver them at the proper rates or in response to particular stimuli. Furthermore, unlike implantable devices such as drug eluting stents that can only deliver drugs for a few years, these cell-based drug producing devices have the potential to last a lifetime.

It is generally considered that delivering therapeutic agents at or near the entrance to coronary arteries would be particularly useful in certain clinical situations. Such delivery methods could then exploit the natural capillary system to perfuse the drug to the entire heart. This could in turn potentially reduce the amount of drugs needed significantly and may also ameliorate undesired side effects known for systemic administration. In another approach, during surgical operations, deployed degradable microcapsules with tuned drug release profiles could be injected into the myocardium adjacent to the coronary arteries. Alternatively, resorbable patches could be adhered over the main coronary arteries and the therapeutic agent would then diffuse into the vessel and be transported to the entire organ.

In addition, a delivery patch could also be adhered to local areas, such as one doped with angiogenic treatment placed on an infarct zone.

In the future, combinatorial therapies could also be extended beyond current clinical practice such as drug eluting stents and pacing leads. This is an area of great opportunity for local drug delivery advancements. For example, ventricular assist devices could incorporate the ability to passively or actively deliver a variety of therapies. As such, their possible approaches and advantages may improve the use of these devices, e.g., when they are being used as a bridge to transplant or recovery.

It should be noted that the direct injection of drugs, proteins, or cells into the myocardium has also been proposed as a method of local delivery [28–31]. More specifically, these could be localized in areas of infarct or near atherosclerotic plaque deposits to aid in restoration of normal function. To date, it is noteworthy that positive results have been observed with injections of adenoviruses encoding for heat shock protein [28] or growth hormone [29], [30] in rabbit and rat models, respectively. Furthermore, clinically, gene transfer by direct injection of plasmid DNA coding vascular endothelial growth factor (VEGF) into ischemic myocardium has promoted angiogenesis [31].

It should be described for completeness that transmyocardial laser revascularization has been applied clinically to patients with inoperable coronary artery disease and often used in conjunction with CABG. This procedure utilizes a laser to perforate the walls of the heart in areas of poor perfusion. The channels created act as conduit for blood and, during healing neovascularization, and also considered to improve perfusion. Perhaps this approach, if considered an option, could be supplemented with adjuvant use of local therapeutic agents to quicken the vascularization process, such as VEGF, or other therapeutics to potentially restore normal function.

2.2. Alternative local delivery methods

To date, numerous drug pumps and other devices and methods for delivering treatment to a localized area or region of the body have been shown to be successful. As mentioned previously, there is a considered difference between local delivery and targeted delivery of treatments. Additionally, it is also possible that various therapeutic approaches incorporate one or both of these methods, in order to maximize the beneficial effects of the therapy and minimize the adverse side effects.

One such method, which has been studied significantly, is to create a polymer or biological scaffold in which the drug/protein has been embedded. Subsequent release is then dependent upon either degradation of the scaffold or diffusion of the drug out of the scaffold. Currently there are clinical devices available, such as the Gliadel® wafer, which is impregnated with a chemotherapy drug and used following surgical resection of cancerous tissue within the brain [32], [33]. Note that these drug delivery platforms have been made from a number of different polymers, synthetic or natural. Ultimately it is considered that whichever material is used, it must be biocompatible and able to dispense the drug at appropriate rates for the particular treatment. Currently, such products have been developed relative to treatments for cancers, which have included polymer structures for subcutaneous or intramuscular placement. More recently, similar scaffolds have been created for the treatment of cardiac diseases, but these are still within the research phase of the design.

Myocardial patches, often made of a gel, collagen, or other biocompatible material, are typically impregnated with stem cells or protein growth factors meant to diffuse into the heart to promote myocardial growth and revascularization. These are placed locally on infarcted areas of the heart. Alternatively, the scaffolds could be designed to promote growth within their structure, becoming a functioning part of the myocardium. If the device/scaffold is made such that it requires stem cell infiltration in an *in vitro* setting, it can be incubated with the particular cells needed prior to implantation onto the cardiac structure [34]. Both of these methods illustrate how tissue engineering approaches could be utilized to locally deliver drugs or therapies to the heart, however there are other mechanical devices that also allow a physician to deliver drugs directly to the site of interest.

2.3. Localized injections and drug pumps

When discussing localized treatment of tissue, a method to deliver the treatment to a specific region of interest is essential. Various methods have been reported in the literature, from simplistic methods of direct injections of the drug to the localized area to be treated to the use of more complex microelectromechanical systems (MEMS). The method for direct injection of a treatment into a specific diseased area is a fairly simplistic idea; however, the means to deliver a needle and treatment to the heart may pose a significant challenge. Current research is investigating injections into the myocardium via angioplasty balloons to reduce the occurrence of restenosis. More specifically, small pores or openings within a catheter deliver gene therapy or alternative drug treatments to the diseased cardiac cells [35], [36]. Likewise a given drug can be coated directly onto the exterior surfaces of a balloon, i.e., when the angioplasty is performed, the coating rubs off on the wall of the vessel to provide therapy. Recently, Scheller and colleagues demonstrated that such a device was able to decrease the incidence of restenosis significantly [37]. Stents themselves can also be thought of as a method for localized delivery of a drug to a specific location. This approach has been well developed and tested; drugs like paclitaxel have been coated onto the outside of a coronary stent to minimize restenosis that can occur at sites of stent implantation [38].

Other treatments that might be administered to a patient may need to be localized, but cover a greater area than a single location along an artery or vein. For those purposes, devices such as MEMS or osmotic pumps could perhaps be utilized to slowly deliver treatment to a specific site continuously or intermittently and with varying rates; i.e., delivery could last from days to months. When considering drug pumps, they generally fall into one of two categories, passive or active. The passive pump approach can be thought of as being similar to the gels or wafers discussed previously; however instead of the drug being embedded within the polymer, it would be contained within a chamber that would be opened once the polymer had been degraded enough to release it. To date, several designs have been implemented including multiple wells in a row with differing polymer closures to release at different times, as well as multiple chambers to release two different types of drugs simultaneously. As one could imagine, the only limitations to these types of designs are the properties of the polymers and the size of the device [32], [39].

One specific design described as a passive system is fairly unique- the use of osmotic pressure to push out the drug from a syringe-like device. These work on the principle that water will diffuse one way across a semipermeable membrane and increase the pressure on one side, thereby pushing out the drug slowly [39]. These types of devices have also been modified slightly to create pulsatile drug delivery pumps, i.e., in one case, a membrane was set up and had immobilized glucose oxidase which converted glucose to gluconic acid [40]. This results in an ionic change in the membrane, and the electrostatic repulsion of the membrane causes an expansion and increased delivery of insulin. This has the added ability to adapt to the specific needs of patients at various times of the day, depending upon glucose levels within their systems [40].

Another type of the MEMS approach for agent delivery is to release a bolus from a small reservoir; initially these devices relied on an electrochemical dissolution of a gold membrane blocking a reservoir of a solution. However, a number of published studies to date have reported that this approach could not be performed reliably, so it was modified to a localized melting of the gold membranes by resistive heating [32]. Another approach of an active delivery pump has been employed for patients with chronic pain, e.g., a pump with a reservoir filled with a pain medication can be implanted with a catheter leading directly into the spinal column or other neuronal targets. It should be noted that more recently the ability to refill these devices has been greatly improved and this is an advantage over MEMS devices that cannot refill, however the size of the former devices are currently much greater [41]. These types of pump systems have their own specific purposes, yet both intend to deliver a drug treatment to a localized area within the body to help reduce the effects of the drug on other organs or nearby healthy tissue.

2.4. Ultrasound and lipisomal delivery approaches

Another delivery technique is encapsulating agents for release in specific areas. As opposed to the local delivery pumps described above, where a drug is released into a specific location within the body, generally these packaged therapies can be administered intravenously with targeted release. In these cases, the drug will circulate throughout the entire body, but importantly the targeted drugs have been altered in a way to make them: 1) released at a specific site, 2) preferentially bind within the diseased area, 3) be more readily taken up by the target cells, 4) preferentially released slowly over time, or 5) any combination of these attributes. Ultimately the aim is to increase the effectiveness of the treatment while decreasing the toxic systemic effects of the drug. These approaches can be considered compatible with localized delivery, especially in the setting of thoracic surgery. For instance, a targeted drug could be infused into the coronary arteries, compounding the targeted design with local delivery.

Another specific way that investigators have been able to achieve targeted delivery is by using liposomes that encapsulate the drug, relying on active or passive targeting of tissues to be treated. First, it can act passively, relying on various cells to uptake the liposomes, e.g., reticuloendothelial cells, which can be found concentrated within the liver and spleen. Thus if the treatment was designed specifically for cells within the liver or spleen, a passive approach might be quite acceptable. It should be noted that this same approach has been discussed within nanoparticle delivery as well, taking advantage of the fact that the vasculature within tumors can be porous, allowing the nanoparticles to accumulate within the tumor region. It is still important, however, to aim to limit peripheral exposure, since such liposomes may still be taken up within the liver and other filtering organs [39], [42].

More specifically, an active targeting paradigm could be achieved by placing a recognition sequence on the outside of the liposome, to develop ligand-receptor interactions that will in turn bind the carrier to the targeted cells. As such, these could be targeted to specific proteins or to biomarkers that are upregulated in specific tissues, like tumors or portions of the myocardium responding to ischemia or heart failure [2], [3]. One needs to consider that these modified liposomes may still be taken up by the liver, spleen, or other non-targets; however, some specified modifications of the developed lipid layers may minimize uptake in these structures [42].

Another reported means that treatments may be delivered to target specific cells is via microbubbles aided by ultrasound disruption. More specifically, the microbubbles can be formed by air or other types of gas and introduced into the bloodstream similar to those techniques utilized in ultrasound imaging with contrast. Note that air bubbles are more readily dissolved into the blood following introduction into the venous system, giving them a shorter lifespan. By using perfluorocarbon gases, the lifespan of the delivery bubbles increase and they can also be coated with a variety of materials including polymers, lipids, or proteins which will further increase the lifespan. These longlasting microbubbles can then be disrupted by focused ultrasound—a trigger that can be applied nearly anywhere in the body [4–6]. It is considered that the ballistics of the cavitation not only disrupt the integrity of the bubble, but it will also momentarily disrupt the plasma membranes of the target cells, allowing for the drug and/or microbubbles to be passed through [43]. While this approach has resulted in detrimental effects on cardiac mechanical function [44], it has been shown to effectively increase absorption of certain drugs [43]. Alternatively, the capsules can be designed to release their therapeutic payload with a slight increase in temperature that can be triggered by local heating [45].

3. Pericardial delivery

It has been noted that the pericardium provides a unique space that holds a vast potential for localized drug delivery. For example, such pericardial approaches may range from: 1) the delivery of preconditioning therapies during surgical preparation, 2) providing for therapies that promote vascular genesis after CABG, and 3) the prophylactic administration of antiarrhythmic agents in order to prevent post-operative AF. We believe that the possible treatments for the myocardium are numerous and will provide a few specific examples below, following a review of pericardial anatomy.

3.1. Anatomy of the pericardium

The pericardium is made up of two connected structures. The innermost layer is serous membrane which is inseparable from the epicardial surface, and is called the "visceral pericardium." The continuous serous membrane is folded in on itself and the single layer also makes up the inner surface of the parietal pericardium. The single layer of mesothelial cells is indistinguishable from the fibrous outer layer (Figure 2). Together, the parietal and fibrous layers make up the outer layer, or "parietal pericardium." This is the most prominent layer of the pericardium and is what we generally think of when we discuss the pericardium.

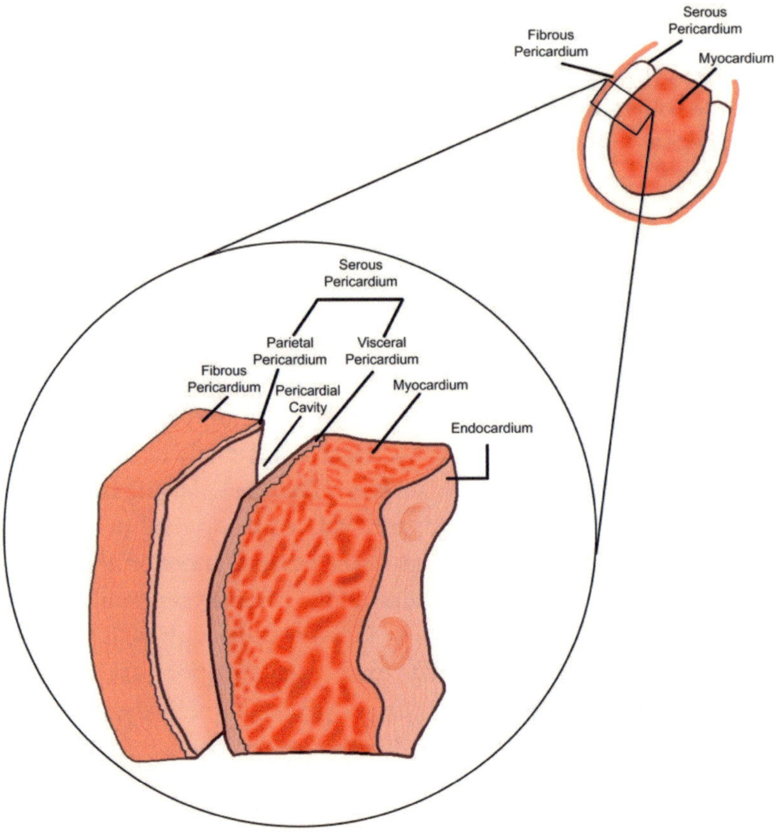

Figure 2. Schematic of the layers of the pericardium. The upper right shows a schematic diagram of the serous and fibrous pericardium with respect to the heart. The expanded cross-section view shows the attachment of two layers of the serous pericardium (visceral and parietal) to the myocardium and fibrous pericardium, respectively.

The healthy pericardium contains 20-60 mL of pericardial fluid. This fluid, an ultrafiltrate of the plasma [46], surrounds the heart, with the majority concentrated in the pericardial sinuses and atrioventricular grooves. This fluid normally drains into the lymphatic system at a relatively slow rate, measured to be a volume equivalent to every 5-7 hours in sheep [47]. However, as pericardial fluid pressure increases, such as in the case of cardiac tamponade, investigators have found that not only does lymphatic drainage increase [48], but fluid may pass through the pericardium and enter the pleural space [49].

Though the volume of pericardial fluid is not evenly distributed, it is generally found to be well mixed due to the motion of the heart; thus agents can be considered to be quickly and evenly dispersed throughout [47]. Even though there is only a relatively small amount of fluid circulating around the ventricles, this aforementioned mixing action will help maintain even distribution of any additions to the pericardial fluid epicardially, thus maintaining consistent gradients relative to the myocardium. While the parietal pericardium is generally considered as non-compliant, the overall pericardial space can accommodate moderate increases in the amount of fluid by filling in the pericardial sinuses. However, once this reserve volume space is filled, pericardial pressure quickly increases with added volume, i.e., symptomatic tamponade is elicited (Figure 3).

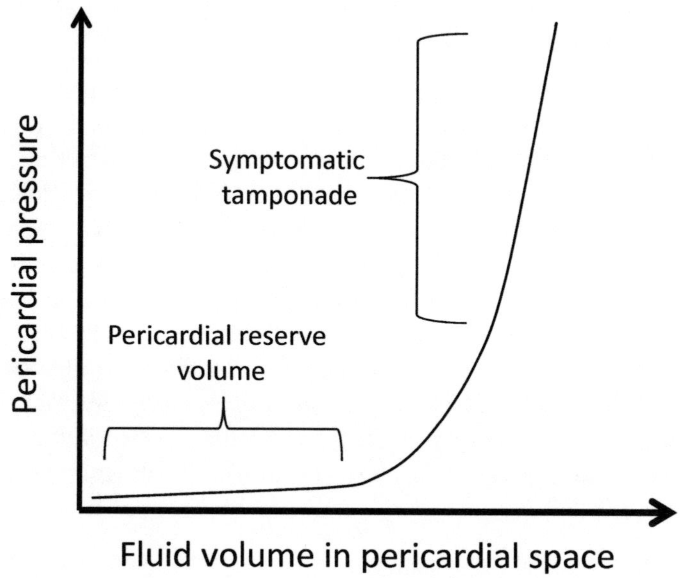

Figure 3. Percardial pressure vs. pericardial volume. As pericardial fluid volume increases, the pericardial reserve volume is filled. Once the reserve volume is full, pressure within the pericardium rapidly rises causing cardiac tamponade and functional depression.

3.2. The basic physiology associated with the pericardium

The fibrous (parietal) pericardium is 1-3 mm thick in healthy humans, and as noted above, is considered as minimally or non-compliant. In fact, because of these features, multiple bioartificial replacement heart valves are made with leaflets of either bovine of swine pericardium. As such, this tough layer has the primary function to physically constrain the heart. While this may not have a large influence at rest, during physical exertion, cardiac filling becomes limited by the pericardium. Further, it has been noted that an intact pericardium also increases cardiac chamber interdependence, i.e., increased pressure in one chamber affects other chambers because the total volume is restricted by the pericardium. A more detailed review can be found in the Handbook of Cardiac Anatomy, Physiology, and Devices [50].

Typically during cardiothoracic surgery, the pericardium needs to be opened to obtain direct myocardial access, and at the end of a procedure the pericardium is not typically closed. This in turn reduces the risk of post-surgical cardiac tamponade, as pressure cannot build up easily in an open pericardium. However, the lack of a barrier between the heart and the healing incision site typically leads to scarring and epicardial fusions within this wound site. Typically, this has minor consequences—that is until a subsequent open-heart procedure needs to be performed — and both the initial incisions and heart access are complicated by these additional fibroses. It has been suggested that a barrier placed between the sternum and myocardium would potentially limit the buildup of subsequent adhesions and make reentry less risky. While synthetic barriers such as the absorbable CovaCard (BIOM'UP, Lyon, France) are being developed [51], the native or graft pericardium also may provide a natural and available option.

Relative to physiological consequences, in addition to reducing reoperative complications, the closure of the pericardial sac following cardiac surgery has been proposed to reduce long-term cardiac performance and aid in maintaining diastolic function and ventricular geometry, as well as reduce right ventricular dysfunction [52], [53]. Additionally, one could also consider that a closed pericardium may also provide a reservoir space for subsequent pericardial therapies. Yet, one reported limitation to pericardial closure is that it can acutely reduce cardiac indices and stroke work [54]. More specifically, Rao et al. corroborated that these functions were reduced one hour post-operatively in patients who had pericardial closure ($P<0.001$). However, they also reported no significant differences in function between patient groups at 4 hours or 8 hours post-operatively. While increased risk of cardiac tamponade still exists with full closure, it has been reported that fenestrated techniques and pericardial drainage tubes have been used to mitigate the consequences of pericardial effusions [55], [56].

In summary, the pericardial space potentially provides a natural barrier and is well suited for localized drug delivery. Thus if pericardial access could be easily and reproducibly obtained, the possibilities of long- and short-term treatment include: antiarrhythmic therapies, delivery of agents to reduce cellular injuries at reperfusion, and/or use of angiogenic proteins to promote revascularization and regrowth specifically within infarcted regions.

3.3. Cardioprotective agents

To date within the US, ischemic heart disease and myocardial infarctions remain as leading causes of clinical morbidity and mortality. Their occurrence often leads to congestive heart failure, which in turn causes further reductions in coronary flow and necrosis in the myocardium, and leads to further functional impairments. It is generally considered that compared to other body tissues, myocardial cells have poor regenerative abilities, a fact that has focused much research on methods for reducing trauma and/or myocardial death, as well as methods for improving repair and regeneration.

It has been reported that the local infusion of nitric oxide donors could promote local vasodilation without major systemic effects [57]. Additionally, the administration of VEGF and other angiogenic agents into the myocardium have been associated with several benefits that include: increased collateral vessel development, increases in regional myocardial blood flow, improved myocardial function in the ischemic regions, and/or increased myocardial vascularity [31], [58–60].

Relative to cardioprotective agents, our laboratory has observed that intrapericardial delivery of omega-3 polyunsaturated fatty acids can dramatically reduce both infarct sizes and ventricular arrhythmias associated with ischemia. More specifically in this study, acute ischemia was induced for 45 minutes followed by 180 minutes of reperfusion, while the omega-3 fatty acid docosahexaenoic acid (DHA) was delivered to the pericardial space prior to ischemia as well as during the initial period of reperfusion. Importantly during the ischemic period, ventricular arrhythmias were reduced 50% (which in the control hearts required defibrillation and caused 20% mortality). Upon completion of the reperfusion, the hearts were excised and ischemic damage was measured; hearts treated with DHA had a similar area at risk, but a 57% reduction in normalized infarct size was seen [61]. Ongoing research in our lab also suggests that omega-3 fatty acids may reduce susceptibility to AF during cardiac surgery.

Most recently, investigations in our laboratory have explored the pericardial delivery of specified bile acids noted to have anti-apoptotic benefits. These molecules are upregulated within hibernating black bears, and reports by others have suggested that ursodeoxycholic acid may be beneficial in reducing AF within myocytes [62]. In these ongoing studies to determine potential beneficial effects within a large animal model, we specifically deliver a taurine conjugate of ursodeoxycholic acid within a formed pericardial cradle (the pericardial space) and periodically induce AF. Preliminary results have suggested that these molecules are effective in reducing the times a given heart will elicit AF, i.e., without having to give this therapy intravenously and thus potentially have undesirable systemic side effects (unpublished data).

3.4. Antiarrhythmic agents

Antiarrhythmic drugs are commonly known for their narrow therapeutic ranges and severe side effects. It has been previously suggested that delivery of these agents to the pericardial space would allow for myocardial diffusion while lowering undesired plasma drug concentrations [63], [64]. In other words, such local delivery allows for higher doses of this class of agents to be safely administered to control focally the heart rhythm—an application that could be especially applied during cardiothoracic surgery. To date, the intrapericardial delivery of antiarrhythmic agents has been attempted with numerous agents, e.g., esmolol [63], solatol [65], atenolol [65], ibutalide [66], procainamide [67], [68], digoxin [67], amiodarone [69], arachadonic acid [70], nitroglycerin [57] and L-arginine [71] have all been shown to have electrophysiological effects when delivered to the pericardial space in various animal models. Additionally, in those studies that also measured plasma concentrations, there was minimal crossover of the delivered agent into the bloodstream [67–69]

To date, despite these reported successes in treating arrhythmias in various animal models, the clinical practice of intrapericardial (IP) delivery is not widely employed. Possible reasons include: 1) the lack of experience (no large clinical trials), 2) difficulties with access and removal of agents, and/or 3) unknown potential complications with this delivery route. It is important to note that one of the described major concerns with pericardial delivery is that it relies primarily on trans-epicardial diffusion to reach the myocardium. In other words, while the thin atria and superficial sinoatrial node may be easy to treat via these mechanisms, the effects of possible ventricular drug gradients are not well defined. Further, it has been hypothesized that moderately soluble or lipophilic molecules will not be evenly transported across the thicker ventricles, causing various degrees of electrophysiological changes through the depth of the myocardium, creating a scenario where the epicardium and endocardium are not conducting and/or contracting at similar rates. This electrical heterogeneity theoretically carries the possibility of initiating, rather than inhibiting, arrhythmias [68].

In our lab, we have investigated the pharmacokinetics and pharmacodynamics of IV and IP delivery of metoprolol [7]. While the β-blocker is typically used to treat angina and hypertension, it is also used to treat tachycardias. With a tachycardic swine model, IV delivery of metoprolol was faster acting compared to IP, but only by several minutes. While the reductions in heart rates were similar for both delivery techniques, these effects were sustained longer after IP delivery. Importantly, IV delivery was accompanied by significant reductions in contractility, while IP delivery elicited minimal effects. In other words, these findings indicated that IP delivery of metoprolol may have similar bradycardic effects compared to IV delivery, but without the reduced contractility. The other important finding in this study was the minimal pericardial crossover of metoprolol within blood, as well as the slightly increased half-life of the drug [7].

3.5. Clinical pericardial access

Access to the pericardial space for the delivery of therapies outside of cardiothoracic surgical procedures may pose many difficulties. However, multiple minimally invasive procedural methodologies are under development. For example in the trans-atrial approach, access to the pericardium is achieved via a catheter coming up through the femoral vein into the right atrial appendage, where it then punctures through this thin myocardium to gain access into the pericardial space. To date, success with this approach has been demonstrated in canines and swine [72]. Alternatively, a subxyphoid access procedure has been suggested

[73]. While this method is often used to drain the pericardial space during episodes of cardiac tamponade, the minimal separation between the fibrous pericardium and the epicardium make this approach more difficult when there is not a substantial amount of intrapericardial fluid present. Several access tools have and continue to be developed to aid in subxyphoid access using minimally invasive approaches. For instance, the PeriPort™ (Cormedics, TX) system is designed to initially enter the thoracic space through a subxyphoid incision, where it uses a vacuum on the distal end to grip the pericardium and separate it from the heart's epicardial surface. Once the pericardium is pulled into the vacuum chamber, a retractable needle pierces the pericardium and allows for a near tangential entrance of a guidewire. Such designed access tools should enhance the safety and simplicity of pericardial access and also have potential to increase the widespread use of localized therapies to treat pericardial and cardiac diseases. Nevertheless, during cardiothoracic surgery, a simple syringe or perfusion pump is all that is clinically needed to deliver pericardial therapies. Thus the hurdles to add localized pericardial delivery of drugs concurrent to surgery are much less compared to pericardial therapies on their own.

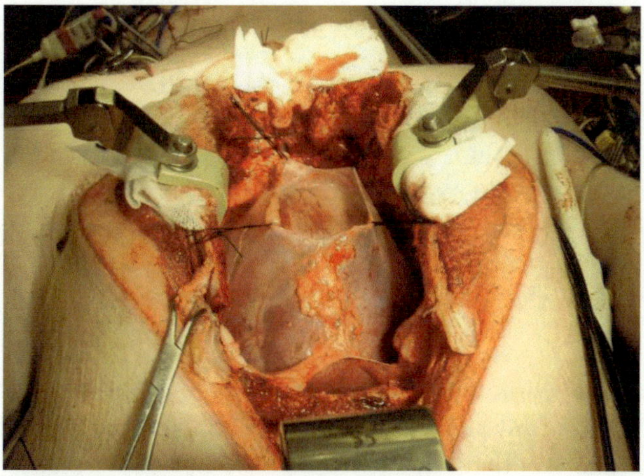

Figure 4. Methods of pericardial access include the pericardium as a reservoir. Pictured here is a pericardial cradle in a swine model.

3.6. Protocols

As noted above, the pericardial delivery of molecules, cells, nanoparticles, etc., becomes simplified with surgical access (Figure 4). Without the requirement of added procedures and incisions, the pericardial delivery of therapeutics can be administered with minimal additional equipment, time, or complications, leading to numerous clinical scenarios that may benefit from the use of pericardial delivery. While some of these applications, as described below, have been tested in pilot studies in animals, future clinical studies have yet to be developed to confirm efficacy.

In one such application, a common first choice of donor vessel for a CABG procedure is the internal thoracic artery. Thus, while the surgeon initially frees and prepares this vessel for subsequent grafting, the pericardial administration of either a prophylactic antiarrhythmic or angiogenic agent could be infused into the pericardium. Once the artery has been prepared and the pericardium is further opened, the drug has a chance to partially diffuse into the myocardial tissue. Additional drugs could also be added through direct myocardial injection to promote revascularization or prevent post-operative arrhythmias. Alternatively, a procedure that requires access from the anterior surface of the heart may make use of the reservoir created by the remaining pericardium to treat the posterior myocardium during the procedure.

Another important approach to consider is the post-operative administration of drugs, which could be accomplished via surgically placed pericardial drainage catheters. More specifically, with the placement of pleural drainage catheters and temporary pacing leads at the end of a procedure, the addition of a catheter leading into the pericardium is sometimes included [74]. This catheter, whether through the main lumen or a second lumen, could hypothetically allow for continued access to the pericardial space and delivery of appropriate antiarrhythmic, antibiotic, or other therapies to the myocardium. Therapies with such devices have been attempted with success in a porcine model [75].

As mentioned above, multiple techniques exist for low or no tension pericardial closures [56], [76], [77]. In addition to reoperative benefits, the planned closure of the pericardium can create a useful reservoir for localized treatment. While the most common clinical reason for non-closure is to reduce the risk of cardiac tamponade, this could be mitigated with the placement of the aforementioned specially designed drainage/therapy delivery catheter. We also believe that with full pericardial closure and access via the pericardial drain, a delivered therapy would reach all surfaces of the heart.

Another clinical situation/option for localized drug delivery might be during cardiopulmonary bypass procedures. To arrest the heart and often throughout the procedure, cardioplegia solutions are perfused through the coronary vessels. Whether antiegrade or retrograde, this perfused solution cools and protects the heart by minimizing metabolism. It has been considered that myocardial damage can be further reduced by introducing cardioprotective agents via this delivery route [78–80]. It is important to note that in this unique situation, any administered drug reaches the entire myocardium via the capillaries, but will have no access to other tissues until after cross clamping is released. In other words, high transmural and widespread myocardial concentrations can be achieved with remarkable speed and accuracy while minimizing side effects.

Similarly, organ transplantation offers ultimate accessibility in localized drug delivery. A typical transplant, includes explant, transportation and re-implantation. Because of the recovery of multiple organs, localized delivery is a viable option where the effects can be greatly enhanced after re-implantation function. Not only are options such as pericardial delivery still available since the heart is typically the last organ removed, but IV therapies just prior to cross-clamping become targeted.

Next, the times between explant and implant can range from under six hours for the heart to up to 24 hours for the liver or kidney. During these times, the heart is often in stagnant cold storage. However, ideas and methods for continuous perfusion during the hypothermic period are well established, e.g., continuous hypothermic perfusion of the heart was first applied only a year after the first successful human heart transplant [81]. Since then it shown that it is possible to keep large mammalian hearts viable for up to 48 hours in baboons and swine [82], as well as improve function compared to non-perfused hearts [83]. While continuous hypothermic perfusion is not used clinically with heart transplantation, it should be noted that the Organ Care System (Transmedics, Andover, MA) gained investigational device exemption status in 2007, and a clinical trial is currently underway. This continuous perfusion during transport before implant provides another opportunity for localized therapies, as they could be simply added to the perfusates.

4. Limitations and conclusions

Localized delivery methods such as those into the pericardial space are not without potential limitations. Without direct access to the bloodstream, an administered agent at a target tissue, such as in the pericardial space, must diffuse into the target tissue to increase concentrations. While this may ultimately limit the depth or distance a given therapeutic agent (drugs, cells, nanoparticles, etc.) might be able to migrate in a significant quantity, it is also one of the major advantages of localized therapies.

Some areas for localized treatments, especially within the myocardium, may be considered as relatively difficult to access. However, with a large number of cardiac surgeries currently being performed and an increasing number of catheter procedures being developed and implemented, these therapeutic methods could piggyback on planned procedures with few added complications or risks. Finally, novel therapeutic deliveries, drugs, or other interventions may need to gain additional approval in order to become indications for localized delivery.

Cardiothoracic surgeries may facilitate novel opportunities for local drug delivery, such as overcoming the hurdle to obtaining pericardial access. Such clinical procedures also provide opportunities for localized injections or coronary infusions. The future opportunities for such therapies are not limited to the duration of the operation; by leaving a pericardial drainage catheter with delivery features, physicians could also incorporate subsequent therapeutic delivery. In some cases, implantable drug pumps or biodegradable patches could provide therapy to the patient beyond their ICU stay. The emerging field of localized therapy delivery shows great potential, but future human studies are needed to verify the positive results observed in pre-clinical studies. Nevertheless, the unique access afforded by cardiothoracic procedures may speed up implementation of these promising local and target therapeutic delivery methods, thus placing surgeons at the cutting edge of novel delivery approaches.

Author details

Christopher Rolfes, Stephen Howard and Ryan Goff
Departments of Biomedical Engineering and Surgery, University of Minnesota, Minneapolis, MN, USA

Paul A. Iaizzo*
Departments of Biomedical Engineering, Surgery, Integrative Biology and Physiology, University of Minnesota, Minneapolis, MN, USA

5. References

[1] Center for Drug Evaluation and Research and Food and Drug Administration, "Guidance for Industry: Bioavailability and Bioequivalence Studies for Orally Administered Drug Products - General Considerations," 2003.

[2] S. P. Jones et al., "Leukocyte and endothelial cell adhesion molecules in a chronic murine model of myocardial reperfusion injury Leukocyte and endothelial cell adhesion molecules in a chronic murine model of myocardial reperfusion injury," *Group*, 2012.

[3] B. J. Lestini et al., "Surface modification of liposomes for selective cell targeting in cardiovascular drug delivery," *Journal of Controlled Release*, vol. 78, no. 1-3, pp. 235-47, Jan. 2002.

[4] J. R. Lindner and S. Kaul, "Delivery of drugs with ultrasound," *Echocardiography (Mount Kisco, N.Y.)*, vol. 18, no. 4, pp. 329-37, May 2001.

[5] C. M. H. Newman and T. Bettinger, "Gene therapy progress and prospects: ultrasound for gene transfer," *Gene Therapy*, vol. 14, no. 6, pp. 465-75, Mar. 2007.

[6] D. Vancraeynest et al., "Myocardial delivery of colloid nanoparticles using ultrasound-targeted microbubble destruction," *European Heart Journal*, vol. 27, no. 2, pp. 237-45, Jan. 2006.

[7] E. S. Richardson, C. Rolfes, O. Woo, W. Elmquist, D. Benditt, and P. A. Iaizzo, "Cardiac response to the intrapericardial delivery of metoprolol: targeted delivery compared to intravenous administration," *Journal of Cardiovascular Translational Research*, vol. 5, no.4, pp535-40, Aug. 2012.

[8] G. M. McKhann, M. A. Grega, L. M. Borowicz, W. A. Baumgartner, and O. A. Selnes, "Stroke and encephalopathy after cardiac surgery," *Stroke*, vol. 37, no. 2, pp. 562-71, Feb. 2006.

[9] A. C. Breuer et al., "Central nervous system complications of coronary artery bypass graft surgery: prospective analysis of 421 patients," *Stroke*, vol. 14, no. 5, pp. 682-87, Oct. 1983.

[10] D. Barbut and L. R. Caplan, "Brain complications of cardiac surgery," *Current Problems in Cardiology*, vol. 22, no. 9, pp. 449-80, Sep. 1997.

---

* Corresponding Author

[11] A. J. Furlan and A. C. Breuer, "Central nervous system complications of open heart surgery," *Stroke*, vol. 15, no. 5, pp. 912-15, Oct. 1984.

[12] E. E. Tseng et al., "Neuronal nitric oxide synthase inhibition reduces neuronal apoptosis after hypothermic circulatory arrest," *The Annals of Thoracic Surgery*, vol. 64, no. 6, pp. 1639-47, Dec. 1997.

[13] E. E. Tseng, M. V. Brock, and C. C. Kwon, "Quantitative analyses of intracerebral excitatory amino acids and citulline following hypothermic circulatory arrest," *Surgical Forum*, vol. 48, pp. 297-9, 1997.

[14] D. C. Harmon, K. G. Ghori, N. P. Eustace, S. J. F. O'Callaghan, A. P. O'Donnell, and G. D. Shorten, "Aprotinin decreases the incidence of cognitive deficit following {CABG} and cardiopulmonary bypass: a pilot randomized controlled study," *Canadian Journal of Anaesthesia*, vol. 51, no. 10, pp. 1002-9, Dec. 2004.

[15] J. P. Mathew et al., "A multicenter risk index for atrial fibrillation after cardiac surgery," *The Journal of the American Medical Association*, vol. 291, no. 14, pp. 1720-9, Apr. 2004.

[16] C. V. Egleston, A. E. Wood, T. F. Gorey, and E. M. McGovern, "Gastrointestinal complications after cardiac surgery," *Annals of The Royal College of Surgeons of England*, vol. 75, no. 1, pp. 52-6, Jan. 1993.

[17] B. Andersson, J. Nilsson, J. Brandt, P. Höglund, and R. Andersson, "Gastrointestinal complications after cardiac surgery," *British Journal of Surgery*, vol. 92, no. 3, pp. 326-33, Mar. 2005.

[18] G. M. Sreeram, I. J. Welsby, A. D. Sharma, B. Phillips-Bute, P. K. Smith, and T. F. Slaughter, "Infectious complications after cardiac surgery: lack of association with fresh frozen plasma or platelet transfusions," *Journal of Cardiothoracic and Vascular Anesthesia*, vol. 19, no. 4, pp. 430-4, Aug. 2005.

[19] M. C. Engoren, R. H. Habib, A. Zacharias, T. A. Schwann, C. J. Riordan, and S. J. Durham, "Effect of blood transfusion on long-term survival after cardiac operation," *The Annals of Thoracic Surgery*, vol. 74, no. 4, pp. 1180-6, Oct. 2002.

[20] B. D. Spiess, "Transfusion of blood products affects outcome in cardiac surgery," *Seminars in Cardiothoracic and Vascular Anesthesia*, vol. 8, no. 4, pp. 267-81, Dec. 2004.

[21] J. F. Rey et al., "Feasibility of stomach exploration with a guided capsule endoscope," *Endoscopy*, vol. 42, no. 7, pp. 541-5, Jul. 2010.

[22] G. Kósa, P. Jakab, G. Székely, and N. Hata, "{MRI} driven magnetic microswimmers," *Biomedical Microdevices*, vol. 14, no. 1, pp. 165-78, Feb. 2012.

[23] B. Laulicht, N. J. Gidmark, A. Tripathi, and E. Mathiowitz, "Localization of magnetic pills," *Proceedings of the National Academy of Sciences of the United States of America*, vol. 108, no. 6, pp. 2252-7, Feb. 2011.

[24] R. Hovorka et al., "Overnight closed loop insulin delivery (artificial pancreas) in adults with type 1 diabetes: crossover randomised controlled studies," *British Medical Journal*, vol. 342, p. d1855-d1855, Apr. 2011.

[25] R. Hovorka et al., "Manual closed-loop insulin delivery in children and adolescents with type 1 diabetes: a phase 2 randomised crossover trial," *Lancet*, vol. 375, no. 9716, pp. 743-51, Feb. 2010.

[26] S. Weinzimer, G. Steil, K. Swan, J. Dziura, N. Kurtz, and W. Tamborlane, "Fully automated closed-loop insulin delivery versus semiautomated hybrid control in pediatric patients with type 1 diabetes using an artificial pancreas," *Diabetes Care*, vol. 31, pp. 934-9, 2008.

[27] E. Renard, "Implantable closed-loop glucose-sensing and insulin delivery: the future for insulin pump therapy," *Current Opinion in Pharmacology*, vol. 2, no. 6, pp. 708-16, Dec. 2002.

[28] S. Okubo, O. Wildner, M. R. Shah, J. C. Chelliah, M. L. Hess, and R. C. Kukreja, "Gene transfer of heat-shock protein 70 reduces infarct," *In Vivo*, pp. 877-881, 2001.

[29] V. Jayasankar et al., "Targeted overexpression of growth hormone by adenoviral gene transfer preserves myocardial function and ventricular geometry in ischemic cardiomyopathy," *Journal of Molecular and Cellular Cardiology*, vol. 36, no. 4, pp. 531-8, Apr. 2004.

[30] V. Jayasankar, L. T. Bish, T. J. Pirolli, M. F. Berry, J. Burdick, and Y. J. Woo, "Local myocardial overexpression of growth hormone attenuates postinfarction remodeling and preserves cardiac function," *The Annals of Thoracic Surgery*, vol. 77, no. 6, pp. 2122-9; discussion 2129, Jun. 2004.

[31] D. W. Losordo et al., "Gene therapy for myocardial angiogenesis," *Online*, pp. 2800-4, 1998.

[32] N. M. Elman, Y. Patta, A. W. Scott, B. Masi, H. L. Ho Duc, and M. J. Cima, "The next generation of drug-delivery microdevices," *Clinical Pharmacology and Therapeutics*, vol. 85, no. 5, pp. 544-7, May 2009.

[33] R. De Souza, P. Zahedi, C. J. Allen, and M. Piquette-Miller, "Polymeric drug delivery systems for localized cancer chemotherapy," *Drug Delivery*, vol. 17, no. 6, pp. 365-75, Aug. 2010.

[34] J. Leor, Y. Amsalem, and S. Cohen, "Cells, scaffolds, and molecules for myocardial tissue engineering," *Pharmacology & Therapeutics*, vol. 105, no. 2, pp. 151-63, Feb. 2005.

[35] D. Brieger and E. Topol, "Local drug delivery systems and prevention of restenosis," *Cardiovascular Research*, vol. 35, no. 3, pp. 405-13, Sep. 1997.

[36] P. Barath, A. Popov, G. L. Dillehay, G. Matos, and T. McKiernan, "Infiltrator angioplasty balloon catheter: a device for combined angioplasty and intramural site-specific treatment," *Catheterization and Cardiovascular Diagnosis*, vol. 41, no. 3, pp. 333-41, Jul. 1997.

[37] B. Scheller et al., "Treatment of coronary in-stent restenosis with a paclitaxel-coated balloon catheter," *New England Journal of Medicine*, vol. 355, pp. 2113-24, 2006.

[38] L. A. Guzman et al., "Local intraluminal infusion of biodegradable polymeric nanoparticles," *Heart*, pp. 1441-8, 1996.

[39] R. Langer, "New methods of drug delivery," *Science*, vol. 249, no. 4976, pp. 1527-33, Sep. 1990.

[40] J. Kost, T. Horbett, B. Ratner, and M. Singh, "Glucose-sensitive membranes containing glucose oxidase: activity, swelling, and permeability studies," *Journal of Biomedical Materials Research*, vol. 19, no. 9, pp. 1117-33, Nov-Dec. 1985.

[41] A. Michael, E. Buffen, R. Rauck, W. Anderson, M. McGirt, and H. V. Mendenhall, "An in vivo canine study to assess granulomatous responses in the MedStream Programmable Infusion System (TM) and the SynchroMed II Infusion System®," *Pain Medicine*, vol. 13, no. 2, pp. 175-84, Feb. 2012.

[42] Y. H. Bae and K. Park, "Targeted drug delivery to tumors: myths, reality and possibility," *Journal of Controlled Release*, vol. 153, no. 3, pp. 198-205, Aug. 2011.

[43] R. J. Price, D. M. Skyba, S. Kaul, and T. C. Skalak, "Delivery of colloidal particles and red blood cells to tissue through microvessel ruptures created by targeted microbubble destruction with ultrasound," *Online*, pp. 1264-7, 1998.

[44] T. Ay et al., "Destruction of contrast microbubbles by ultrasound: effects on myocardial function, coronary perfusion pressure, and microvascular integrity," *Circulation*, vol. 104, no. 4, pp. 461-6, Jul. 2001.

[45] D. E. Meyer, B. C. Shin, G. a Kong, M. W. Dewhirst, and A. Chilkoti, "Drug targeting using thermally responsive polymers and local hyperthermia," *Journal of Controlled Release*, vol. 74, no. 1-3, pp. 213-24, Jul. 2001.

[46] A. Gibson and M. B. Segal, "A study of the composition of pericardial fluid, with special reference to the probably mechanism of fluid formation," *Journal of Physiology*, vol. 277, pp. 367-77, 1978.

[47] B. Boulanger, Z. Yuan, M. Flessner, J. Hay, and M. Johnston, "Pericardial fluid absorption into lymphatic vessels in sheep," *Microvascular Research*, vol. 57, no. 2, pp. 174-86, Mar. 1999.

[48] Z. Yuan, B. Boulanger, M. Flessner, and M. Johnston, "Relationship between pericardial pressure and lymphatic pericardial fluid transport in sheep," *Microvascular Research*, vol. 60, no. 1, pp. 28-36, Jul. 2000.

[49] B. L. Pegram and V. S. Bishop, "An evaluation of the pericardial sac as a safety factor during tamponade," *Cardiovascular Research*, vol. 9, pp. 715-21, 1975.

[50] E. S. Richardson, A. J. Hill, N. D. Skadsberg, M. R. Ujhelyi, Y.-F. Xiao, and P. A. Iaizzo, "The Pericardium," in *Handbook of Cardiac Anatomy, Physiology and Devices, second edition*, 2009, pp. 125-36.

[51] A. Bel et al., "Prevention of postcardiopulmonary bypass pericardial adhesions by a new resorbable collagen membrane," *Interactive Cardiovascular and Thoracic Surgery*, vol. 0, pp. 1-5, Jan. 2012.

[52] R. Shabetai, *The Pericardium*. 2003, pp. 1-85.

[53] M. Watkins and M. LeWinter, "Physiologic role of the normal pericardium," *Annual Review Medicine*, vol. 44, pp. 171-80, 1993.

[54] G. D. Angelini et al., "Adverse hemodynamic effects and echocardiographic consequences of pericardial closure soon after sternotomy and pericardiotomy," *Circulation*, vol. 82, no. 5, pp. IV397-406, Nov. 1990.

[55] H. Ekim, V. Kutay, A. Hazar, H. Akbayrak, H. Basel, and M. Tuncer, "Effects of posterior pericardiotomy on the incidence of pericardial effusion and atrial fibrillation after coronary revascularization," *Medical Science Monitor*, vol. 12, no. 10, pp. 431-4, 2006.

[56] F. Kargar and M. H. Aazami, "Rotational pericardial flap: an alternative tension-free technique for pericardial closure," *The Journal of Thoracic and Cardiovascular Surgery*, vol. 134, no. 2, pp. 510-1, Aug. 2007.

[57] K. Kumar et al., "Potent antifibrillatory effects of intrapericardial nitroglycerin in the ischemic porcine heart," *Journal of the American College of Cardiology*, vol. 41, no. 10, pp. 1831-7, May 2003.

[58] R. J. Laham, M. Rezaee, M. Post, X. Xu, and F. W. Sellke, "Intrapericardial administration of basic fibroblast growth factor: myocardial and tissue distribution and comparison with intracoronary and intravenous administration," *Catheterization and Cardiovascular Interventions*, vol. 58, no. 3, pp. 375-81, Mar. 2003.

[59] D. F. Lazarous et al., "Pharmacodynamics of basic fibroblast growth factor: route of administration determines myocardial and systemic distribution," *Cardiovascular Research*, vol. 36, no. 1, pp. 78-85, Oct. 1997.

[60] R. A. Tio, J. G. Grandjean, A. J. H. Suurmeijer, W. H. van Gilst, D. J. van Veldhuisen, and A. J. van Boven, "Thoracoscopic monitoring for pericardial application of local drug or gene therapy," *International Journal of Cardiology*, vol. 82, no. 2, pp. 117-21, Feb. 2002.

[61] Y.-F. Xiao, D. C. Sigg, M. R. Ujhelyi, J. J. Wilhelm, E. S. Richardson, and P. A. Iaizzo, "Pericardial delivery of omega-3 fatty acid: a novel approach to reducing myocardial infarct sizes and arrhythmias," *American Journal of Physiology. Heart and Circulatory Physiology*, vol. 294, no. 5, pp. H2212-8, May 2008.

[62] M. Miragoli et al., "A protective antiarrhythmic role of ursodeoxycholic acid in an in vitro rat model of the cholestatic fetal heart," *Hepatology*, vol. 54, no. 4, pp. 1282-92, Oct. 2011.

[63] R. Moreno, S. Waxman, K. Rowe, R. Verrier, and C. von Schacky, "Intrapericardial [beta]-adrenergic blockade with esmolol exerts a potent antitachycardic effect without depressing contractility," *Journal of Cardiovascular Pharmacology*, vol. 36, pp. 722-7, 2000.

[64] T. J. van Brakel et al., "Intrapericardial delivery enhances cardiac effects of sotalol and atenolol," *Journal of Cardiovascular Pharmacology*, vol. 44, no. 1, pp. 50-6, Jul. 2004.

[65] T. J. van Brakel et al., "Intrapericardial delivery enhances cardiac effects of sotalol and atenolol," *Journal of Cardiovascular Pharmacology*, vol. 44, no. 1, pp. 50-6, Jul. 2004.

[66] A. Vereckei, J. C. Gorski, M. Ujhelyi, R. Mehra, and D. P. Zipes, "Intrapericardial ibutilide administration fails to terminate pacing-induced sustained atrial fibrillation in dogs," *Cardiovascular Drugs and*, vol. 18, no. 4, pp. 269-77, Jul. 2004.

[67] T. M. Kolettis et al., "Intrapericardial drug delivery: pharmacologic properties and long-term safety in swine," *International Journal of Cardiology*, vol. 99, no. 3, pp. 415-21, Mar. 2005.

[68] M. R. Ujhelyi, K. Z. Hadsall, D. E. Euler, and R. Mehra, "Intrapericardial therapeutics: a pharmacodynamic and pharmacokinetic comparison between pericardial and intravenous procainamide delivery," *Journal of Cardiovascular Electrophysiology*, vol. 13, no. 6, pp. 605-11, Jun. 2002.

[69] G. M. Ayers, T. H. Rho, J. Ben-David, H. R. Besch, and D. P. Zipes, "Amiodarone instilled into the canine pericardial sac migrates transmurally to produce electrophysiologic effects and suppress atrial fibrillation," *Journal of Cardiovascular Electrophysiology*, vol. 7, no. 8, pp. 713-21, Aug. 1996.

[70] T. Miyazaki and D. P. Zipes, "Pencardial prostaglandin biosynthesis prevents the increased incidence of reperfusion-induced ventricular fibrillation produced by efferent sympathetic stimulation in dogs," *Online*, pp. 1008-19, 1990.

[71] L. Fei, A. Baron, D. Henry, and D. P. Zipes, "Intrapericardial delivery of L-arginine reduces the increased severity of ventricular arrhythmias during sympathetic stimulation in dogs with acute coronary occlusion," *Circulation*, vol. 96, pp. 4044-9, 1997.

[72] R. L. Verrier, S. Waxman, E. G. Lovett, and R. Moreno, "Transatrial access to the normal pericardial space and therapeutic interventions," *Online*, pp. 2331-3, 1998.

[73] A. P. Mannam "Safety of subxyphoid pericardial access using a blunt-tip needle," *American Journal of Cardiology*, vol. 89, no. 7, pp. 891-3, 2002.

[74] S. Eryilmaz et al., "Effect of posterior pericardial drainage on the incidence of pericardial effusion after ascending aortic surgery," *The Journal of Thoracic and Cardiovascular Surgery*, vol. 132, no. 1, pp. 27-31, Jul. 2006.

[75] E. S. Richardson, B. Whitson, and P. Iaizzo, "A novel combination therapy for post-operative arrhythmias," *Journal of Medical Devices*, vol. 3, no. 2, p. 27511, 2009.

[76] V. Rao, M. Komeda, R. D. Weisel, G. Cohen, M. A. Borger, and T. E. David, "Should the pericardium be closed routinely after heart operations?," *The Annals of Thoracic Surgery*, vol. 67, no. 2, pp. 484-8, Feb. 1999.

[77] G. Bhatnagar, S. E. Fremes, G. T. Christakis, and B. S. Goldman, "Early results using an ePTFE membrane for pericardial closure following coronary bypass grafting," *Journal of Cardiac Surgery*, vol. 13, no. 3, pp. 190-3, May 1998.

[78] H. Hwang et al., "Ranolazine as a cardioplegia additive improves recovery of diastolic function in isolated rat hearts," *Circulation*, vol. 120, no. 11, pp. S16-21, Sep. 2009.

[79] R. M. Mentzer et al., "Adenosine as an additive to blood cardioplegia in humans during coronary artery bypass surgery," *Society*, pp. 38-43, 1997.

[80] J. A. Coles, D. C. Sigg, and P. A. Iaizzo, "The potential benefits of 1.5% hetastarch as a cardioplegia additive," *Biochemical Pharmacology*, vol. 69, no. 11, pp. 1553-8, Jun. 2005.

[81] E. Proctor and R. Parker, "Preservation of isolated heart for 72 Hours," *British Medical Journal*, vol. 4, no. 2, pp. 296-8, Jan. 1968.

[82] W. N. Wicomb, D. Novitzky, D. Cooper, and A. Rose, "Forty-eight hours hypothermic perfusion storage of pig and baboon hearts," *Journal of Surgical Research*, vol. 40, pp. 276-84, 1986.

[83] T. Ozeki et al., "Heart preservation using continuous ex vivo perfusion improves viability and functional recovery," *Circulation journal*, vol. 71, pp. 153-9, 2007.